FIGHTING
FOR OUR
FUTURE

FIGHTING
FOR OUR
FUTURE

*How Young Women Find Strength,
Hope, and Courage While Taking
Control of Breast Cancer*

BETH MURPHY

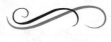

MCGRAW-HILL

NEW YORK   CHICAGO   SAN FRANCISCO.   LISBON
LONDON   MADRID   MEXICO CITY   MILAN   NEW DELHI
SAN JUAN   SEOUL   SINGAPORE   SYDNEY   TORONTO

The **McGraw·Hill** Companies

Library of Congress Cataloging-in-Publication Data

Murphy, Beth
    Fighting for our future how young women find strength, hope, and
courage while taking control of breast cancer / by Beth Murphy.
        p. cm.
    Includes bibliographical references and index.
    I   SBN 0-07-140925-4 (hardcover : alk. paper)
    1. Breast—Cancer—Popular works.   2. Young women—Diseases—Popular
works. I. Title.
·RC280.B8 M85 2003
616.99'449—dc21   2002011266

1 2 3 4 5 6 7 8 9 0 DOC/DOC 0 8 7 6 5 4 3 2

ISBN 0-07-140925-4

The purpose of this book is to educate. It is sold with the understanding that the author
and publisher shall have neither liability nor responsibility for any injury caused or
alleged to be caused directly or indirectly by the information in this book. While every
effort has been made to ensure the book's accuracy, its contents should not be con-
strued as medical advice. Each person's health needs are unique. To obtain recommendations appropriate to your particular situation, please consult a qualified health care
professional.

National Alliance of Breast Cancer Organization® (NABCO®) is a registered trademark
of the National Alliance of Breast Cancer Organization. All other trademark products
or organizations mentioned are used in an editorial fashion only and to the benefit of
the trademark owner, with no intention of infringement of the trademark. Where such
designations appear in this book, they have been printed in all caps or initial caps.

This book is printed on recycled, acid-free paper
containing a minimum of 50% recycled de-inked fiber.

"Hope" is the thing with feathers—
That perches in the soul—
And sings the tune without the words—
And never stops—at all—

— Emily Dickinson

To the women of the Young Survival Coalition
who provide hope to all young women fighting breast cancer

Contents

Foreword *by Ann Curry*   ix

Introduction *by Dr. George Siedge*   xi

Preface   xiii

Acknowledgments   xv

CHAPTER 1
Young Women with Breast Cancer
A Life Worth Fighting For   1

CHAPTER 2
"I Didn't Even Know What to Ask"
Negotiating the Medical Process, from the First Sign
of Trouble through Establishing a Diagnosis   20

CHAPTER 3
"No One Told Me It Would Be Like That"
Measuring Options, Making Choices, from Surgery
through Treatment   48

CHAPTER 4
"Can I Still Run the Marathon?"
Fitness, Diet, and Taking Care of Your Body   87

CHAPTER 5
"This Empowers Me"
Alternative, Complementary, and Integrative
Approaches to Healing   108

CHAPTER 6
"I See the Pain in Their Eyes"
Getting Support from Family, Friends, and Community   139

CHAPTER 7
"I was Just Starting to Like My Body"
Coping with Body Image, Dating, Sex, and Intimacy   164

CHAPTER 8
"Do I Want Another Breast?"
The Pros and Cons of Reconstruction   182

CHAPTER 9
"This Is My Miracle Baby"
Dealing with Fertility, Pregnancy, and Breast-Feeding   209

CHAPTER 10
"I Want to Dance at my Son's Wedding"
When You've Got Children at Home   230

CHAPTER 11
"I Wanted to Be Taken Seriously"
Workplace Issues   249

CHAPTER 12
"I Just Try to Focus on the Now . . ."
When Cancer Recurs or Metastasizes   267

CHAPTER 13
"I Was Looking for a Way to Fight"
A Guide to Getting Active   285

Notes   299

Resources   305

Index   315

Foreword

I will never forget the fear in my sister's voice the day that she told me, "I have breast cancer." There was no making sense of it. She was a young, healthy mother of three beautiful children. How could she get this disease at age 40? Aren't mammograms advised only for women over the age of 40? Isn't age breast cancer's number one risk factor?

Since that day I have learned that more than 10,000 young women—undergraduates planning college courses, professionals planning new careers, brides planning weddings, mothers-to-be planning baby showers, women planning lives—are diagnosed every year.

Beth Murphy's book *Fighting for Our Future* is an invaluable contribution for young women diagnosed with breast cancer. So many of them are told that they are *too young* for the disease. Even their doctors don't believe they can get it, so the doctors may overlook symptoms until the cancer's spread. We now know that young women (premenopausal women, typically 40 and under) have more aggressive cancers and are more likely to be initially misdiagnosed—and that younger women are more likely to die from breast cancer. Yet, because the disease is more common in older women, young women are often called "anecdotal" and made to feel that the extra challenges they face are not worthy of attention. The despair—and shock—that they go through can seem overwhelming. But there is hope, and it's here, in these pages.

Young women face unique issues simply because of their age. Fertility, premature menopause caused by chemotherapy, young families, body image, dating, confronting mortality so early in life, problems with peer support, and intense feelings of isolation—these issues and so many others, Murphy tackles and explains, providing information that's been difficult to obtain before now. For years, the medical community has focused on older women; so the younger women have fewer support services, networks, and medical information. Older women, for example, have specific guidelines to follow to better catch breast cancer early, when chances of survival are greatest. But young women have no clear guidelines about what they *should* do for early detection.

While giving voice to those who need to be heard, Beth Murphy helps young women understand and cope with the unique and difficult issues they face. She explores the frustration young women experience because of the prevailing attitude that young women don't get breast cancer. She outlines the gaps in research. And she proves that raising awareness about young women with breast cancer is both positive and necessary.

Ignorance does not protect young women from breast cancer. It only justifies waiting longer to see a doctor or accepting being told you're *too young* for the disease. Doing either can cost young women their lives.

For the first time, the wisdom and experience of the young provide comfort and hope to other young women, to their families, and to health-care professionals, letting them know what it means to live with—and survive—breast cancer. These are powerful voices, powerful testimonials. Not just of the women themselves, but of their families, caregivers, partners, and friends. This book gives voice to all those touched by breast cancer.

Like the spirit of young women you will meet here, this book is an outgrowth of women and men, doctors and patients, families and children supporting one another. Saying, over and over again: *We can get through this. We can go beyond this. We can fight for our future.*

And we can win.

Ann Curry
of NBC's *Today* show

Introduction

Survival. As a medical oncologist, I spend a great deal of my life talking to my patients about it. When the patient is a young woman, the word has an even deeper resonance, especially when I, the physician, have to admit that science does not hold all her answers.

I remember one particular woman in her late twenties. As we discussed various alternatives, she became indignant. Was that all, she asked, that medical science had to offer to such a young woman with two daughters at home?

That moment has remained with me years after initially meeting that young woman. Her response was not terror or fear but indignation: Why couldn't we do better? I considered it then, as I consider it now, an appropriate response; we *should* be indignant about our inability to do better.

For breast cancer *is* different in young women—different because the patients are different and different because the nature of the disease is different. The young woman with breast cancer must deal with issues such as fertility and pregnancy, effects of therapy on sexuality, and the onset of premature menopause and its consequences. She is more likely to have an inherited predisposition for breast cancer, and must face the prospect that she may have passed a breast cancer gene on to her children. She is faced with cancers that frequently act differently, and more aggressively, than those she might have faced had she developed a breast cancer two decades later. By virtue of her age, she is likely to be at a different and more vulnerable point in career development. Her children are younger and (as often occurs with young children) demand more of her than she may be able to give because of the physical and emotional effects of therapy. She must face difficult body image issues, and the reality of her own mortality, all the time surrounded by healthy, active peers. She must worry about the stresses placed on fragile relationships with significant others.

The book that you are about to read represents what I consider to be a unique resource. It examines breast cancer in young women through the lives of—young women. We live with young women through their diagnosis, through their therapy, and through the many issues they face in dealing with the universe of problems that are associated with breast cancer. Unlike many texts that I have read on breast cancer over the years, this one is suffused with humanity: It never forgets that breast cancer is a disease that happens to individuals, real living women with real lives outside the caverns of the medical system. We hear the voices of real women facing real challenges.

One of this book's real sources of excellence, to my thinking, is its sophistication in realizing that we don't have all the answers, that patients and their physicians are faced, at every turn, with questions and decisions for which we lack final answers. Sometimes, indeed, we are faced with questions for which there are no answers at all. Yet it confronts these issues forthrightly and intelligently, offering the reader a balanced understanding of where we are today. By its appreciation of the subtleties of current medical issues, it offers the young woman with breast cancer real options that she might not otherwise have. I learned from it, and I am sure that you will as well.

Finally, this book gives one a good understanding of the evolution of therapy. Breast cancer therapy is work in progress. Therapeutic advances are incremental rather than sweeping. That recent years have seen real advances comes through loud and clear. At the same time, this book articulates a challenge: We must do better. The exciting thing is that given the real increase in our understanding of the biology of breast cancer (and in particular the biology of young women's breast cancer), we can look forward to a day when this disease may be considerably less frightening. That day cannot come too soon.

George Sledge, M.D.
Indiana University Cancer Center

Preface

There are times in a journalist's career when a story becomes so meaningful that the very act of telling it fundamentally changes the way you view yourself and your role in the world.

This is one of those times.

My mission as a documentarian has always been to give a voice to voiceless populations. Often this means traveling to war-torn countries, documenting human rights abuses, and focusing on refugees, war crimes, and relief work. This time, however, the cameras capture a neglected population right here at home: young women with breast cancer.

While researching *Fighting for Our Future,* the Lifetime Television documentary, I heard time and time again young women express the same truth: They felt alone in the breast cancer community and neglected by the medical community. While the documentary would succeed in raising awareness for the unique issues young women face, I became motivated by a responsibility to do more to help newly diagnosed young women, their loved ones, and their caretakers understand the journey they are about to make.

This book is designed to give young women a tool that has never before existed. If you have recently been diagnosed, or know someone who has, you will notice one central message exists here: *You are not alone.* And while you will be able to find very practical information and advice from doctors and peers, you will also notice that this material can give you a voice in the medical, research, and breast cancer communities and inspire a climate in which you can partner with doctors and politicians to effect change if you so choose.

What is so striking to me is that this is the first time in history young women with breast cancer are united—and truly changing the face of breast cancer in America. They are the women of the Young Survival Coalition, who serve as the intellectual and emotional inspiration for this work. I consider it an honor to have been allowed into their lives to witness the dogged determination that drives them, capture the energy that exemplifies their work, and enjoy the laughter that permeates their spirit.

Acknowledgments

This work would not have been possible without the help of many individuals, organizations, and institutions. The Young Survival Coalition deserves primary recognition for the earnestness and devotion they dedicated to this project. In particular, I want to thank YSC founders Roberta Levy-Schwartz, Joy Simha, and Lanita Hausman for their courage, strength, and wisdom and for the countless hours spent sharing their stories and insights with me. They serve to embody everything being communicated here. Also, the YSC Task Force of Cynthia Rubin, Michele Przypyszny, Jennifer Levinson, Jeannine Salamone, Francie Coulter, Randi Rosenberg, Jody Rosen Knower, and Lori Atkinson proved to be an invaluable resource and sounding board. Special thanks also to Tracy Hill, Lisa Muccilo, and Kelly Douglas for opening their homes and hearts to me. To them, and all the young women and families who've shared their stories with me, I say, "Thank you." You have all influenced this project in meaningful ways.

I am especially grateful to my agent, Jeff Kleinman, of Graybill and English, for his round-the-clock work ethic and willingness to go beyond the call of duty. I owe a great debt to Nancy Hancock of McGraw-Hill; she is a terrific editor whose vision and editorial perspicacity shaped these chapters in the most profound ways. I am also grateful to the exceptional McGraw-Hill staff: Ruth Mannino, Meg Leder, Lynda Luppino, Eileen Lamadore, and Lydia Rinaldi. Special thanks is reserved for Rachel Kranz for her talent and dedication. Her knowledge and skills brought this book to life and added a depth that would not have otherwise been possible. This entire editorial and marketing team is ultimately responsible for making the book what it is.

I'd also like to thank the medical advisory panel who gave their expertise freely and graciously, with special thanks to doctors Bert Petersen, Jeanne Petrek, and George Sledge for the many late-night and weekend calls and emails.

I am also grateful to Ann Curry and Traecy Smith of the *Today* show for their generosity and spirit and to Lifetime Television for its extraordinary commitment to breast cancer awareness. In particular, I'd like to thank Carole Black and Mary Dixon for their support and Rosemary Sykes, Dorian Winship, and Bill Brand for their enthusiasm.

Roche Pharmaceuticals, Lorad Medical, Margaret McCormick, and Jack Cumming have my unending gratitude for their belief in the value of this work and their commitment to support it.

There are numerous other individuals who assisted with or contributed to this project in various ways. In particular, my mother, Mary Brundage, and mother-in-law, Jane Murphy, who read the manuscript and offered the kinds of insights only lifelong English teachers could; my father, Howard Brundage, who provides wisdom; my sisters, Bonnie Cummings, Briana Brundage, and Brita Brundage, who have always been a source of strength and inspiration; Michael Cummings and Jim, Mike, and Maureen Murphy for their support; Kevin Sullivan, Bill Schlosser, Michelle Milne, Kevin Belli, Ralph Fasano, and Patrick Roche for their hard work and humor; and, most of all, my husband, Dennis, whose love and support make my life's work possible.

CHAPTER 1

Young Women with Breast Cancer

A Life Worth Fighting For

Shirley Williams, diagnosed with breast cancer at age 30: "I can't believe I was diagnosed almost 40 years ago. I'm 68 years old now. My surgery was in 1964 on Christmas Eve. I'll never forget it. You won't believe this when I tell you—are you sitting down? All right, then. They told me I had 10 days. That I would only make it 10 days. Well, here I am—38 years later. Not only did I make it through, but I've had an amazing life. I have loved living my life. And I would like my life to be an inspiration to others—and I think it should be. All these young women who are diagnosed today need to know that I'm here. Your doctor may not be able to tell you about a 40-year survival rate, but I sure can. I lived it."

Nalini Yadla, diagnosed with breast cancer at age 22: "It's odd. I don't feel like a strong person. But if I looked at myself from someone else's perspective, I would say, 'Yeah, I am overcoming things that most people will never even have to face.' I just see myself as someone trying to do the best I can. Is there any alternative? I can't give up. I won't give up. I definitely don't feel like a superhero or anything. I just see every day as a tremendous opportunity to appreciate my family and friends—to appreciate life itself. Does that make me heroic?"

Joy Simha, diagnosed with breast cancer at age 26: "Hope is an amazing and powerful thing. And, by God, if I can give that to someone, then that's amazing. I never thought I'd be able to date again. I never thought I'd fall in love or that anyone could fall in love with me. And I certainly

1

never thought I'd be able to have a baby. Look at me now. A wonderful husband, and a beautiful baby boy. We named him Anand—which means happiness. Yes, it's pretty incredible."

"But I'm Too Young for Breast Cancer!"

If you're like most young women, these may have been your first words upon hearing of your diagnosis. Randi Rosenberg, who was diagnosed at age 32, remembers having that reaction from the very beginning—even on the day her gynecologist found the lump. "I asked her, 'What do you think? Do you think I should go for a mammogram?' And her response was, 'Well you probably have fibrocystic breasts. I wouldn't worry too much about it. You're too young for breast cancer.' And those words just sort of echoed. I thought, 'Perfect. Absolutely right. I am too young for breast cancer.' And I didn't worry about it. And I wasn't actually diagnosed until a full year later."

Randi's experience is one that many young women share. The perception that young women *can't* and *don't* get breast cancer often leads to an initial misdiagnosis. "There is no young woman with breast cancer whom I know of who hasn't heard those words," says Roberta Levy-Schwartz, who was 27 and single when she was diagnosed. "I heard them. Everybody has heard those words: 'Don't worry, you're *too young.*'"

Given that fact, it's understandable that you find yourself asking, "How can I possibly have breast cancer? Isn't that something you get in your fifties and sixties?" And it's true; the average age for a woman diagnosed with breast cancer is 64. Breast cancer is shocking at any age, but if you're under 40, it helps to realize how many women there are out there who are just like you. "It's not my grandmother's disease. It's not my mother's disease. It's my disease," says Lanita Hausman, who was diagnosed at age 32.

Now you've discovered that you have breast cancer, and suddenly your world changes. You have to understand what your diagnosis means, what kinds of treatment options are available, and how long you can expect to spend in treatment and recovery. You may be wondering how this diagnosis will affect your career, your dating life, your marriage, your children, your parents. You might already have started calling your insurance company or looking for a second opinion.

If you're like most young women with breast cancer, you may already have discovered a rather disheartening fact: Virtually all of the information on the disease that is readily available is geared to older women.

In a way, that's not surprising. After all, women aged 40 and under make up about 5 percent of the total number of U.S. women with breast cancer. It makes sense that doctors would be more familiar with the needs and concerns of the other 95 percent. You can understand, too, why most of the pamphlets, brochures, and books on coping with cancer assume that you're in a decades-old marriage, that your children are grown, that you're at the peak of your career if not actually approaching retirement— instead of being a woman in your twenties and thirties who in many ways is just getting started with your life.

Well, take heart. You are not alone. There are more than 250,000 women in the United States just like you, diagnosed with breast cancer at age 40 or younger. And, sadly, more than 10,500 women in this age group will be diagnosed with breast cancer this year.

In a way, that's the bad news—that so many young women are facing this disease. But it's also the good news, because as more young women are diagnosed with breast cancer, they are also starting to come together and to speak out for themselves and for one another. Through political organizations and as individuals, to their doctors and to their families, within the breast cancer community and in the halls of Congress, young women are speaking up. They're identifying the issues that are important to them, and pushing for funding and research to address their special needs. They're forming support groups and political organizations, so that they can find one another, share information, and offer support. And they've pulled together a formidable body of medical information specifically geared to young women like themselves.

Thanks to the young women who have broken this ground, you now have access to vastly more medical information. You also have access to emotional information—the hard-won wisdom and experience of young women who, despite the challenges of breast cancer, have gone on to affirm their new body images, reconnect to their sexuality, continue with their careers, and raise their children. This book is designed to share their work, their discoveries, and their stories with you. Between these covers, you'll find the latest medical knowledge about young women with breast cancer, based on interviews with doctors and scientists who are doing cutting-edge research in the field—and who, in some cases, are breast cancer survivors themselves. You'll also find a host of practical information: how to find a breast surgeon, pointers for dealing with your insurance company, suggestions for coping with coworkers and bosses, even tips on how to throw a head-shaving party. You'll read about the kinds of breast reconstruction that are available, what role exercise and diet can play in your recovery, and the latest facts about fertility and pregnancy as they affect breast cancer survivors. You'll also find information that can help you through this difficult experience: the latest on alternative and complementary treatments, spiritual approaches to illness, advice from young mothers on child-rearing during chemotherapy, and a look at your legal rights on the job.

Perhaps most important of all, you'll hear the voices of other young women with breast cancer as they describe the full range of their experiences, from discovery and diagnosis to treatment and recovery. You'll hear from a mother who dreams of dancing at her son's wedding, a lawyer who made partner 21 days before her diagnosis, a woman who fell in love during chemotherapy, and an amateur sports enthusiast who plans her surgeries around her volleyball schedule. You'll hear from women aged 22 to 68, coming from places as varied as Casper, Wyoming, and West Palm Beach, New York City and Fergus Falls, Minnesota. You'll also find a Resource Guide at the end of the book that can point you to more books, articles, Web sites, and organizations.

If your primary concern is mastering the voluminous amounts of medical information necessary to fully understand your condition and choose a treatment, you may want to check out some of the many books available that focus on the medical aspects of breast cancer. *Dr. Susan Love's Breast Book* is an excellent resource, as is *Breast Cancer: The Complete Guide,* by Yashar Hirshaut, M.D., and Peter Pressman, M.D. This book won't attempt to duplicate their encyclopedic range of scientific information—although you will find a great deal of important medical information here, particularly specific explanations of the unique issues faced by young women. And, of course, this book is no substitute for talking to your doctor. Certainly you and your physician must be partners if your treatment is to be effective, and any medical concerns you have should be discussed with your doctor.

What you will find here—and nowhere else—is all the basic information about breast cancer as it relates to young women. This book was created for you with your concerns in mind. It's intended to be your survival guide and your support group. You can read it from cover to cover or skip around, according to your needs. Either way, you'll have at your disposal the vital information that you as a young woman need in order to cope with breast cancer.

Your loved ones, friends, and caregivers will also find this book a useful tool for understanding your physical, emotional, and spiritual experience. And they, too, will meet people like themselves in these pages. They'll hear from a husband who shaved his head to overcome feelings of helplessness during his wife's treatment, a mother who wants nothing more than to take her daughter's place, and a doctor who believes it's not enough to treat the breast cancer—he must heal the patient.

On your journey through breast cancer, you're likely to encounter many unexpected twists and turns as you navigate this unfamiliar territory. So think of *Fighting for Our Future* as your guidebook. We can't tell you what your journey holds, but we can help you prepare yourself for the trip.

Breasts, Sexuality, and Being a Woman

Breasts. Every woman starts out with two. In fact, for many of us, when our breasts first start growing is when we first realize that we *are* women. From Victoria's Secret ads to MTV, from the bosomy *Cosmo* model to the jiggly lifeguards on *Baywatch*, breasts seem to hold the secret of feminine sexuality.

Girls with attractive breasts are encouraged to see their bodies as giving them power over men, while girls whose breasts are "too small," "too big," or otherwise not up to the mark are enticed with the correctives offered by cosmetic surgery, padded bras, or special exercises. We may love defining ourselves by our breasts, feeling sexy, womanly, powerful, or content; or we may resent the role that breasts play in our lives—interfering with athletic activity, drawing unwanted attention from boys and men, marking us as female in a world that often seems to value men more. Whatever our own relationship to our mammary glands and the flesh that surrounds them, we know that breasts are an important part of our identity, in others' eyes if not in our own.

Kathryn Kash, Ph.D., Psycho-Oncologist, Beth Israel Cancer Center, New York City

There's no question that femininity and sexuality in our society are directly connected to breasts. You don't have look any further than the billboards on the side of the highway or the latest magazine covers to see how female sexuality is all around us. And for young women who are in the prime of their lives, their sexuality is an important part of their sense of self. And what the young woman with breast cancer experiences is in stark contrast to the world around her. It's very confusing and very isolating.

One of the first things I try to do is normalize patients' feelings and reactions. Often women think they're the only people who feel this way, and they're not the only ones.

Feminist author and activist Ellen Leopold agrees that we "over-involve breasts in every aspect of our culture." Leopold is the author of *A Darker Ribbon: Breast Cancer, Women, and Their Doctors in the Twentieth Century,* which is a cultural history of breast cancer treatment and activism. She is struck by the way in which breasts have taken on a cultural importance that is far beyond their personal meaning to any young woman:

> Breasts have become sex objects, sources of nourishment—they play all these roles that feed into each other as well as into cultural ideas. The national symbol of France is Marianne, the female figure with exposed breasts and the French flag—she's the symbol of the republic. I think this political imagery is very revealing, that a nation would have this body organ playing a very visible and central role.

As a result of both their own feelings and the social pressures that Martin and Leopold describe, young women can be particularly overwhelmed by a threat to their breasts. According to Dr. Kash, who studies the emotional effects, "The overriding concern among the doctors is trying to save somebody's life. But when you're in your twenties and thirties, your sense of femininity and sexuality is very important. It's right up there with trying to save your life."

Ernie Bodai, M.D., Director of Breast Surgical Services at Kaiser Permanente in Sacramento and the advocate responsible for the breast cancer stamp, puts it even more succinctly. "Society has put today's young women in a tough situation," he says. "Breasts are considered the ultimate sign of sexuality." But where does that leave a young woman with breast cancer?

Breast Cancer Treatment and Activism: A Brief History

One response to society's problematic messages about breasts has been for women to come together, to offer one another support. Through a variety of groups and movements, women have worked together to create new self-definitions and new responses to breast cancer. One such group is the Young Survival Coalition (YSC), an organization founded by three young breast cancer survivors to encourage young women to speak to one another and to the medical community, demanding research and attention to their particular needs. And the YSC draws on a 40-year history of breast cancer activism in which women challenged both the medical establishment and society itself.

In the 1960s, the standard of care for breast cancer was the radical mastectomy, pioneered by Dr. William Halsted of Johns Hopkins at the beginning of the century, a highly disfiguring operation in which the cancerous breast was completely removed, along with nearby lymph nodes and the two chest wall muscles on the affected side. Halsted advocated early detection of breast cancer, followed by an immediate radical mastectomy, with the idea that as soon as cancer was detected, it had to be "rooted out" as thoroughly as possible. Despite opposition from such pioneering physicians as Bernard Fisher, who focused less on local control of breast cancer than on eliminating possible metastatic disease through systemic treatments like chemotherapy, Halsted's approach was widely adopted by the U.S. medical community (though his methods received for less acceptance in Europe). In 1968, close to 70 percent of U.S. breast cancer patients were receiving essentially the same radical mastectomy that Halsted had introduced at the turn of the century. And breast cancer mortality rates in the United States had not changed.

During this period, breast cancer was a largely taboo subject in which women had virtually no voice. Almost all doctors at that time were male, and patients operated in a system in which both male and medical authority went largely unchallenged. Shirley Williams, diagnosed with breast cancer at age 30 in 1964, vividly recalls how silenced she felt by the prevailing atmosphere: "My entire cancer experience has been in the closet. It wasn't something in the sixties that you talked about. And if you did, you didn't have a job. I worked for the New York City Department of Corrections. When I had my last mastectomy, I stayed out of work for 2 weeks, and then I went back to teach my class. They still don't know to this day. There are very few people who do know about it."

The sense of women as passive and silent was enhanced by the protocol of the time. A woman would normally be put under anesthesia for a biopsy—and then, if the biopsy indicated cause for concern, she would be given an immediate radical mastectomy. It was not considered necessary to consult with the woman about this decision; indeed, the female patient was literally unconscious while the (mostly male) physician made this decision for her.

By the early 1970s, however, the feminist movement had begun, and women were beginning to speak up. They were challenging authority in all sorts of arenas, and a large and vocal women's health movement was demanding more information on birth control, abortion rights, and new practices in gynecology, and calling on women to take a more active role in their own health care.

At the same time, prominent women were beginning to go public with their diagnoses of breast cancer. Former child star and then U.N. Ambassador Shirley Temple Black, First Lady Betty Ford, vice-presidential wife Happy Rockefeller, and NBC news anchor Betty Rollin were making their breast cancer stories available to a mass audience, with Rollin's first-person account of her experience, *First, You Cry*, becoming a bestseller. Although these women were not closely linked to the women's liberation movements of the time and none of them were associated with the women's health movement, their speaking out helped to create a climate in which breast cancer could finally be talked about.

A more activist approach was taken by Rose Kushner, diagnosed with breast cancer in 1974. When Kushner, an outspoken journalist, found a "tiny elevation" in her breast, she went straight to the library, where she discovered that even among surgeons, Halsted's technique had been called into question. Her major reference was a book by surgeon George ("Barney") Crile, Jr., *What Women Should Know About the Breast Cancer Controversy*, in which Crile challenged the prevailing notion that early detection and immediate radical surgery was the best way to treat cancer. Crile's writing of this book was itself a radical move, for by going outside the medical establishment and taking his case directly to the public, he violated an unwritten code of his profession. He reached many women, however, including Rose Kushner, who insisted that her family surgeon perform only a biopsy and then stop and discuss the results with her.

As a journalist, Kushner chose to write about her experiences, but her work went far beyond the first-person accounts that had previously dominated public discussion of breast cancer. Kushner's *Breast Cancer: A Personal History and Investigative Report*, which appeared in 1975, included the results of her research in England, Scotland, Scandinavia, and the Soviet Union, where radical mastectomies were far less popular than in the United States. Kushner pointed out that European doctors, working for national health systems, had long since adopted simple rather than radical mastectomies as their standard treatment and that they generally performed far fewer operations per capita than their U.S. counterparts. U.S. doctors, by contrast, were reimbursed for radical mastectomies at three times the rate for simple mastectomies—and so they tended to recommend the more expensive operations and perform more surgery generally.

Although Kushner considered herself a civil libertarian rather than a feminist, she expressed her views in language that the women's movement was to recognize and appropriate: "No man is going to make another man impotent while he's asleep without his permission," Barron H. Lerner quotes her as saying. "But there's no hesitation if it's a woman's breast."[1]

Kushner's work continued to be controversial. Leopold writes that Kushner's willingness to speak out "laid the groundwork for what would eventually become the modern culture of breast cancer."[2] Although Kushner died of metastatic breast cancer in 1990, she left behind the National Alliance of Breast Cancer Organizations (NABCO), which she

Roberta Levy-Schwartz, Diagnosed at Age 27

The story of me getting diagnosed is a little bit strange. I went to a primary-care doctor, who found an abnormal pap smear and said everything else was fine. And I was uncomfortable with his recommendation that I come back in 6 months, so I went to an ob-gyn about 2 months later. He said the pap smear was fine, everything else was fine, but did I know I had a lump in my breast? He recommended I see a breast surgeon. I was busy trying to find a breast surgeon who could see me on a Friday when I was in town, so I wouldn't have to completely rearrange my week!

I finally found somebody, and he said it was nothing, just a fibroadenoma, which is quite normal for young women and nothing to worry about. He did recommend that I have it taken it out, though, because it would keep growing and I wouldn't like how it looked.

At that point I really wasn't worried, and I preferred not to do the surgery. But I happened to bring my mother to that appointment, and she was sitting in the corner with a white face saying, "Take it out. Take it out."

So I made the appointment to have the thing removed. They diagnosed it the day of my surgery. The doctor called me back into his office and told me I had breast cancer.

The only thing going on in my mind was, how soon could I get back to work? And I remember looking at the doctor and going, "Breast cancer? But I'm 27!" And then I laughed at him, saying, "You gotta be joking. You told me it was a fibroadenoma"—as if we'd had a contract.

But I think that I knew it was fairly serious. I found myself only dealing with what he'd said at 2 A.M., when the room was black— when everything was dark—and it was dead quiet—and I didn't know how long I was going to be living for.

Now it's 4 years past my diagnosis. I'm married to Lee; I've gotten pregnant and become a mother. And now I have to look at the future in a different way, because I can't live with the possibility that I won't be here for my child's fourth birthday, or her fourteenth. I'm going to be here for a good long time.

had formed with Ruth Spear, Nancy Brinker, and Diane Blum in 1986. That same year, NABCO executive director Amy Langer, a breast cancer survivor, joined with breast surgeon Susan Love, M.D., and other activists to form the National Breast Cancer Coalition (NBCC), whose goals were to increase funding for research, widen access to screening and treatment, and promote women's participation in health policy decisions. Dr. Love continues to be a major voice in the breast cancer community, as does the NBCC.

Breast Cancer in Young Women: A Different Kind of Disease

Ironically, because breast cancer is such a big problem among women over 40, the chances of its striking younger women tend to be ignored. If you're in your thirties, your chances of getting breast cancer are 1 in 249, according to figures provided by the American Cancer Society. If you're in your twenties, the risk is 1 in 2044. It's not surprising that doctors discount the possibility of breast cancer in young women.

Yet, as we've seen, one-quarter of a million U.S. women ages 40 and under have breast cancer—a sizable number by any standard. When Randi Rosenberg, diagnosed with breast cancer at age 32, attended the American Association for Cancer Research annual conference in 2002, she met a young woman from Scandinavia who asked her how many young women in America had breast cancer. "I told her, '250,000,'" Randi reports, "and her jaw dropped to the floor. She said, 'That's almost half the population of my entire country!'"

> **Jeanne Petrek, M.D., Breast Surgeon, Memorial Sloan-Kettering Cancer Center, New York City**
>
> *I think there's a big difference in the lives of young women with breast cancer versus older women who develop the disease. The older woman sees her peers dealing with health issues. Conditions like breast cancer, hypertension, and diabetes are things associated with being older. Whereas the younger woman has all the expectations of health. And certainly her peers are healthy.*
>
> *I find my young patients also have many more demands on their time. Young patients have different lives, different things are important to them, and breast cancer behaves differently in them. That's why it's important to study them.*

Aquatia Owens, Diagnosed at Age 32

My life is great today. Even when I have bad days, I think it's a great day. I wake up every morning and I'm glad I'm alive. Literally. I'm planning my wedding now, and I'm just so happy to have the experience of getting married; that I'm here to be able to plan a wedding.

Every day on my way to work there's a song I listen to, and one of the lines says, "Look where you are now, compared to where you've been." And that sums it up for me, because a few years ago, I didn't even know if I was going to see tomorrow. I didn't know if I'd ever have a chance to get married, or even celebrate another birthday. So many great things have happened to me since my illness.

The Need for a Screening Tool

Thomas Kolb, M.D., is a New York City-based radiologist specializing in breast cancer detection, with a special focus on high-risk younger women. He is an experienced administrator of mammograms, which are the diagnostic screening tool used to find breast cancer—in women over age 40. But Dr. Kolb will be the first to say that "mammography is not foolproof." It turns out that breast density is the most important factor in whether mammograms find cancer or not. And young women, says Dr. Kolb, tend to have dense breasts. The dense breast tissue common in young women makes mammogram results difficult to interpret because, as Dr. Kolb explains, "On a mammogram, both breast density and cancer tumors appear as white masses, making it hard to distinguish between the two."

So Dr. Kolb is investigating a promising new technique: a combination of sonograms/ultrasounds and mammograms as a screening tool for younger women. "With a sonogram, a breast cancer tumor appears as a black mass, which differentiates it from the white breast density," he says. Preliminary studies suggest that this technique has great potential, at least for high-risk women—women who have a family history of breast cancer or have some other reason to suspect that they may be prone to the disease. Dr. Kolb's work is an indication that there is potential for improving the accuracy of breast cancer detection in young women and that some specialists, at least, are beginning to take young women's concerns more seriously.

A More Aggressive Type of Breast Cancer

Many researchers believe that breast cancer is somewhat more aggressive in younger women than in women who have gone through menopause. Researchers speculate that because young women have higher levels of estrogen than postmenopausal women, they may be facing greater risks. Estrogen is known to feed some tumors, and some researchers believe that it generally promotes breast cancer, making the disease more likely to spread throughout the body.

Research on this question is still in its infancy. But many top U.S. specialists—including Dr. Susan Love, a breast surgeon who is widely recognized as a national expert on breast cancer; George Sledge, M.D., professor of medicine and pathology at the Indiana University Cancer Center; and Robert Taub, M.D., an oncologist at New York Presbyterian Hospital in New York City—agree that breast cancer cells seem to divide more rapidly in younger women and that the disease is more likely to spread. Their concerns are borne out by the difference between the 5-year survival rate in young women with breast cancer—82 percent—and that in older women—86 percent.[3] Fortunately, both younger and older women have access to a wide variety of treatments. And young women are even more likely than their mothers and aunts to supplement their standard medical care with alternative approaches such as acupuncture, nutrition, and herbal medicine. Although many doctors are skeptical of these alternatives, many see young women's interest in them as a promising sign, suggesting that young women are willing to embrace a wide variety of approaches in their quest for health. (For more about alternative approaches to treatment, see Chapter 5.)

The Urgent Questions You're Asking

After your diagnosis, you're likely to have the following questions on your mind, now or in the future. Here's how this book can help you answer them:

- *How has breast cancer changed my relationship to my own body?* As a woman in your teens, twenties, or thirties, you may still be exploring your body image, your sexuality, and your sense of yourself as a woman—and your breasts are probably a central part of that identity. You may find yourself working through initial feelings of despair and betrayal to redefine your physical self and your womanhood. To find out how other young women have coped with the loss of a breast and all the other changes in body image that breast cancer brings, see Chapter 7.

- *How do I mobilize the emotional support I need from my friends and family?* Your concerns may include parents who worry about your health, friends and siblings who don't expect to encounter a serious illness in someone their age, and perhaps a new spouse, girlfriend, or boyfriend with whom you haven't yet faced tragedy or hardship. How do you create the support network that you need—and how can your partner and loved ones find their own sources of support? To examine this issue more thoroughly, look at Chapter 6.

- *How has breast cancer affected my sexual life and/or my dating life?* Sexual intimacy can be a charged issue for breast cancer survivors of any age. But if you are a young woman, your marriage or partnership is likely to be newer, or maybe you're still out on the dating scene. Figuring out how your new body will perform sexually, having the courage to see yourself as attractive, and recreating your sexual identity will be your special challenges. Luckily, other young women have been there before you. They share their stories—and their reasons for hope—in Chapter 7.

- *What about the effects of pregnancy on breast cancer?* Again, this is a question that older women rarely face, but younger women often do. One in every 3000 pregnancies is accompanied by a diagnosis of breast cancer within the year, and some one-third of young women with breast cancer were diagnosed within a year of being pregnant.[4] As a young woman with breast cancer, you may be concerned about preserving your fertility, protecting your current pregnancy, or making responsible decisions about childbearing in the future. For a thorough discussion of these questions, see Chapter 9.

- *How do I continue to raise my children?* If you have children, you have probably already begun to wonder how to help them through this difficult time. And then there are the practical problems: finding the physical energy to chase a toddler when you're recovering from chemo, deciding how to explain "cancer" to your kids. To hear from other moms who have coped before you, look at Chapter 10.

- *How do I manage at work?* Maybe you've found your niche in the working world, or perhaps your work identity is still in flux. Either way, as a young woman, you probably still feel you have something to prove in the workplace, as you explore your work identity, deal with office politics, figure out your professional goals, and strive for recognition and respect. Throw breast cancer and chemo into the mix, and suddenly you have a whole host of new problems to deal with: taking time off for treatments, keeping up with your duties or negotiating new arrangements, deciding what you can and can't manage, maintaining the respect you've earned. Moreover, breast cancer requires you to focus on your breasts and on your femininity, which may run counter to the professional image you were previously trying to promote. To learn how other working women have handled their careers—and for a review of your rights on the job—check out Chapter 11.

- *What are my options for prosthesis and cosmetic surgery?* Perhaps one of the fastest-growing specialties in U.S. medicine is plastic surgery, and physicians now report excellent results from new techniques in breast reconstruction. Whether you're a sports enthusiast or a mother with small children, there are a variety of things that may influence your decision. Check out your options in Chapter 8.

- *What are the long-term effects of radiation, chemotherapy, and tamoxifen?* These standard treatments for breast cancer have been studied in older women, who have shorter life spans and different hormonal levels. But how do they affect those under 40, especially over the longer time span that they are expected to survive? Doctors, too, have many unanswered questions about this issue. For a review of current studies and advice from young survivors, see Chapter 3.

- *What effects will chemotherapy, radiation, and tamoxifen have on my fertility?* We know that these standard breast cancer treatments can have profound effects on women's fertility, but sometimes the resulting sterility is only temporary, whereas in other cases it becomes permanent. Can you protect your fertility—and if so, how? For a discussion of the latest thinking on this question, see Chapter 9.

- *Will I undergo premature menopause—and if so, what can I expect?* Premature menopause sometimes occurs as an unintentional result of chemotherapy, or it may be deliberately induced through a procedure known as ovarian ablation. Young women with breast cancer face a temporary or sometimes permanent loss of fertility, along with hot flashes, vaginal dryness, and other symptoms that can accompany menopause. To learn more about chemotherapy and ovarian ablation, see Chapter 3. For tips on how to restore your sexual vitality if you do undergo menopause, check out Chapter 7. And to find out about how to protect your fertility, see Chapter 9.

- *What effect do diet, exercise, smoking, and other lifestyle choices have on my treatment and recovery?* Researchers are just beginning to address these issues, especially as they relate to young women.

Luckily, several significant studies dealing with exercise, diet, and alternative approaches to nutrition, including phytohormonals (vegetable sources of hormones) and soy, are already in progress. For our latest understanding of diet, fitness, and weight as they relate to breast cancer, look at Chapter 4. To learn more about alternative approaches to nutrition, including a soy-rich diet and macrobiotics, see Chapter 5.

- *What kinds of alternative and complementary treatments have been shown to be effective?* Proponents of such treatments as acupuncture, herbal medicine, and macrobiotics have argued that these approaches can either help to combat cancer or help to ease the effects of chemotherapy and radiation, especially in conjunction with standard medical techniques. But which treatments really make a difference,

Lisa Muccilo, Diagnosed at Age 27

I was really shocked to be diagnosed, even though I had the family history. My mother had breast cancer when she was 48, and my grandmother had breast cancer too. So I always knew it was a possibility. But I just assumed that I couldn't get it at 27, that for me it would come later. I had that invincible young feeling. I just couldn't imagine getting it so young.

I started going to meetings to connect with other breast cancer patients, but most of the people there were my mom's age and they were sitting around talking about their grandchildren. I was thinking, "Wow, I'd love to have some grandkids. Wouldn't I be so lucky if I could live long enough to have grandchildren. I don't even have children yet, never mind grandkids." I felt totally out of place. Then I went to a meeting of the Young Survival Coalition. I was so relieved to see that I wasn't the only one who was young. The women there were all young, all in various stages of treatment. They were all young and strong, and knew great things would come of trying to do something to raise awareness about young women with breast cancer. They were all very passionate, and I knew immediately that this was where I belonged.

I think it's so important for women going through the same things to connect. That means young women connecting with other young women, and young women with metastatic disease connecting with other young mets patients. You just can't imagine how much it helps to connect with someone who knows exactly how you feel; it's what gives me hope and strength and the courage to fight.

and which are simply fads? Find the latest scientific opinion on alternative and complementary medicine in Chapter 5—along with some suggestions for drawing on your spiritual resources and the powerful mind/body connection.

- *How can I cope with recurrence (the return of cancer) or metastasis (the spread of cancer to other parts of the body)?* Recurrence and metastasis are frightening for women of any age—and, statistically, they're not very likely possibilities for you. But when young women face these issues, they have unique concerns. If you or a loved one is facing recurrence or metastasis, or if you want more information, you can turn to Chapter 12 to hear the stories of survivors who have confronted these challenges for themselves.

- *What kind of spiritual approaches are meaningful to me?* Women of all ages may be spiritually active, of course, but as a young woman, you may find it especially challenging to find meaning in an illness that is so unexpected and so rare. Yet many young women have reported finding unexpected meaning and even joy as a result of their breast cancer diagnoses—meaning that goes on to shape the rest of their lives. For more on spiritual approaches to cancer and the quest for meaning, see Chapter 5.

Speaking Out for Young Women: The Story of the Young Survival Coalition

Despite the increasingly large, visible, and vocal breast cancer community, young women with breast cancer remained virtually invisible for many years. As the testimonies at the beginning of this chapter showed, young women were often told they were simply "too young" to have breast cancer.

Then, in 1998, three young breast cancer survivors got together, almost by accident, and went on to form the YSC. Lanita Hausman had a family history of cancer—a paternal aunt had been diagnosed with the disease at age 29, with a serious recurrence at age 43. Lanita asked for a mammogram when she herself was only 26. Her first gynecologist categorically refused to give her the test "until you're at least 35." Lanita switched to another doctor, but the mammograms didn't reveal any problems. At age 32, Lanita discovered her cancer because of an irritation around the nipple that wouldn't go away. Eventually, not a gynecologist but a dermatologist diagnosed her condition. What she thought was "runner's nipple" was actually Paget's disease of the breast, a rare form of cancer that usually first appears as a scaly, red rash affecting the nipple and sometimes the areola, the dark area of the skin surrounding the nipple.

Although Lanita was diagnosed with ductal carcinoma in situ (DCIS) and no cancerous cells had spread into the surrounding breast tissue, when she heard that she had cancer in one breast, she chose a bilateral mastectomy without a moment's thought, telling the doctor, "Take two, they're small." The operation was successful, and because Lanita's disease had been caught so early, she didn't need chemotherapy. She went on to fulfill her longtime dream of running in the New York Marathon, and life seemed to have gotten back to normal. On some level, though, Lanita was aware that she hadn't yet processed her experience.

Roberta Levy-Schwartz had no family history of breast cancer and was shocked when she got her diagnosis at age 27. Like Lanita Roberta went on to have a mastectomy, but she was also treated with chemotherapy. While still in treatment, she fell in love with Lee Schwartz, who eventually became her husband.

A consultant for a public health agency where Lanita worked, Roberta was used to researching medical problems and taking charge of situations. So much so, that when she and Lanita reminisce about how unlikely their incredible friendship is, they find themselves laughing in disbelief. "I didn't really like her," says Lanita bluntly. "Which is so funny now, because she is one of my best friends in the world."

When Lanita first got Roberta's call, she was taken back. She remembered Roberta very well—and not at all fondly. A year earlier, when Lanita had been coping with her own diagnosis, Roberta had come storming into her department, frustrated by the fact that her computer problems were being ignored.

"Where's Jackie?" she'd practically shouted. "I've been calling her for half an hour, left about a million messages—but nothing! I think it's rude no one returns my phone calls! This is unacceptable!"

Look, Lanita felt like saying, you think you're having a bad day? I've just been diagnosed with breast cancer, and my boss is quitting her job! Let's talk about a bad day, shall we? Lanita had held her peace, but she'd also held a grudge. Now that Roberta was calling for help, though, she couldn't help but respond. Yes, she told Roberta, they could meet for lunch. Why not?

The two women started to talk. Roberta found herself opening up, sharing how upset she was, how scared she was that she was going to die. To her astonishment, she found that it helped to talk. Lanita was also surprised to discover that talking to Roberta stirred up long-buried emotions. "I realized that I'd never mourned anything," was how she described it later. "I never mourned my breast. I never said goodbye to the life I didn't have any more. I just got through it. When I met Roberta, it was like a chance to go through it all over again. This time, with feeling."

Both women were struck by how similar their experiences with doctors had been. They'd both heard doctors say "Don't worry" and "Young women just don't get this disease." They were both upset by the discovery that no organizations seemed to be addressing the issues that were most important to them. Roberta convinced Lanita to attend a few meetings of SHARE, a New York-based group whose flyers talked about self-help and women's education. Once again, they were struck by the similarities of the young women's stories, although both women were looking for more than SHARE's support-group atmosphere. At SHARE, however, Roberta met Joy Simha, diagnosed at age 26, and eventually introduced her to Lanita.

Before Joy got her diagnosis, she'd been having the time of her life. She was working happily as a video producer, she loved her Greenwich Village apartment, and she'd just begun to discover her body. Uncomfortable with her body image for most of her life, Joy had finally made the decision to go to Weight Watchers, lose her unwanted weight, and start working out. For the first time in her life, she was happy with her body and her appearance. When she discovered a lump through a breast self-exam, she never expected it to be cancer. Nor did her doctors, who treated Joy's discovery casually at first. When Joy finally got the cancer diagnosis, she remembers she plunged into depression.

"It was really hard to get out of bed," she recalls. "I just wanted to lie there in bed and let breast cancer get me, just give into it. I didn't want to go through chemo or surgery or any of the horrible things you have to do. I just wanted to roll over and let it get me. And then I realized I could let it get me in the bed or I could give it a good fight."

Joy went on to have surgery and chemotherapy. One year after treatment was over during a routine follow-up visit, her oncologist noticed that she seemed more depressed than when she was in treatment and offered to prescribe antidepressants. "No," Joy responded, "that's not it. I am frustrated because I have no way to fight."

So when Joy met Roberta and Lanita, the three women began, almost casually, to talk about possible responses to the way young women were treated in the medical and breast cancer communities. They knew women who were losing their battle with breast cancer, and this kept the mission urgent. They considered various approaches: lobbying, advocacy, educating young women, urging doctors to do more research. One day Roberta said there had been enough talk and insisted on calling an actual meeting of young breast cancer survivors. Lanita and Joy agreed, and a couple of months later, the Young Survival Coalition held its first meeting, a pot-luck brunch attended by 14 other young survivors.

The group went on to launch a Web site so that young women with breast cancer could find one another, as well as access basic information about their condition. Dozens, then hundreds, then thousands of women began connecting through the Web site and registering to join the new organization.

If you, a loved one, or a patient you're treating has been recently diagnosed, finding a voice in the breast cancer community may help you or her connect with other young women. That alone can make getting involved a rewarding experience. In 2001, the first national conference specifically geared to the needs of young women was held in Philadelphia. It's now an annual event cosponsored by the YSC and Living Beyond Breast Cancer, an organization focused on posttreatment issues. It's one place young women can come to hear the latest research and quality-of-life information they need to make decisions about their treatment and futures. In 2002, 500 young women with breast cancer attended, making it the largest gathering of young survivors under one roof.

In the recent past, gatherings of young women with breast cancer were unheard of—particularly on this scale. But the more vocal they've become, the more likely they are to experience the sheer relief of coming face to face with other young women with breast cancer.

"I didn't think I'd find anyone my age in my area that I could talk to," says Kelly Douglas of Indianapolis, diagnosed at age 24. "I don't want to sit here and be upset about having cancer. I want to do something against it. I want to be either learning or doing something politically—or something just to educate people. I think I have a lot to offer the breast cancer community, and I think right now, especially, my bald head is really going to have an impact."

Tracy Pleva Hill was diagnosed at age 32. To her, connecting with other young women was a revelation. "I'd always felt like I'd never been challenged in my life," she says. "I grew up in a nice middle-class family, my parents were great, I went to a good school, graduated from college, got married, got a house in the 'burbs,' found a nice job. Never had any major hardships. I felt like I was waiting my whole life for something like this. Isn't that strange? I felt like I was waiting my whole life to be challenged."

"And this was something that I could do. I'm going through this, and I'm going to help other people go through it, and I'm going to make sure that somewhere down the line, no more women have to go through it at all. Because having breast cancer changes your life forever."

CHAPTER 2

"I Didn't Even Know What to Ask"

Negotiating the Medical Process, from the First Sign of Trouble through Establishing a Diagnosis

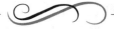

When Kelly Douglas was diagnosed with breast cancer at age 24, the first thing that struck her was how much she didn't know. "There are so many things that are general for anyone who develops breast cancer, but I think you often don't know the questions to be asking that are specific to young women," she says.

Kelly had an advantage in that her husband, Mark, was a nurse practitioner who had cared for people with cancer, but even Mark had never seen a breast cancer patient as young as Kelly. "Your classic patient is not in her early twenties," he points out. "So this involves greater looking, without always finding. We had to very quickly get over the shock that she was being diagnosed at 24, and focus on getting the best answers for us at this stage in our life."

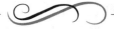

Roberta Levy-Schwartz had worked for years as a consultant to a health-care agency. So when she was diagnosed at age 27, she too knew more than most people about health issues—and she too soon realized how little she knew.

"So I did what I do with just about everything in life—I started researching the hell out of it," Roberta recalls. "I went immediately to the bookstore, pulled out 15 books on the subject, and started taking notes. And literally, between the time I was diagnosed and the time I

went back to do the lumpectomy, I had picked out the type of breast cancer I wanted—I had actually highlighted the one I thought would be best! You know, fewer side effects, easiest to treat—stuff like that. As if I had a choice!"

❧

Charnette Messé was 31 years old when she was diagnosed with breast cancer—and the next day she found out that she was pregnant. As Charnette was to discover, breast cancer is the most common kind of cancer during pregnancy, occurring as often as one in every 3000 pregnancies,[1] and many researchers believe that the high estrogen levels of pregnancy can set off a latent breast cancer. (For more on pregnancy and breast cancer, see Chapter 9.)

Although Charnette would eventually learn those statistics, at the time, she was completely shocked. "I had developed a little pimple on my breast," she recalls. "That went away. Then another one came right near the same spot. And then the whole half of my breast turned red and hot. When the pimple went away I developed a lump under my arm. I thought Terms of Endearment right away. When I saw my doctor, she found five palpable lumps under my arm. There was one huge one and then four smaller ones. She swore up and down that it was from the rash draining. I said, 'What about cancer?' She said, 'I don't think it's cancer.' I said, 'What if it is cancer?' And she said, 'Well, then it's already spread.' I said, 'I want a mammogram.' She said, 'I really don't think it's cancer. You're too young. I'd like to watch it for 2 months.' I said, 'No, I want a mammogram.' I demanded it. And she hesitated, and then said, 'Okay, and we'll do an ultrasound too.'"

The next day, Charnette got a call at home, confirming that she had cancer. The following day, she recalls, "My chest was hurting. So, I went to see another doctor. She did a blood test that morning and then called me in the evening. She said, 'Charnette, you're pregnant.'"

Working Your Way through the Treatment Process

As Kelly, Roberta, and Charnette found out, working your way through the treatment process can be a bit overwhelming, to say the least. Because serious illness is scary and upsetting, uncertain and painful, you will probably find yourself drawing on all your intellectual, emotional, and spiritual resources.

Most young women who have been through the process, though, find that there are three things that can make an enormous difference:

1. *Arm yourself with knowledge.* The more you know, the better your chances of making the decisions that are right for you. You'll have more productive conversations with your physician, and a better sense of what's likely to be ahead. Of course, you'll never be able to know everything about your illness and its treatment—even the top researchers in the world acknowledge that too many important questions remain unanswered, especially for young women. But at least you can understand what the unknowns are and the range of possible outcomes.

2. *Draw on your support systems.* From your earliest appointments, it's helpful to have someone else in the room, listening and perhaps even taking notes. Many people simply stop hearing anything after the word *cancer* has been spoken, so bringing a friend or family member to listen for you and with you can make a huge difference. Not going through the experience alone may be even more important. Knowing that you are loved and cherished, that you have a network of friends and family who will work through this experience with you, will make you stronger, physically as well as emotionally. (For more on support systems and loved ones, see Chapter 6.)

3. *Find your own meaning in the experience.* The people who emerge the strongest from life's tragedies seem to be the ones who manage to accept the circumstances and go on from there, looking for whatever meaning they can find or make from their experience. Some people become part of a group that fights back against cancer, so that other women won't need to face the same pain. Others find meaning in a renewed appreciation of life, or a deeper commitment to their loved ones, or a better understanding of their own resources, or involvement in another way to make the world a better place. Finding your own way through this difficult experience can be enormously helpful. (For more on emotional and spiritual responses to having breast cancer, see Chapter 5.)

In this chapter and the next, you'll find the basic information that you need. You can read about every step of the process, from your first suspicion that there's something wrong to your final decisions about treatment. This chapter will focus on initial diagnosis and on dealing with your insurance company. Chapter 3 will take you from decisions about surgery through recovery from the various postsurgical treatments available: chemotherapy, hormonal treatments, and radiation therapy.

Rosanne Drogonski, Diagnosed at Age 31

I had been feeling run-down for about 2 months. I had a fever, and I was tired. I figured it was a cold. Or flu. Or mono. Then I realized that my armpit was really sore. When I touched it, I felt swollen lymph nodes. I then found more in my neck. And then it happened . . . I found the lump. For about a month, I ran around asking all my friends to "feel this . . . what do you think it is?" But when I saw it in the mirror through my sports bra during a kickboxing class, I knew that whatever it was, it had to go.

Luckily, my doctor took it much more seriously than I did. The surgeon palpated my breast and said, "It's good-sized and you're young, so it's probably nothing to worry about."

He stuck a needle in the lump to drain it [but there was no fluid]. . . . I asked him if he had any idea what to do. He said, "You need surgery."

Then he went outside the room and shut the door, and I could hear him whispering outside. I tried not to be paranoid. I tried to imagine that I was not the topic of conversation and that they were just talking about their weekend plans. I overheard him say, "I'm going to run this to pathology myself." That was when the anxiety set in.

When he came back in the room, he told me that he had sent some tissue to be biopsied. While we were waiting for the results, he told me to go make mammogram and sonogram appointments for Monday. I started to feel a little dizzy. Tears were stinging my eyes as I headed off toward radiology. I was starting to get worried, but I wasn't sure exactly what it was that I was worrying about. . . . Then he told me that it might mean cancer.

I just looked at him like he was crazy. This was not possible. I could feel myself breathing faster and I could hear voices inside my head screaming . . . I am young. I am vibrant! I am so healthy! I just had my annual exam 6 months ago and she didn't feel any lumps! I'm barely a B cup, for God's sake! I eat well and work out religiously! Oh, and did I mention I am young?

Did I Cause This?

Before we start our journey through the process, let's get one thing out of the way: *No one knows what causes breast cancer.* You didn't *ask* for breast cancer. And no matter how you live, what you eat, what type of personality you have, or who your family is, breast cancer is not your fault.

You may choose to see breast cancer as your *responsibility*. You may decide that there are things you can do that will give you a better chance of overcoming it, or open you further to healing energies, or generally support your physical health, or enable you to find more meaning in this experience. That's terrific, and much of this book is designed to help you do just that. But to decide that you "caused your own illness" or that "breast cancer is your fault" is not helpful, especially because it tends to drain your energy and sap your self-love just when you most need those inner resources.

While doctors don't know what causes cancer to develop in breast tissue, they do have a number of theories, suspecting that some combination of genetic factors, lifestyle, and the environment may increase women's risk for the disease. Eric Winer, M.D., is one of America's leading breast cancer specialists and the director of breast oncology at Dana-Farber's Gillette Centers for Women's Cancer in Boston. He explains that while some types of cancer behave in a relatively uniform and regular manner, breast cancer operates in a wide variety of ways. In fact, the single term *breast cancer* actually refers to many different types of diseases. That's why different women often have vastly different responses to the same treatments. Dr. Winer refers to breast cancer as "a crowd with 100

Randi Rosenberg, Diagnosed at Age 32

I was just filled with so many emotions when I got my diagnosis. When my gynecologist called me and asked me to come into the office first thing Monday morning, somehow I knew instinctively what I was going to hear. So I had a lot of trepidation, butterflies, just feeling ill, that whole morning. When we actually went to the office to talk to her, I was with Andrew, who's now my husband. The doctor looked into my eyes and said, "I'm sorry to tell you, but you have breast cancer." And as soon as the words came out of her mouth, I felt myself floating out of my body and hanging on the ceiling looking down at the situation.

I honestly don't remember all that much about what I was thinking or feeling. I'm pretty sure I was numb. I switched onto autopilot, where I spent the next several months. We walked from my doctor's office to the hospital. As we went in, the sight of a young bald woman walking very slowly and deliberately in our direction made my stomach turn. I thought, "Oh, my God! That's a cancer patient! That's what's going to happen to me."

faces," as opposed to, say, pancreatic cancer, which can be more easily compared to a single person.

So in the end, breast cancer is still one of life's mysteries. Understanding that you cannot control how this illness occurred, you'll probably find it more useful to focus on what you *can* control—your own physical, emotional, and spiritual response to the disease.

At the First Sign of Trouble

You've probably already heard that if you've got a breast lump, nipple discharge, unusual breast pain or inflammation, or anything else that leads you to suspect a problem, you should go to your gynecologist and have it checked out. Alternatively, you can try to convince your insurance company to let you see a breast surgeon, someone who specializes in treating breasts.

Given that many women's breasts are lumpy and that young women in particular are prone to breast-area acne, it can be hard to know which kinds of breast changes might signal the need for a visit to the doctor. Susan Love, M.D., the renowned breast surgeon and breast cancer activist, offers some surprisingly simple advice in this matter. Trust your instincts, she says, and if you suspect that something is wrong, insist that your doctor pay attention:

> It's sometimes really hard to tell which lumps are significant and which are not. The ones that need to be checked out are what we call dominant lumps—a lump that persists and doesn't go away with your menstrual cycle. A dominant lump will always be there, and it will feel different from the rest of the breast tissue. I think women get a sixth sense about a lump that is abnormal. And when you have that sense, that's when you should push for a biopsy. And if the doctor refuses, then you should insist on a second opinion. It's up to you to push, and if the doctor dismisses you, it's time to find another doctor.

For women over 40, a mammogram would be the next logical step. Unfortunately, as we saw in Chapter 1, mammograms aren't as effective for younger women because their breasts tend to be too dense. However, Thomas Kolb, M.D., a New York City–based radiologist specializing in breast cancer detection who works extensively with high-risk younger women, believes that a combination of mammography and ultrasound can be remarkably effective. He recently completed a study of more than 27,000 women, 13,000 of whom had dense breasts and were screened with mammography and ultrasound. In those cases, screening mammography caught only 47.6 percent of cancers. A combination of mammography and ultrasound, however, found 97 percent of all breast cancer cases in these same women, who were generally younger.[2] Dr. Kolb also found that mammography plus ultrasound was far more effective than mammography plus physical examination in diagnosing breast cancer in earlier stages. So if you consider yourself at risk for breast cancer, whether because of a problem you've found (at which point you need a diagnostic tool) or because of your family history (when you'll need a screening tool), you might press your doctor to do both an ultrasound and a mammogram.

The Search for a Screening Tool

Young breast cancer activists are urgently seeking a screening tool that can better detect breast cancer in young women. Unfortunately, given that the vast majority of young women don't have breast cancer, it's unlikely that researchers will ever develop such a tool. While a combination of mammography and ultrasound can be prescribed for young women who seem to be at risk, giving that test or any other to the general population of women under age 40 raises the concern that there would be too many false positives, and that healthy young women would find themselves going on for further unnecessary, frightening, and expensive tests and treatment.

"Any time you have a situation where the condition is rare, the big concern with screening is, 'What's going to happen to all the people who *don't* have the disease?'" says Beverly Rockhill, professor of epidemiology at University of North Carolina, Chapel Hill. "There are too many people who potentially face unnecessary biopsies and risky treatments who don't have the disease."

Questions to Ask a Technician before Beginning Any Procedure

- Please tell me, step by step, what you are going to do and what I will feel.

- Will the procedure hurt? Will I feel any pain later?

- Can you numb my skin? Can you give me some kind of pain relief so that I can be more comfortable during the procedure?

- Can I take any pain medication after the procedure?

But young women with breast cancer fear that the opposite is true. "There aren't too many unnecessary biopsies happening. That's not the problem. The problem is, young women aren't being biopsied enough," says Cynthia Rubin, president of the YSC.

In the absence of a screening tool, young women need to rely on clinical breast examination (CBE), a physical examination performed by a health-care professional, and breast self-examination (BSE), a physical examination that a woman performs on herself. In fact, according to the YSC Membership Profile, one of the best existing sources of data on young women with breast cancer, some 83 percent of the group's members first found their cancer themselves (at least 43 percent through breast self-examination).

The Debate over BSE

In recent years, the medical and breast cancer communities have engaged in a fierce debate over BSE. When the notion of women examining themselves first came into prominence in the 1970s, both women health-care activists and medical professionals praised the idea; women would be using their personal knowledge of their own bodies as an effective health-care tool. In theory, women knew their own breasts better than anyone else, and they would be best able to detect any changes in shape or unusual lumps that might signal cancer.

But there's one serious problem with relying on breast self-examination as a screening tool: There is simply no current scientific evidence to indicate that breast self-examination actually saves lives or enables women to detect breast cancer at earlier stages. And there are data showing that breast self-examination greatly increases the number of benign breast lumps that women find, resulting in increased anxiety, more visits to the doctor, and unnecessary biopsies.

The problem is that once breast cancer has advanced far enough for a woman to be able to feel a lump in her own breast, she's already had the cancer for as many as 8 to 10 years, according to Dr. Susan Love. Perhaps breast self-examination will enable a woman to find the lump a month or two before it would otherwise be discovered accidentally, by her lover, her doctor, or herself, but for women over the age of 40, that slightly earlier detection time seems to make very little difference in the long run.

Beth Lesnikoski, M.D., a breast surgeon at the Dana Farber Cancer Institute, is not necessarily opposed to BSE. But she says that designing a study to demonstrate the effectiveness of BSE is virtually impossible, because BSE's benefits are so small—if indeed they exist at all. "If there is

Rosanne Drogonski

First I had the ultrasound. The tech was an older woman who seemed completely put out by my existence. She asked me why I was there, and I'm quite sure she rolled her eyes when I told her I had a lump in my breast. I guess she thought I was wasting her time. She was kind of rough at first, but as the exam continued and she asked me more questions, she got nicer. She softened up even more when it appeared that the lump was solid, meaning it was probably not a cyst. Meaning things were not looking good.

A few days later I had the mammogram. The tech walked out into the lobby that, except for me, was empty. She looked around. She called my name. She looked past me, above me, and through me. As I stood up to go with her, she gave me a funny look. She said my name again, questioning, staring at me in disbelief. "Girl, you are much too young to be in my waiting room," she said as she exited with me in tow. When I left, she said she would pray for me. She looked like this pretty little angel in pink scrubs and black braids. I believed her when she said it.

a difference in survival, it may be too tiny to study, perhaps one or two in hundreds of thousands of women," she says.

The controversy heated up in June 2001, when the Canadian Task Force on Preventative Health Care published an article in the *Canadian Medical Association Journal* recommending that doctors stop routinely advising women to do breast self-exams. Although the article specified that the recommendation applied only to women aged 40 to 69, who had been most widely represented in the study, the results were widely interpreted as applying to women of all ages. In fact, the task force explicitly avoided recommendations for women younger than 40 or older than 70, saying that it lacked sufficient evidence.[3]

As we've seen, younger women are not getting the routine mammograms that are recommended for women in their forties, fifties, and sixties, and their breast cancers tend to progress far more quickly and aggressively than those experienced by older women. So for younger women, BSE may indeed be a useful screening tool; without more studies, it's impossible to know. And the YSC immediately spoke out against the Canadian report, arguing that for younger women, who could not rely upon mammography alone, BSE could not be discounted. Randi Rosenberg elaborates on the YSC's position:

Young women have no existing methodology for detecting breast cancer besides monthly BSE and annual clinical examination. We agree that BSE is not a very effective method for breast cancer detection in younger women because cancer detected by BSE is already at a later stage, and we know that early detection and treatment access are the keys to survival.

Therefore, Randi says, the YSC continues to recommend both monthly BSE and annual clinical examinations for young women beginning at age 18, as well as mammograms beginning at age 40 (or earlier if suggested by your physician).

Having a Biopsy

Once a problem has been detected, the next step is to do a biopsy, an analysis of living tissue. There are five types of biopsies available. Two of them involve removing small samples of tissue via needle: a *fine-needle biopsy*, which removes only a tiny bit of tissue, and a *core biopsy*, which is done with a slightly larger needle and removes more tissue. One type of core biopsy, called a *stereotactic biopsy*, uses special equipment to pinpoint the location of a tumor that can be seen only on a mammogram. Once the tumor is located, the needle can move quickly in and out of even the smallest lumps. Charnette Messé, who was diagnosed at age 31, said that the process was "like putting your breast in a sewing machine. You're lying on this table, your breast goes through this hole, and then the needle comes in. I didn't have a defined mass, so the needle was just going around and around like a sewing machine."

There's another new device that is sometimes used to perform a breast biopsy: a mammotome system, which uses a small rotating cutter and a vacuum to remove a larger sample. Because the sample is larger, the diagnosis will be more reliable, and there will be less chance that your doctor will have to order another sample because of uncertain results.

In other cases, your doctor may choose an *incisional biopsy*, in which part of the lump is removed, or an *excisional biopsy*, in which all of the lump is removed. In fact, though, these procedures are rarely done for diagnostic purposes. Of course, any lump that is removed from your body for any reason will probably be biopsied to determine whether it is malignant or benign.

Kelly Douglas, diagnosed at age 24, looks back almost fondly at the biopsy portion of her journey, although, she says, it was difficult at the time. "It's funny to look at everything now," she says. "Just the de-

Questions to Ask Your Doctor about Your Biopsy

- What kind of biopsy will you be doing?
- If my biopsy results are unclear, will you need to do another, more extensive biopsy for follow-up?
- How much tissue are you planning to remove? Will it leave a dent or scar in my breast?
- How long will the procedure take? Will I be awake during it?
- Is this procedure painful?
- Can I have a friend or family member with me during the procedure?
- Are you calling for both frozen section and permanent section, or just a permanent section?
- How can I make sure I hear the results of the frozen section, if I decide I want to?
- How can I make sure I get to see the tissue that is removed, if I decide I want to?
- How long will it take to get the results?
- Will I get the results over the phone, or should I make an appointment now?
- If the biopsy comes back positive, what's the next step? If it's negative, what's the next step?
- How long will it take me to recover?
- Will I have to restrict my activities after the biopsy?

cision to have that biopsy was pretty tough. It was, 'Oh, gosh, I have to have a mammogram.' Then it was, 'Oh, gosh, I have to have a biopsy,' then, 'Oh, gosh, I have to have a mastectomy,' then, 'Oh, gosh, chemo!' And then it's like, 'Oh, a biopsy. No big deal.' It's funny how your perspective changes completely."

Rosanne Drogonski, diagnosed at age 31, was given a mammotome biopsy. "I was awake throughout the entire procedure," she recalls. After the procedure was over, Rosanne insisted on seeing the tissue that had been removed. "It looked just like a meatball," she remembers. I couldn't stop looking at it."

Rosanne knew that there were two kinds of analysis that could be done on the tissue: *frozen section,* in which a thin slice of tissue is frozen and analyzed in about half an hour; and *permanent section,* in which an unfrozen section is analyzed. Because freezing the cells can distort them, frozen section is less reliable, but it has the advantage of taking only half an hour to yield results, whereas permanent section takes a day or two. Although no important medical decision should ever be made on the basis of a frozen section, Rosanne insisted on hearing the results of her frozen section before she left the clinic. She knew she'd have more reliable results in a day or so, but she wanted whatever news she could get as early as possible.

Understanding Your Pathology Report

When your doctor gets the tissue sample pathology report back from the lab, there are three possible results: benign, malignant (cancerous), or unclear. Each of these raises several more questions.

Unclear

If your test results aren't clear, your doctor may order further tests or wait to see how the lump develops. Discuss with your doctor what his or her plan of action is.

Benign

It's possible that your test will indicate that the lump is benign but that you will be diagnosed with *atypical hyperplasia:* abnormal and proliferating breast cells that are not themselves malignant (cancerous) but that may suggest that you're at increased risk for cancer. In the words of Dr. George Sledge, a professor of medicine and pathology at Indiana University Cancer Center, "There's benign and then there's *benign.* Let's say you're a young woman and you have a positive family history and your tumor comes back showing atypical hyperplasia. Even though the tumor is truly benign (it's not cancer), it is a marker for a breast that is at higher risk. That's possibly a patient who might consider breast cancer prevention therapy of some sort, such as tamoxifen." According to the College of American Pathologists, a woman whose biopsy shows atypical hyperplasia has "a moderately increased risk (five times) for developing breast cancer as compared with a woman who has no known significant breast abnormality." While abnormal breast cells increase the risk of breast cancer, not all women with atypical hyperplasia will develop breast cancer.

A benign lump may also be a sign of fibrocystic breast condition, also known as fibrocystic disease, fibrocystic change, cystic disease, chronic

31

Tips for Undergoing a Biopsy

- If you're having a mammotome biopsy, ask them to turn on the machine for a moment before the procedure actually begins. The noise will come as less of a shock if you hear it before you're strapped in.

- Bring headphones and some soothing music that you can listen to during the procedure. Some women like to buy or make visualization or meditation tapes to help them relax.

- Think about bringing a friend or family member. You might need someone to drive you home afterwards. It may also be easier to go through the experience with support.

- Consider bringing something sweet and delicious—hard candies, chocolate, fruit, a popsicle—to have in your mouth during the biopsy. Some people find that focusing on the sensory taste experience helps blunt the discomfort of the procedure.

- Be aware of your feelings about seeing the tissue after it's removed and about finding out the frozen section results. Some women like to be more involved in the process; others want to keep a little distance. Listen to your own feelings and choose the option that's right for you.

cystic mastitis, or mammary dysplasia. This is not actually a disease; it only means that your breast tissues are prone to change, perhaps developing cysts (packets of fluid), fibrosis (scarlike connective tissue), lumpiness, thickening, tenderness, or breast pain. If the lump is not filled with fluid, it's called a solid mass (of which there are many kinds, including cancer, but fibroadenomas are the most common). There is no connection between fibrocystic breasts and breast cancer, except that having such breasts makes mammography less reliable as a screening tool because of the breast density associated with the condition. So again, if you've got dense breasts, you may want to press your doctor to use ultrasound as well as mammography in future exams. According to the American Cancer Society, at least one-half of all women have fibrocystic breasts at some point in their lives—and, of course, this condition is the most common cause of breast lumps in young women, far more common than cancer. Because the condition is related to the menstrual cycle, women with fibrocystic breasts often experience breast tenderness and pain around the time of menstruation. Many doctors suggest wearing supportive bras and lowering dietary intake of caffeine and salt to minimize the symptoms.

Malignant (Cancerous)

If your biopsy reveals that your lump was malignant, you'll have many questions for your doctor. In some cases, your doctor will have had the entire lump removed and then biopsied, in which case you'll want to read your pathology report and follow up with questions until you understand the report completely. You might ask specifically about the *margins* (the area around the lump). If the margins are clear, that means that the tumor has been entirely removed. If there was cancer at the margins, some of the tumor probably still remains in your breast. In either case, you're likely to be given further treatment—radiation, chemotherapy, and/or hormonal treatments—since it's possible that the cancer had spread to another part of your body before it was removed.

Here are some other questions that you might want to ask your doctor about a malignant biopsy:

- What type of breast cancer do I have? (Some of the possibilities include *ductal carcinoma in situ (DCIS), lobular carcinoma in situ (LCIS), inflammatory, invasive ductal, invasive lobular,* and *Paget's disease.* Each type of breast cancer has its own behavior and prognosis, so you'll want to learn as much as you can about your particular kind.)

- What *stage* is my breast cancer (how far advanced is it, or how far has it spread)? (The staging system, numbered 0 through 4, is often referred to as TNM because it is based on Tumor size, Node involvement, and Metastasis. *Node involvement* refers to whether the cancer has spread to the lymph nodes. If it has, it's possible that the cancer has been carried by the lymphatic system to other parts of the body as well. *Metastasis* is the spread of breast cancer to other places, such as the bones, lungs, or liver.)

- Can I have a copy of the pathology report? (Don't take no for an answer on this one!)

- Should I get a second opinion from another pathologist? Why or why not?

- What is the tumor's *grade* (the rate of cell growth)?

- Which lab tests were done on my tumor? What were the results?

- Are these the most accurate tests available?

- What other tests are available?

- Was my tumor *estrogen-receptor (ER) positive* or *negative?* (A receptor is the part of a cancer cell that allows a hormone to attach to the cell and cause it to proliferate. Estrogen-receptor-positive tumors grow more quickly in response to estrogen, so they can be treated with antiestrogen therapies and are considered to be less aggressive. However, younger women are more likely to have tumors that are ER negative, which means that the tumor will require a different type of treatment and is likely to be more aggressive.)

- Was my tumor *progesterone-receptor positive* or *negative?* (This type of tumor is sensitive to another common hormone, progesterone. Again, hormone-sensitive tumors are believed to be less aggressive—and are less common among young women.)

- Was my tumor *HER2neu positive* or *negative?* (HER2neu is the name of an *oncogene*—a gene that is supposed to keep cell growth in check. When HER2neu malfunctions, it can cause cancer. Cancers caused by oncogene abnormalities tend to be more aggressive, but they are amenable to additional treatments.)

- Are there other tests I should have, such as a bone scan or a CT scan? (If your cancer has metastasized, your doctor will want to test for cancer in other parts of your body, such as your bones [tested by a bone scan] or the organs in your abdomen [tested by CT scan]. If your cancer has not metastasized, your doctor may want to get a baseline of some or all of these tests, so that you can be monitored for metastases in the future.)

"The first time I read my pathology report was kind of hard for me," says Kelly Douglas, "because I saw 'estrogen-positive' and 'HER2neu' and things about staging and cell differentiation, and I had no idea what anything meant. And that was the most difficult thing, because you're sitting there reading all this stuff, but you can't apply it yet."

Kathy Burgau, diagnosed with breast cancer at age 26, had a scare when her doctor was doing further tests to see whether her cancer had metastasized to her bones, liver, or brain. "I was waiting for my bone scan," she recalls, "and I could see the doctor pulling my charts—and he showed me that there was a spot on my liver. He said, 'We'll have to do a biopsy on that, too.' So during the bone scan, that's all I was thinking about. I was lying on the gurney bawling my head off. The nurse started crying. She was the same young nurse who did my mammogram. She was scared to death for me and for herself—since I was so young, she realized she could get cancer, too. Then I went up to the doctor, and I found out that the spot on my liver was something caused by my method of birth control. It's not something that's going to cause me any problems. It was such a relief hearing those words, 'It's not cancer.'"

For Kathy, the testing process wasn't over, though; her doctor had also ordered a CT scan of her brain. For that, she said, "They give you a shot, and you get a metal taste in your mouth, and you feel like you wet your pants. But I hadn't. The nurse said everybody asks about that. The shot just makes you all warm down there. You have to go through all this, and nobody really tells you exactly what to expect."

As we discussed in Chapter 1, there's some evidence that breast cancer is more aggressive in young women, with the cells dividing even more rapidly than in older women. In the poetic words of Katherine Russell Rich, diagnosed with breast cancer at age 32 and author of *The Red Devil: A Memoir about Beating the Odds,* "Cancer behaves like a wilding adolescent. Healthy cells grow for a few months, then die off to make way for new ones. Cancerous ones refuse to accept limitations; they defy the body's signals and rules and run away from their home sites, hell-bent on living forever."

Aron Goldhirsch, M.D., professor of medical oncology, director of the Department of Medicine at the European Institute of Oncology, and chair of the Scientific Committee of the International Breast Cancer Study Group, agrees that breast cancer tends to be more aggressive in young women, although he adds, "The reason for this more aggressive behavior is something that hasn't been studied. There is a general belief that it is due to some endocrine aspects, because a young woman has more vigorous hormonal production than an older woman. But none of us are really sure. Nobody has studied this."[4]

Handling a Positive Biopsy

Each woman handles a positive biopsy in her own way. Many report feeling overwhelmed, upset, terrified, angry, or in shock. Some women are too depressed to get out of bed. Others plunge into action mode, making lightning-fast decisions and trying to push through each stage of their treatment as quickly as possible. Some women turn for support to spouses, partners, friends, or family. Still others isolate themselves. Many women bounce from one response to another as they try to develop a coping strategy that feels right.

So the first thing to do when your biopsy comes back positive is to stop, breathe, and get yourself into a place where you can make a truly calm decision. According to Dr. Love, "This is not an emergency. When you're first diagnosed with breast cancer, you are blown away; you are scared and will do almost anything. You get into this sort of magical thinking. You think, 'Maybe if I offer my breasts up, I'll get my life in exchange.' Or, 'If I take chemo, I'll extend my life a few years.' You tend to do almost whatever the doctor says, and you tend to rush into it—because you're scared. Ideally, someone will tell you to slow down and take

Randi Rosenberg

After I got my positive biopsy results, I went in to see the breast surgeon, whom I nicknamed "Dr. OldDude." I was with my future husband, Andrew, and after waiting for what seemed like an eternity, Dr. OldDude examined me for about 10 seconds. When he was done, he said, "Get dressed and meet me in my office." Andrew was already waiting there. I pulled out a pad and pencil, because somewhere I had heard that it was a good idea to write down what the doctor was saying, since you may not be in the best frame of mind to really hear.

I scribbled: "Cancer . . . tumor . . . surgery . . . " Right away the doctor yelled, "PUT THAT AWAY!! Look me in the eye while I'm talking to you!" Whoa, I thought. I'm just trying to make sure that I understand everything that you're telling me. He kept yelling. "I don't want to talk to the top of your head, I want to look at you as I'm explaining your options!" Suddenly, instead of a young woman who's just had the pleasure of being told she has cancer, I felt like a schoolgirl whose daddy just yelled at her for misbehaving. He was talking a mile a minute as he proceeded to tell me what was wrong and what I needed to do about it. The first thing he said was, "You'll need a lumpectomy," but all I heard was, "You'llneedalumpectomy." And that's how the whole conversation went.

He wanted me to have my surgery within the week.

I said, "Isn't that a bit soon? What about a second opinion?"

He said, "With cancer, you need to move quickly. The next availability is Wednesday, but I already have four surgeries that day. Thursday morning, then. You can get a second, third, or fourth opinion if you like, but they'll all tell you exactly what I've told you. I've seen thousands of these cases."

I walked out of that office with my head spinning. Holy cow! What just happened in there? The experience officially catapulted me onto autopilot! There was no way in hell I was going back to see that guy ever again, let alone trusting him to perform major surgery on the pristine temple that is my body!

Questions to Ask Yourself about Your Test Results

- *Whom do I tell?* You may want to make two lists: *people who need to know right away* and *people you'll tell later.* Give yourself some time to think carefully about who should be on each list. Some of your loved ones may simply not offer the support you need at this time. Perhaps they live far away, or they're ill themselves, or they just don't handle crises well. Let your instincts be your guide, because now is when you'll want to start identifying your "inner circle" of support—the friends and family who will provide the emotional stability and reality-based perspective that you're going to need over the coming months. You're probably in for some surprises—good friends who melt away in a crisis, a coworker or neighbor who comes through in amazing ways. But it is important to begin with what you know now about those closest to you, sharing your news with the people whose love and support can help sustain you.

- *When do I tell?* The best answer to this question is, "When you feel like it." Another good answer is, "When it will help *you.*" Kathryn Kash, Ph.D., is a psycho-oncologist who helps cancer patients deal with emotional issues. Dr. Kash points out that you may have to distinguish between people who are genuinely able to offer you support and those who require support from *you.* While you may eventually tell people in both categories, save the people in the second category for a time when you can more easily handle their response. Some people also respond better once they know that you've decided on a plan of action. And there may be some people whose opinions you don't want to take into account—so tell them after you've already made your decisions.

- *How do I tell?* Don't put yourself in the position of having to call five or six people every night to report on each doctor you've seen and each opinion you've gotten. Figure out a way to inform people close to you while also conserving your emotional and physical energy. Roberta Levy-Schwartz had a strong network of good friends who actually formed a phone tree. She only had to call a single friend and the news would spread to everyone.

a deep breath, and you'll have a chance to get a second opinion and some more information and really choose what is best for you."

Dr. Love points out that although you've just found out about it, "The breast cancer is not going to spread that afternoon or the next day. Whatever has happened, has happened, and there is time to look at the options, to get a second opinion, to see what studies are available before you embark on a program."

The YSC also advises young women to slow down and make careful decisions regarding a breast cancer diagnosis.

> Stop, react, adjust, make a game plan. Allow yourself moments alone to just sit and let it sink in as much as it can—get away to places that make you feel good. Don't necessarily do anything yet. Moments alone will allow you to get your head clear enough to understand what is happening to you, determine who you need to share your news with, in what order, how and when. And, begin to make lists of all the questions you want to ask your doctor and all the people who can possibly help you or might know something about your new disease.[5]

Getting a Second Opinion

As Randi found out, the first doctor you see is not always the right one for you. If you don't feel that you're being treated with the respect you deserve, if you're not getting answers to your questions, or if your doctor just doesn't "feel right," don't be afraid to get a second opinion, or even a third.

Dr. Sledge believes strongly that a patient should never feel uncomfortable about getting a second opinion. "Remember," he says, "it's your life. It's not the doctor's life. There are doctors who are offended if the patient asks for a second opinion. In my mind, that's good evidence that you need a new doctor." In fact, says Dr. Sledge, a doctor who's offended by your search for another opinion is probably "unwilling to listen to anyone else's opinion. Or else he is so pretentious, he thinks he is never going to learn anything—and the patient is never going to learn anything—from someone else. Doctors should not only not be offended, they should routinely offer to let patients have a second opinion. And patients should never feel uncomfortable about that. It's not about the doctor or the doctor's feelings. It's about you, your feelings, and your life. If your doctor makes you feel bad about asking for a second opinion, that's evidence that you really do need a second opinion."

Tips on Getting a Second Opinion

- Call ahead to find out what materials the second doctor will need: mammograms, accompanying reports, reports of tests, tissue slides of the tumor, the pathology report, x-rays, imaging studies, radiology reports, and your medical history. If possible, make several copies of everything, in case you need more opinions. Make sure you always have your own copy.

- Be prepared with a list of specific questions about your condition to ask the second physician.

- Put together a list of all the tests and procedures related to your breast cancer diagnosis and treatment that you've had, the places they were done, and their dates, as well as a comprehensive list of any medication you are currently taking.

- Try to get a specific treatment plan from every doctor you consult. That way, you can compare the plans that are right for you.

Finding the Doctor Who Is Right for You

During your experience with breast cancer, you'll often have to find the right physician or health-care professional. You'll probably need a breast surgeon, a medical oncologist (a specialist in cancer), a radiation oncologist, and a plastic surgeon (if you choose to have breast reconstruction, see Chapter 8). Some women further seek a physical therapist (see Chapter 4), a nutritionist (see Chapter 4), a practitioner of alternative or complementary medicine (see Chapter 5), a psychotherapist (see Chapter 5), or other types of specialists for particular conditions or concerns.

It can feel a bit overwhelming to go on a doctor hunt when all you want to do is solve your medical problem and get on with your life. But choosing a doctor whom you trust and with whom you can work is key to your treatment and recovery. Even if you are on a managed-care health plan, you will probably be able to choose from among a list of specialists—or you may be able to negotiate with your insurer about who will treat you.

The best way to find the right specialist is simply to ask everyone you know: your regular practitioner, other doctors you encounter, family, friends, and coworkers. You never know who may have had a friend or family member with breast cancer. It's also useful to talk with other breast cancer survivors, especially young women who may share your perspective and values. Breast cancer organizations often provide referrals as well.

Questions to Ask a Prospective Doctor

- How much experience have you had with my type of breast cancer?
- What are your procedures for scheduling an appointment? For an emergency?
- If I need someone after office hours, will I be in touch with you or with someone else?
- How comfortable are you with sharing information with your patients? If I have questions, can you find time to explain things to me?
- (If this is a concern for you:) What are you feelings about alternative or complementary medicine? About nutrition? I plan to work with specialists in those fields. How can we integrate that work into my work with you?
- If I need a specialist, can I find one through your office?
- What else do you think I should know about working with you? What do you expect from me as your patient?

Questions to Ask Your Surgeon(s) about Your Treatment

- What procedure do you recommend? Why?
- How many of these operations have you done?
- How long will I be in the hospital?
- What kind of follow-up care do I need?
- How long will it take me to recover? When can I go back to work? When can I start caring for my children again?
- What will it cost?
- What will my insurance cover?
- What else do I need to know?

In the course of your search, certain names are likely to come up again and again. These are probably the people you want to consult. Arrange to meet your top two or three choices and talk to them for 15 minutes or so. Doctors are busy people, of course, but meeting with prospective patients is part of their work, so prepare yourself with a list of questions and put your instincts on alert. You're looking for someone whose judgment you trust, someone who is honest and good at sharing information. Ideally, your doctor or someone from his or her office will be accessible 24 hours a day, via a service or pager. Given the amount of time you and your doctor will spend together and the crucial decisions the two of you will make, it's also important that your doctor be someone who can view you as a person, not just a patient. And, of course, you want someone who has a lot of experience dealing with your particular form of breast cancer.

Different people have different styles, and so do different doctors. What one woman views as helpful, another woman might see as patronizing. What one woman thinks of as informative, another woman might experience as information overload. Try to choose a doctor whose style matches your own, so that the two of you can work together effectively as partners in your health care.

Coping with All the Information

"I liken it to drinking water out of a fire hydrant," says Mark Douglas, Kelly's husband. "You have all this information at your fingertips. You log onto the Internet and type in 'breast cancer,' and there are millions and billions of entries." As Mark's simile suggests, the sheer volume of information can sometimes be overwhelming. Somehow, you have to find a way to learn all that you need to know without being flooded with so many facts and figures that your brain simply shuts down in protest.

Tips for Dealing with Internet Resources

- Find out who is responsible for the site. It might be a foundation or a pharmaceutical company, a government agency or a research institute. Whatever it is, you'll want to know, because each different organization will have its own slant. Ultimately, you'll have to decide: Is this a credible organization?

- What are the references for the information? And how current are the references? You don't want references from 1988. You want to see that the information being provided is current and that the citations are credible. Remember, anyone can build a Web site and promote propaganda.

- What other sites does this site link to? Does it take you to the National Cancer Institute, the American Cancer Society, breast cancer support groups, or other sites that you know and respect? Linking with other reputable sites adds credibility and shows that the sponsor of this site has nothing to hide.

- Look for a site that allows you to ask questions and receive responses.

- If you see information that contradicts what your doctor has advised, do not assume that your doctor isn't telling you the right thing. Every case is different, and each case has subtle nuances that cannot necessarily be addressed on an Internet site.

- If reading something on the Internet makes you question the approach of your health team, you should definitely print it out and discuss it with your doctor. This gives you an opportunity to verify that this site is credible, as well as an opportunity to be reassured about the treatment you're choosing. The more comfortable you are with the recommendations you're getting from your physician, the stronger you'll be—mentally, physically, and emotionally—to handle what's ahead.

- Don't forget: If the site isn't specifically focused on young women, the information may not apply to you.

Suggested by Bert Petersen, M.D., surgical oncologist, Beth Israel Cancer Center, New York City.

Remember, as Dr. Winer explained, breast cancer is not one disease, but many. And there is no standard treatment for breast cancer—every woman needs something different, particularly if she's age 40 or under. So you may indeed hear different opinions from different doctors. You may even be presented with a range of options by a single doctor. Somehow, you'll have to sort through all the information. Take your time as you master this new material, and make your decision calmly.

Dealing with Insurance Companies

It's not a medical issue, but it could be one of the most important aspects of your health care: dealing with your insurance company. While this chapter won't tell you everything you need to know about this crucial and often frustrating necessity, it will give you a brief overview. Remember, though, that everyone's policy is different, so you will need to talk to your own insurance company to find out exactly how your policy works and what it covers. For more on work-related insurance issues, including what happens when you change jobs or when your employer switches insurance companies, see Chapter 11. For more information on insurance issues in general, as well as for support and guidance concerning any part of your dealings with insurance companies, contact the Patient Advocate Foundation. (For contact information, refer to the Resources section.)

Types of Providers

Although insurance companies have set up many different systems, these systems basically fall into two categories: *fee-for-service* and *managed care*. With a fee-for-service plan, you're generally allowed to choose your own doctors and treatment facilities; you pay them yourself, and then you get back some percentage of the cost. You pay a fee called *coinsurance* (often 20 percent of the total), and the insurance company reimburses the rest. Usually there's a *deductible*—an amount that you have to pay before the insurance company's percentage kicks in. Of course, the insurance company will decide whether to approve the procedures and costs that you submit, so if you've got a fee-for-service plan, you'll need to work with your provider to make sure ahead of time that your costs will be reimbursed.

Under *managed care,* you're covered in advance for a range of services, but you can go only to doctors and facilities that belong to your managed-care plan. You may also be charged a *copayment* for each service, such as $10 per doctor visit. Usually, under managed care, you can make an appointment with your *primary-care physician*—your regular doctor—but you must get a referral for all other services, including oncologists, radiologists, breast surgeons, and other specialized care that you'll need for your breast cancer. You'll usually be given a choice (a list of specialists that are part of the plan), although sometimes you'll be assigned to a particular specialist.

Most managed-care plans put tight restrictions on their referrals. You aren't simply referred to an oncologist; you're allowed a specific number of visits or a specific time period within which visits are approved. If your needs extend beyond that initial referral, as they almost certainly will, you usually have to go back to your primary-care physician and get another referral. In theory, you can do this over the phone, but sometimes the primary-care doctor insists on actually seeing you and reviewing your case before referring you back to the specialist.

Lisa Muccilo, diagnosed with breast cancer at age 27, has seen her cancer recur five times and become metastatic. For her, the need to get a referral from a primary-care physician has been a particularly frustrating burden. "Once you've been diagnosed with cancer, if you feel anything is wrong, you're going to go to your oncologist," she points out. "Even for aches and pains." At one point, Lisa had used up all her oncologist referrals, but the billing office didn't notify her at the time. When the bills came, she discovered that 2 months of her treatment hadn't been covered, and she had to try to get her insurance company to approve them after the fact. Meanwhile, she had to go back to her primary-care physician for another referral.

> I called my primary-care office, and, of course, you have to deal with the secretary. And she says, "You have to come in." I told her I really wanted the referral done over the phone. She said, "No, you haven't been here in over a year; you have to come in." I said, "You don't understand; he's not going to look at me, I'm being treated for metastatic breast cancer." She said, "No, I'm sorry, we can't do a referral."
>
> So I said, "I can't let this get to me. Just go to the doctor's office and get it done." It's time out of the day, time out of work, and it's annoying, but I just wanted to be done with it. I get there, and I wait and wait. Finally, I go into the room, and the nurse asks me, "What are you here for today? Tell me about the problems you're having." I said, "Well, I have metastatic breast cancer. I'm here for a referral." "Oh." Then the doctor comes in. He says, "So, why are you here today?" I said, "Well, I have metastatic breast cancer—I'm here for a referral." He was like, "I can't believe they made you come in for this." He said, "I'm really sorry."

Lisa finally resolved her insurance problems in a creative way: Her father agreed to take over all dealings with the insurance company on her behalf. "It was so stressful, dealing with insurance," she says. "I just couldn't do it. I turned it over to my dad, which is the best thing I ever did." Lisa feels that it's a huge burden for her father, too—"It is monumental," she says. "My dad has a whole file cabinet that is now filled"— but she believes that the relief from the stress has made an enormous difference in her own health. If the idea of getting out of the insurance hassle appeals to you and you don't have a loved one who is ready to volunteer, you may actually be able to hire someone to take on this task, a service that has become available in some cities in response to the rise of managed care. Check your local papers for ads, do an Internet search, or place a help wanted ad of your own.

Coping with the Bureaucracy

Whatever type of insurance coverage you have, you may find that your insurance company is not sympathetic to your situation. After all, its mission is to hold down costs and, if it's a for-profit company, to make a profit for its shareholders. Your mission is to get the best health care you can. Sometimes these two missions come into conflict. Perhaps you aren't

Tips for Dealing with Your Insurance Company

- Buy a notebook and make it the insurance notebook. Have a blanket rule: Everything gets written down.
- Be preemptive. Ask questions before they turn into problems.
- Get to know the person in your doctor's office who is responsible for authorizations. Form an alliance with this person. This person will be able to explain to you what you need to know about getting precertifications (approvals before the fact for certain procedures).
- Confirm for yourself that every procedure has been approved. Write down who in your insurance company told you it was approved.
- Get the first and last names of everyone and record the date you spoke to them. If they tell you that they have a policy that won't allow giving a last name, tell them you want to talk with a supervisor. Even if they tell you the call is being recorded "for quality assurance," don't assume that there is any record of it. Keep your own records.
- Get a confirmation number whenever possible.
- Ask for a social worker in the doctor's office or in the hospital. Sometimes they can help you.
- Ask a family member or friend for help. People are always saying, "I want to help." This is a very concrete way they can do that. You just have to ask them.
- If you have an HMO, find out the policies for the office of your primary-care physician. Remember, you're going to be dealing with the office staff just as much as, if not more than, with the doctor, and you have to find a practice whose policies you can live with. If you don't like the way your doctor's office is run, consider switching doctors.
- Ask your insurance company to assign you a case manager. Tell your insurer you'd like to deal with one person who understands your complicated situation so that you don't have to start fresh with every new conversation.
- Find out if the oncologist you've chosen is also a primary-care physician in your HMO. Sometimes specialists are listed as primary-care physicians. They may be listed in a confusing way, but you can find out by asking your insurance carrier or doctor's office. That's something you can shop around for—to make sure your oncologist and your primary-care physician are the same person, so you don't need a referral.

Elizabeth Tarr is Director of the New York chapter of the American Cancer Society's Reach to Recovery, a program that provides support to breast cancer patients. She offers these recommendations for dealing with an insurance company.

satisfied with any of the doctors to whom you've been referred. Maybe you want a treatment that the insurance company doesn't think is necessary. Or perhaps you're interested in an experimental treatment, either because you and your doctor have decided that conventional treatments aren't useful in your case or because these treatments have already failed. According to the National Cancer Institute, experimental treatments that are part of an approved clinical trial are supposed to be covered by insurance, but as Debu Tripathy, M.D., an oncologist at the University of California–San Francisco, warns, "Some patients have a difficult time getting experimental treatments because their insurance company won't pay for the drugs or for the patient to be treated at the site of the trial." Therefore, it may take some convincing before the insurance company agrees that such a treatment is necessary. While the medications in an experimental treatment are covered by the group that's conducting the experiment, the associated costs—hospital admission, follow-up, blood work—must be paid for by either you or your insurance company, and these costs are not covered by most plans.

It's also important to know whether your insurance company requires precertification for certain tests and procedures. If precertification is required, your doctor's office must get approval from the insurance company *before* the test or procedure; otherwise, it will not be covered. While your doctor's office will most likely be responsible for obtaining precertification, you'll want to make sure you ask about it, because mistakes can be costly. If you're not happy with an insurance company's decision, you have several options. You can work with someone in the company to reverse the decision. You can take your case through the insurance company's appeals process. Sometimes going to a state legislator is helpful. In some cases, it may be worthwhile to sue and/or to take your case to the media. Figuring out the appeals process and your range of options can be another source of stress, but it may be worth it if it makes the difference between staggering medical bills and getting the coverage you deserve. Again, the Patient Advocate Foundation is available to advise you as you figure out what options are available and how to pursue them.

Elizabeth Tarr points out that dealing with the health-care system is particularly hard for young women, who generally don't have much experience with either health problems or the medical community. Nor are they used to dealing with managed care, which did not exist when they were growing up. "It's not easy," Tarr says. "The rules are constantly changing. You think you've got it figured out—and it changes. It's a world no one ever wants to get to know—and now you have to get to know it at the worst possible time."

If You Don't Have Insurance

- Contact the Patient Advocate Foundation and ask for *The National Financial Resource Guidebook for Patients: A State-by-State Directory*, a guidebook for patients seeking financial relief for a broad range of needs, including health care.

- An independent insurance broker may be able to help you get your own insurance at a reasonable rate.

- Many communities have HMOs that can be joined by individuals. You can often get comprehensive coverage for an affordable individual fee. Many HMOs offer an annual open enrollment period, during which you must be accepted regardless of your health or medical history.

- You may be able to get group insurance through a fraternal or professional organization, such as those for teachers, social workers, or realtors.

- If you are unemployed or in a low-income bracket, you may be eligible for Medicaid.

- Negotiate fees with your doctor if your only option is self-pay.

Making the Right Decision—for You

Now that your diagnosis is complete, it's time for you to choose a course of treatment—a decision that's discussed in detail in Chapter 3. You may feel a bit overwhelmed as you navigate between your doctor's opinions, your loved ones' ideas, and your own responses. Remember that, ultimately, there is no "right decision." There's only the right decision for you. Take your time, learn what you're able to, and make the wisest choices you can, based on your own instincts. Then trust yourself. Having confidence in the decisions you've made will be enormously helpful to your treatment and recovery—and, paradoxically, will actually make it easier for you to change course, should that be necessary.

CHAPTER 3

"No One Told Me It Would Be Like That"

Measuring Options, Making Choices, from Surgery through Treatment

Susan Kolevsohn, a 22-year-old breast cancer survivor from Atlanta, Georgia, thought she was prepared for her mastectomy. Her doctor had even talked her through the process. As Kolevsohn said, "He wanted me to wake up feeling whole." Kolevsohn had opted for immediate reconstruction—a single operation that would remove her breast (a mastectomy) and replace it with a new one before she woke up.

"'Whole' was a misconception," Kolevsohn says now. "As soon as I woke up, I remember I was petrified. I couldn't feel my chest. No one told me it would be like that. I was hysterical. I thought I'd died. I didn't know what was happening. I said something about it to my gynecologist, and she said, 'What did you expect?' It was shocking."

When Kathy Burgau of Fergus Falls, Minnesota, was diagnosed with breast cancer at age 26, she was prepared for just about everything—except losing her hair. Although she'd known intellectually that it might happen, the actual hair loss, which occurred about 2 weeks after she began chemotherapy, was quite a shock.

"I had already cut off 6 inches of my hair—it was now at shoulder length," she recalls. "And it was just coming out in hunks. When my husband, Perry, got home from work, I said, 'You're shaving my head.' He sat me down and started shaving it. Perry's mom took pictures. Then I got in the shower to get all the little hairs off me. I couldn't wear my contacts during chemo because it hurt to wear them. So I had my glasses

off, and I couldn't see all that well, and I'm covered in whiskers. I saw all this hair in the tub—longer hair. And I got down on my hands and knees and realized it was my pubic hair. I just never expected that.

"I got out of the shower, and my husband said, 'You look like a 12-year-old.' I said, 'Well, you're the one robbing the cradle.' I had no hair anywhere. Not in my armpits, not on my arms. My eyelashes and eyebrows were gone. I couldn't believe what had happened."

⁓

Randi Rosenberg, diagnosed with breast cancer at age 32, felt that she had a good relationship with all her doctors and was able to get good answers to all her questions. But she soon discovered that there were many questions that she had never thought to ask—such as what were the side effects of tamoxifen, a hormonal treatment that her oncologist had prescribed for her after her chemotherapy.

"Honestly, when I first started taking tamoxifen, I really noticed a lot of bizarre changes," Randi recalls. "I kind of likened it to going through puberty again—which was just really strange. There were intense mood swings. I would be gloriously happy, and then the next minute a Captain & Tennille song would come on the radio and I would burst into tears—sobbing for no apparent reason. Then anger. It was just this roller coaster of emotions. The other thing I noticed was that I was breaking out—I had a really bad case of acne, just like junior high school. It was rough." Nothing would have made it easy to be on tamoxifen, Randi says—but it would certainly have been easier if she had been better prepared for what the drug might be like.

Continuing through the Treatment Process

If you have been recently diagnosed with breast cancer and you're reading this book, this chapter will educate you about the multitude of issues you may face during the treatment process. If you have already been through the treatment process, however, you may want to skip this chapter, as the information provided may not be relevant to you at this stage, or may even be upsetting if you are not prepared to relive your treatment experience.

As Susan, Kathy, and Randi found out, it's hard to be prepared *enough* for the range of experiences you'll have during your breast cancer treatment. Some things you simply can't prepare for, but in other cases, knowing what to expect can make a crucial difference to your sense of security and well-being. So in this chapter, you'll find out at least some of what to expect as far as surgery and the treatment after surgery are concerned.

This part of the process begins after your biopsy comes back. Based on the pathologist's report, your doctor will recommend a course of treatment, usually surgery to remove the cancer from the breast and perhaps also the lymph node area, followed by systemic treatment, such as chemotherapy and hormonal therapy, to keep the cancer from spreading and to attack any cancer that has already spread. Sometimes radiation therapy is recommended after surgery, to ensure that any cancer that still remains in the breast area has been rendered inactive.

You may be given a relatively open choice, or you may be strongly urged to choose a particular option. Either way, the final decision is yours—and the more you know, the better decision you'll make.

If you want more information about how these treatments might affect your fertility or your pregnancy, turn to Chapter 9. If you'd like to know more about breast reconstruction—which you can usually have either during your mastectomy or in a whole separate procedure—check out Chapter 8. And if you'd like to learn more about participating in a clinical trial (an experiment designed to help us learn more about which treatments are effective), see the discussion later in this chapter. Many women find that taking part in clinical trials is a meaningful way to turn their own experiences into at least some measure of help for other young women.

And, of course, you'll hear from young women who have gone through surgery, chemotherapy, hormonal treatments, and radiation, as they share their stories and offer their advice.

Sorting through Your Surgical Options

Lumpectomy, or "Breast Conservation Surgery"

In this procedure, the surgeon removes only the cancer itself, along with as much surrounding tissue as is needed to get the "clear margins" that indicate that the tumor is gone. The amount of breast scarring or deformity you experience will depend on the size of your breast and the size of the lump removed. Women with smaller breasts may lose so much in the lumpectomy as to defeat the idea of "conserving the breasts." Women with larger breasts may find that their breasts look pretty much the way they did before the surgery. A lumpectomy is almost always followed by radiation treatment. Usually, a lumpectomy is done with a local anesthetic. The whole procedure takes 2 or 3 hours. You'll probably be able to leave the hospital that day, but some doctors prefer their patients to spend the night.

Mastectomy

A mastectomy is a removal of the entire breast. In most cases, having a mastectomy means that you'll spend one night in the hospital. If you decide to have reconstructive surgery at the same time, you'll probably spend two to five nights in the hospital. (For more on breast reconstruction, see Chapter 8.)

There are several different types of mastectomy. A *total* or *simple* mastectomy removes the entire breast but leaves most of the lymph nodes and surrounding muscle. It will leave you completely flat. If you are especially thin, your chest may even be a bit concave. When the surgery is completed, your doctor will insert one or two tubes (called *drains*) under the skin to help drain the fluid that accumulates at the surgery site. Although you may regain some feeling in some parts of your chest, the area around the scar will always be numb.

Risks from a total mastectomy include *lymphedema,* a chronic swelling of the hand and/or arm that occurs when the lymph system under your arm is blocked, either by scar tissue from the surgery or because the lymph nodes under your arm have been removed. Lymphedema may also limit your arm's range of motion and make you more vulnerable to infection and cellulitis, a redness around the surgery site that may have to be treated with antibiotics. Another common risk is *paresthesia,* a numbness and tingling, if the nerve under the arm was severed during lymph node removal.

In some cases, you may have a *radical mastectomy,* the complete removal of the breast along with the chest muscles on either side. Although this used to be the standard treatment for breast cancer, it is now performed only when there is extensive cancer that has spread to the muscles of the chest wall. More common than the radical mastectomy is the *modified radical mastectomy,* in which the entire breast and the lining over the chest muscles are removed, but not the chest muscles themselves. Complications of both procedures also include limited mobility and lymphedema. Generally, this procedure leaves you with weaker arm and shoulder muscles and far more limited mobility than the simple mastectomy.

According to Dr. Bert Petersen, a surgical oncologist and director of the Family Risk Program at Beth Israel Cancer Center:

The radical mastectomy of the past is only done when there is very, very extensive local disease—and even then we will usually try to shrink the disease with chemo and radiation before going in for surgery. Back in the days when radical mastectomies were done all the time, there was no good chemotherapy. So the radical mastectomy was big at a time when the mentality of treatment was that surgery was the cure. Today we have a multidisciplinary approach. Rather than run for surgery, we try to lessen the need for a radical mastectomy by offering chemo and radiation up front.

Yet another option is a *partial mastectomy,* or removal of a portion of the breast—more than just the cancer, but less than the entire breast. Even though only part of your breast is being removed, you will lose all sensation in that breast, and your two breasts will no longer match. In some cases, your doctor may recommend either a lumpectomy or a partial mastectomy as a first step and then later tell you that a full mastectomy is in fact necessary. If your doctor recommends a partial mastectomy, find out how much of your breast is being taken and why this procedure is suggested, rather than either a full mastectomy or a lumpectomy.

Having a mastectomy—losing a breast—can be a traumatic prospect, but to some women the idea may actually come as a relief. "After I had the biopsy, and I found I had breast cancer, my breast was so swollen," recalls Kelly Douglas, diagnosed at age 24. "It was so painful—it was all nasty colors that skin should not turn, and it was painful, it really hurt. At that point, I was like, 'We've gotta get rid of this. The breast has got to go. It hurts. It's swollen. It looks disgusting, and it's turned on me.' The thought 'I just need to get rid of this thing' made the mastectomy easier."

Lanita Hausman, diagnosed at age 32, went even further. "My breast surgeon was advocating that I have the whole breast removed because it was a ductal cancer, and she didn't know how much it had infiltrated into the ductal system," she explains. "And as the niece of a woman who had breast cancer at 29 and again at 43, I had an idea of what I wanted to do. So when she said, "We ought to take the breast, and here's why," I remember I didn't even look at my husband. I just said, 'Well, take two, they're small.' She looked up and said, 'Don't laugh, or I'll take you seriously.' And I said, 'I am serious.' She said, 'Okay, we'll take both.'"

Lanita was requesting a *prophylactic mastectomy,* a mastectomy done to prevent cancer from developing in the as-yet-unaffected breast. Doctors have mixed feelings about prophylactic mastectomies: Some believe that they are a wise move for high-risk women, whereas others feel that they don't actually help to prevent cancer. Dr. Bert Petersen has gone through an evolution in his own response to prophylactic mastectomies:

When I first went into practice, I was so against prophylactic mastectomy. Then one day I found myself listening to what a young woman was saying in a way that I had never done before. She described what it was like going to bed at night and waking up worried in the morning. This is what she was dealing with every day. She had seen family members young and old be diagnosed with breast cancer and die. It shaped and colored her world. I said, "You know, I never go to bed worrying about that. How arrogant of me to tell her not to do this." So I had to step back and ask myself, "Where else am I not listening to what patients are trying to tell me?"

Removal of the Lymph Nodes

Along with removing breast tissue in either a lumpectomy or a mastectomy, a doctor will typically remove one or more of your adjacent lymph nodes in a procedure known as an *axillary node* dissection. This may be done either as treatment (if your doctor suspects that the cancer has spread there) or as diagnosis (to find out whether the cancer has spread). If no cancer cells are identified in the lymph nodes, the doctors will assume that the cancer has not spread; if the lymph nodes are cancerous, your postsurgery treatment with radiation, chemotherapy, or tamoxifen may be more aggressive. (For more on treatment after surgery, see the discussion later in this chapter.)

The advantage of leaving in as many lymph nodes as possible is that it reduces the chance of lymphedema and is generally less invasive. The advantage of taking lymph nodes, obviously, is that they can give valuable clues as to what kind of further treatment is needed.

In a newer procedure called a *sentinel node biopsy,* only a single lymph node is removed for diagnosis. Some dye is injected into the woman's breast during the mastectomy or lumpectomy, and the first lymph node into which it flows is identified. This first node, the "sentinel," is presumably the first place to which the cancer would flow as well, so if the node tests negative, that's a good sign that the cancer has not spread.

Choosing the Surgery That Is Right for You

Deciding whether you want a lumpectomy, a partial mastectomy, or some version of a full mastectomy can be difficult. On the one hand, a smaller and less invasive operation means that you'll recover faster and risk fewer complications. On the other hand, if you have the smaller operation and the cancer is not completely removed, you may need a second operation.

The size and stage of your cancer will play a major role in your decision. Many young women are not good candidates for lumpectomies because, since there are no effective screening procedures, their cancer was often discovered at a later stage.

Joy Simha, Diagnosed at Age 26

When I was initially diagnosed, the original breast surgeon told me that she would only consider a mastectomy. And she had the benefit of doing the biopsy, so she knew where that tumor was, and knew that it was very centrally located . . . very close to the nipple. So when I went for a second and then third opinion, the second- and third-opinion doctors were saying, "I don't know, maybe we could do a lumpectomy. Let's try a lumpectomy and see if we get clear margins." So the treatment I ended up having was a lumpectomy. And just 2 days after I had the lumpectomy, I got a phone call from my breast surgeon, and she said there was still a little bit of cancer near the nipple and "We're going to have to remove the nipple or give you a mastectomy. We're kind of giving you the choice."

And I asked her, "What do you think is best?" And she said, "If you can stomach it, I think having the mastectomy would be best, because you are more likely to live a cancer-free life without a local recurrence if you have a mastectomy."

And that was all I needed to hear, because I had been living with cancer for a month and that was long enough for me. A month later, mastectomy was a much easier concept to accept. So I chose to have the mastectomy.

Researchers had assumed that, given the choice, most young women would select partial mastectomies rather than full mastectomies, out of concern for their body image. But a recent study at the University of California–Berkeley found that, contrary to expectations, young women were actually having mastectomies more often than older women—an indication of how much more aggressive breast cancer can be in younger women, and perhaps also of greater fear on the part of younger women and their doctors.[1]

According to Dr. George Sledge, a professor of medicine and pathology at Indiana University Cancer Center, these concerns may be warranted. "After they've had a lumpectomy and radiation, younger women do have a higher breast cancer recurrence rate than older women," he says. "However, that's not a reason *not* to consider lumpectomy and radiation. It is a reason—maybe—to consider mastectomy to possibly avoid future problems. But I would never tell a woman that just because she's young, she can't have breast preservation surgery. Those who can't have a lumpectomy usually can't have it for a very good reason. Maybe it's because the tumor is too big, or because they're small-breasted, or they're pregnant—it's not just because they're young."

Questions to Ask Your Doctor about Your Surgery

- What kind of surgery do you recommend for me, and why?
- How much of my breast will be removed?
- Will I be able to have breast reconstruction?
- Should I have my breast reconstruction during the same operation as my mastectomy, or should I wait until later? (For more on breast reconstruction, see Chapter 8.)
- Will you remove any of my lymph nodes? Why or why not?
- Am I a candidate for a sentinel node biopsy? Why or why not?
- How many times have you performed this procedure?
- Can I have chemotherapy before my surgery to shrink the tumor, and then have a lumpectomy rather than a mastectomy? Why or why not?
- What do I need to do to prepare for my surgery?
- Will I have a local or general anesthetic? Do I have a choice? (A local anesthetic is generally less stressful for your body and is easier to recover from. However, some women find it upsetting to remain awake—though sedated—during the operation. Other women find it reassuring to be awake and at least somewhat conscious of the procedure.)
- What side effects should I report to you?
- How long will I stay in the hospital?
- What kind of follow-up care will I need?
- Will I need to miss work? Should I make other arrangements for taking care of my children? For how long?
- Can I see photos of what I will look like after my surgery?

As recommended by the YSC.

Timing Your Surgery According to Your Menstrual Cycle

Some researchers believe that timing your breast cancer surgery according to your menstrual cycle can increase the effectiveness of your surgery. This is quite a contested theory in the medical community, and even those who believe strongly in the efficacy of timing acknowledge that there is room for a great deal more research.

Ruby Senie, Ph.D., professor of epidemiology at Columbia University's Mailman School of Public Health, conducted an extensive study of the link between the timing of surgery and the risk of recurrence. In her investigation of 283 premenopausal women at Memorial Sloan-Kettering, Senie found that the second 2 weeks of the menstrual cycle (the luteal phase) were clearly a better time to have surgery, whereas the first 2 weeks (the follicular phase) were less effective. However, Senie's findings applied only to women with positive lymph nodes. For women with no positive lymph nodes, Senie found, the timing of the surgery didn't matter. The problem is that until women go into surgery, they don't know whether their lymph nodes are positive—so they don't know in advance whether timing is important for them.[2]

Dr. Aron Goldhirsch, professor of medical oncology, director of the Department of Medicine at the European Institute of Oncology, and chair of the Scientific Committee of the International Breast Cancer Study Group, believes that there's some evidence that the timing of surgery might make a difference, although he is reluctant to embrace this idea with too much certainty. But in support of the notion that timing matters, he cites a recent study conducted under the leadership of Richard Love, M.D., president of the International Breast Cancer Research Foundation and professor of medicine at the University of Wisconsin, Madison, involving more than 700 premenopausal women with breast cancer in Vietnam and China.[3] The study found that women whose treatments included a combination mastectomy and oophorectomy (ovary removal) responded differently depending on when in their menstrual cycles the operations took place: 84 percent of those women whose surgery was performed during the second half of their cycle survived cancer-free for 5 years, as opposed to only 67 percent of women who'd had the same operations during the first half of their cycle.

Dr. Goldhirsch thinks that this new study may open promising vistas for breast cancer patients. "Perhaps," he says, "timing matters because hormonal factors in the menstrual cycle either suppress or encourage cancer cell activity: During the first part of the cycle there are only estrogens around, so there is a potential maximal stimulation of any micrometastases that are left behind. In the second part of the menstrual cycle, there is also progesterone . . . and the hypothesis is that the progesterone actually suppresses the micrometastases . . . during the second phase of the monthly cycle."

Dr. Sledge is frankly skeptical of the idea that a surgery's timing plays any role in its success. He says that previous studies, including Ruby Senie's, were based on different procedures from those done today. Dr.

Sledge points out that it's now common for breast cancer patients to have two or three different surgeries. So, he asks, which of those many surgeries should be timed according to the menstrual cycle?

Ruby Senie responds, "I would say, it's when the tumor is removed. But it's true, when we were looking into this question, it wasn't a multi-stage issue."

If you're considering breast cancer surgery, you might discuss the issue of timing with your doctor. New research could help you and your doctor decide whether to take the timing of your surgery into account.

Coping with the Aftermath of Surgery

You may find yourself having strong feelings about looking at the results of your surgery. Consider whether you'd like to be alone or with a loved one when you first look at your postsurgery breast or at your scar. Think, too, about waiting to look until you feel strong enough, both physically and emotionally.

Drains

As we discussed, if you have a mastectomy, your doctor will insert drains under your arm to help remove the fluid that builds up in this area. You (or a loved one) will need to empty the drains each day, and to measure the fluid. When the fluid declines to an acceptable level—something that could take 2 days or 2 weeks—your doctor will remove the drains during an office visit.

Some women find the whole business of the drains traumatic, but Kathy Burgau, an avid softball player diagnosed at age 26, found a way to make them part of a comic moment that helped her bond with her surgeon:

Charnette Messé, Diagnosed at Age 31

By the time I got to the drains, I just had to laugh. Drains are two holes in your side under your arm—near where your breast was. It was awful. The mastectomy was nothing; it was the drains I couldn't take. I wouldn't wish those on anyone or anything. It wasn't bad when they were in, but it was painful to have them taken out. The doctor holds you by the side and just rips them out. Oh, the drains.

It was so funny, because I didn't know about the drains. I thought they were going to cut off my breast and I'd be free to go. That's it. I saw the drains in a book. And I said, "What's this?" He said, "Those are drains." I said, "Okay." I was definitely not free to go.

Questions to Ask Your Doctor after Surgery

- Can I have a copy of my pathology report? (Remember, there will be a pathology report on whatever tissue was removed during your surgery.)

- Will you please review my pathology report with me?

- (If you had a lumpectomy:) Did my tumor have clear margins? If it didn't, what do we do now?

- How many lymph nodes were removed?

- Did any of them contain cancer cells? How many?

- Were micrometastases found anywhere outside my tumor? What does this mean for me? (*Micrometastasis* is the spread of microscopic cancer cells in the body. Because it is undetectable by mammography or ultrasound—the cells are so small that you need a microscope to see them—micrometastasis is usually determined by studying the lymph nodes that are removed during a mastectomy. If a woman does not need her lymph nodes removed for treatment, this means that they are also not available for diagnosis.)

As recommended by the YSC.

My surgeon had a really hard time dealing with me. He didn't know what to say—he had a hard time looking at me. The nurse told me it was because he has two daughters, and looking at me was like looking at them. When he came in to take my drains out, I said, "So do you think I'll be able to throw a softball better without the boob there?" It lightened the moment, and he finally let his guard down.

Treatment after Surgery

The goal of your surgery was to remove the *local* cancer—the cancer that had developed in your breast tissue. The goal of treatment after surgery is to counteract the spread and prevent recurrence of cancer.

In young women, treatment is likely to be more aggressive because their breast cancer tends to be more aggressive, more likely to recur, and more likely to be fatal. According to Dr. Susan Love, "Breast cancer in younger women compared to women who are middle-aged is more aggressive. What does more aggressive mean? It means it's more likely to spread."

"The chance of my cancer coming back is a possibility—and a very scary possibility," says Kelly Douglas, "especially since we found out that the cancer I have is an aggressive cancer. And the fact that it was in my lymph nodes was frightening as well. Because is it just going to show up in my breast next time, or is it going to show up somewhere else? Is it going to be my liver? My brain? That's what's really frightening. That's why we're going through a more aggressive treatment, to make sure we get rid of everything, so I don't have to worry about cancer later on."

Your treatment choices after surgery are chemotherapy, hormonal therapy, and radiation. Chemotherapy and hormonal therapy are called *systemic* because they treat your entire system, and one or both are usually prescribed after a full or partial mastectomy. Radiation can be given after a mastectomy but is more routinely prescribed after a lumpectomy. It is a local treatment, designed to follow up the surgery by eradicating any cancer cells that remain in the breast.

In some cases—especially if your tumor is larger—your doctor may recommend neoadjuvant chemotherapy before surgery. The goals of presurgery treatment are to shrink the tumor and to evaluate which drugs are most effective.

Chemotherapy

In this form of treatment, you'll be given a number of different chemicals, either intravenously or orally, that are intended to move through your bloodstream and destroy any cancerous cells remaining in your body. Chemo works because it keeps cells from dividing. Unfortunately, it doesn't work on just cancer cells; it also stops other fast-growing cells from multiplying, including your bone marrow and hair cells. As a result, you'll probably experience *alopecia*, or hair loss, and a weakened immune system, since your bone marrow produces the white blood cells that help protect you from various ailments, as well as manufacturing your red blood cells and platelets. Your hair will probably grow back within 6 to 8 weeks of completing treatment, and doctors say that your immune system should bounce back in that time as well—especially if you are physically active.[4] However, many women find it painful to lose their hair and find the weakness, nausea, and lowered immune function that chemo often brings to be frightening. So make sure you have the emotional support you need to make it through this difficult time. (For more on emotional support, see Chapter 6. For more on hair loss and other body-image issues, see Chapter 7.)

Proponents of various types of alternative treatments believe that in many cases, these approaches can help ease your passage through chemotherapy by minimizing many of the side effects. The medical evidence for these claims varies widely, and many physicians are generally skeptical about alternative treatments. A growing body of medical opinion, however, welcomes integrative approaches that combine standard and complementary treatments, and such prestigious cancer centers as Sloan-Kettering now have centers for integrative medicine. (For more information on complementary, alternative, and integrative approaches, see Chapter 5.)

You may want to consider visiting your dentist to have your teeth cleaned and any cavities filled before you start chemotherapy. The most important reason for doing this is that your suppressed immune system will be less able to handle the risk of infection from mouth bacteria during treatment. Also, if you develop mouth sores (a common side effect of chemo), dental work will be very uncomfortable.

What Happens during Chemotherapy

Chemotherapy is administered in cycles, usually once every 3 weeks, to give your bone marrow a chance to recuperate between treatments. Your doctor will be aiming for a balance between lowering the number of cancer cells in your body to the point where your immune system can take them on and keeping your immune system healthy enough to do that. So before each chemo treatment, your doctor will take a blood sample to measure your red and white blood cell counts. If your blood counts are too low, your treatment may be postponed.

Because Kelly's white blood count was lower than expected, one of her chemotherapy treatments, originally scheduled for December 20, had to be postponed to Christmas Eve. "I hadn't thought about it at all," says Kelly. "I was really surprised. And it's something I did know—that your blood count has to be at a certain point—but it passes out of your mind because you don't think it's going to apply." The experience reminded Kelly that she could never really count on when her chemo treatments were going to be, regardless of when they were scheduled.

Your chemotherapy may last anywhere from 3 months to a year. During that period, you'll be given a variety of drugs, and the particular ones you are given may change over time. The list below gives some of the most common medications, each of which has its own effects and side effects. Find out from your doctor which of these drugs you'll be given and what you should expect from each. Your doctor should be able to give you drug information sheets that list the standard side effects of each drug used in chemotherapy and explain which symptoms are important to share with your health-care team. Remember, everyone reacts differ-

Joy Simha

Chemotherapy sucks. And I can't say that it doesn't. But, you know what? It's not the end of the world either. I was actually surprised that it wasn't as bad as I thought it was going to be. I think when you read about all the possible side effects, you think, "Oh, no. I'm going to experience every single one of them." But you don't. And as hard as the experience is, there's something that's such a relief about it— knowing that you're sitting there doing everything you can to fight this thing. And before you know it, it's over. It feels like it's going to last forever. But it doesn't. I never want to go through it again, and I don't want anyone else to go through it ever, but I made it through. And I think about that a lot. I made it. And, today, I think I'm a stronger person for having done that. The fear was a lot worse than the reality of it. And as I try new things in life now, that's a very important lesson I take with me.

ently to chemotherapy, and you should not expect your experience to mirror those of the women in this chapter.

- Adriamycin (doxorubicin)
- Cytoxan (cyclophosphamide)
- Methotrexate
- 5-Fluorouracil
- Taxol (paclitaxel)
- Taxotere (docetaxel)

Side Effects

One of the most talked-about aspects of chemotherapy is its side effects. Young women who have been through chemo say that there are days when you'll feel full of energy and days when you'll feel exhausted; days when you feel like eating and days when even the smell of food makes you sick. Common side effects are mouth sores (treated with a saltwater rinse), a metallic taste in your mouth, nausea, and extreme fatigue.

"Tomorrow is my chemo day," said Kelly during one interview. "Last time I was really excited. I was like, 'Yeah! Okay! Let's get the cancer!' I was really kind of pumped. This time I know how sick I got. So I'm saying, 'Okay, I'm going to have chemo and 4 hours later I'm probably going to be puking my guts out. I'm just not looking forward to that.'"

Tips for Beating the Nausea

- Antinausea medications can definitely help you make it through the chemo. Kytril, Zofran, or Anzemet may be choices that your doctor considers or recommends.

- If you don't feel like eating, tempt yourself with your favorite foods.

- Integrate green apples, ginger, and mint tea into your meals. They've been known to help some women beat the nausea.

- Try chewing on fresh greens, including sage, mint, parsley, cilantro, dill, and basil. The act of chewing helps stimulate the appetite, and the vitamins in the greens are good for you, too.

Young women who are on chemotherapy may experience hot flashes as they are thrown into temporary or permanent menopause induced by the chemo. According to Dr. Susan Love, some 57 percent of all premenopausal women receiving chemotherapy have at least a few hot flashes. Although permanent premature menopause is more common among women over 40, who are a bit closer to menopause to begin with, many young women do suffer short- or long-term fertility problems from chemotherapy. (For more on fertility problems and cancer treatment, see Chapter 9.)

Another serious—although rare—side effect of chemotherapy can be heart disease, particularly for women who are taking Adriamycin. Nalini Yadla was a 22-year-old medical student when she was diagnosed with breast cancer. She had to switch her chemotherapy regimen, dropping the Adriamycin she had been taking, when it had toxic effects on her heart.

"We believe that it's dose-related, and is rare with four to six cycles of Adriamycin, but it's possible that there are also long-term cardiac effects that we don't yet know about," writes Dr. Love in *Dr. Susan Love's Breast Book*. "Adriamycin is one of the best drugs we have to treat breast cancer. If it is indicated it should certainly be used. But we should not use it indiscriminately in women who are not . . . high risk."

Dr. Jeanne Petrek, a breast surgeon at Memorial Sloan-Kettering, is also concerned about heart disease and fertility problems resulting from chemotherapy. "Young women have difficulty deciding about chemotherapy," she says. "There are so many serious—albeit rare—complications of chemo, such as cardiac damage." However, she says, cardiac damage has been "pretty well studied," whereas fertility issues have not been. This is one more example, in Dr. Petrek's view, of the lack of information that is specifically relevant to younger women.

"The reproductive issues are unique to this population," she comments. "And at the time of initial detection, diagnosis, and planning treatment, these issues are overlooked not only by the doctor, but by the patient herself. It's only after—maybe 6 months after finishiing treatment—that the patient is distressed. 'How could I have forgotten about this? How could I not have even asked about it?'"

Juanita Lyle is now 58, but she was first diagnosed with breast cancer at age 32, and since then her cancer has recurred three times. Her chemotherapy led her to have menopausal symptoms that lasted for over 20 years, and she agrees with Dr. Petrek that information on the subject was sorely lacking. "I couldn't understand what was going on with my mood swings," she recalls. "I couldn't sleep at night. I would have hot flashes in midwinter. And physically I felt terrible. No one was preparing me for these changes. You could experience this on and off for 20 years. And sure enough, I did. I just got over this 3 years ago."

Kelly Douglas, Diagnosed at Age 24

I'll start the Herceptin in 4 weeks. Until then, it's Taxol. Taxol is so much better than Adriamycin/Cytoxan—it's a world of difference. I can tell you everything it's not. I'm not throwing up. I'm not dead for 3 days after. It's still not great. But it's not as punishing. The one thing about Taxol is, it can be more frustrating. You don't feel good, but you don't feel terrible either. You want to do things, and you start doing things, and then you realize how tired you are. I did the 5K Race for the Cure for the Komen Foundation—I walked it—and I was so tired for days afterward.

My fingers have had a bad time of it, too; they've been getting numb. It was so bad I couldn't open the toothpaste tube or my contact solution bottle. I didn't have treatment last week because my fingers were in so much pain, and my fingernails were changing color. The middle finger was turning blood red and the others were turning purple—it was not very pretty. They said I was getting toxic. You can get too much Taxol and it can cause nerve damage. It's reversible, but some women I've talked to still have neuropathy in their fingers, so I'm a little nervous because I still don't have all the feeling in my little finger.

Another frequent side effect of chemotherapy is popularly known as "chemo brain"—a loss of the ability to think clearly. Although some doctors dismiss this condition as resulting from depression or anxiety, there are studies that give credence to this "chemo-fog" phenomenon. A Canadian study published in the *Journal of Clinical Oncology* found significantly more memory and language difficulties in women who were receiving chemotherapy than in the control group of cancer-free patients. The study concluded that cognitive decline was not explained by differences in age, educational level, menopausal status, or mood.[5] A 1998 study published in the *Journal of the National Cancer Institute,* conducted by researchers at the Netherlands Cancer Institute, also found that certain drugs used in chemotherapy caused memory problems.[6] Other researchers have suggested that there is a link between high-dose chemotherapy and increased mental "dullness."

Randi Rosenberg can testify to the effects of chemo brain. "It was wreaking total havoc on my body," she recalls. "I was having trouble remembering things. I'd ask the same questions over and over, have little slips of the tongue, and put together sentences that made no sense."

Certainly, there are plenty of emotional reasons for you to be feeling anxious and depressed, and depression and anxiety can make you forgetful, easily confused, and just not as sharp as you're used to being. But don't discount the possibility that these responses are primarily physical reactions to your treatment. Again, alternative approaches may help restore some of your temporarily missing brain function. You might consider deep breathing, meditation, and Chinese, herbal, or Ayurvedic medicine. (As always, discuss all treatments with your physician. For more on complementary and alternative treatments, see Chapter 5.)

Making Decisions about Chemotherapy

Dr. Susan Love is strongly opposed to what she calls a "one size fits all" approach to chemotherapy. Just as every young woman's condition is unique, says Dr. Love, so are the choices, trade-offs, costs, and benefits different for each woman. "Young women need to sit their doctors down and get the real story," she says. "And they may not know, they may need to do some research. What is the benefit versus the risk? Are you willing to give up your fertility for a 5 percent reduction in recurrence?" Working with your doctor to decide about chemotherapy can be challenging because no one really knows exactly how the treatment will work or what its effects will be. But finding out from your doctor—and from other sources—what can be known at least allows you to make your own choices based on the factors that are most important to you.

> ## Questions to Ask Your Doctor about Chemotherapy
> - Why do I need chemotherapy?
> - What type of chemotherapy do you recommend? Why? What are the risks and benefits of this type of chemotherapy? What other alternatives are available? What are their risks and benefits?
> - How will I know if the chemotherapy is working?
> - What are the side effects?
> - Are there any long-term side effects?
> - How will the treatment you're recommending affect my fertility? Are there other alternatives that are less likely to cause premature menopause and/or compromise my fertility? (For more about fertility issues, see Chapter 9.)
> - Are there any clinical trials of new approaches to chemotherapy that I should know about? (For more information about clinical trials, see the discussions later in this chapter and in Chapter 13.)
>
> As recommended by the YSC.

Hormonal Treatments

Hormonal treatments include drugs—tamoxifen, raloxifene (still in trial), and aromatase inhibitors—that alter the way your hormones work. Other hormonal treatments—ovarian ablation by surgery or chemicals—stop the natural production of estrogen by your ovaries.

Tamoxifen

A common type of hormonal treatment is medication with some anti-estrogenic substance, usually tamoxifen. Originally used as a birth-control method in England, tamoxifen blocks the effects of estrogen in various parts of the body, including breast tissue, without affecting the body's actual production of estrogen.

Tamoxifen can compromise your fertility if you take it long enough, particularly in combination with chemotherapy, which already tends to weaken your ovaries. Women are routinely prescribed tamoxifen for 5 years. In most cases, women can get pregnant within several months of discontinuing tamoxifen, but if preserving your fertility is of concern to you, be sure to discuss this issue with your doctor. (Again, you'll find more detail in Chapter 9.)

Other possible side effects of tamoxifen include blood clots, pulmonary emboli, uterine cancer (more likely in postmenopausal overweight women), visual problems, depression, nausea and vomiting, and hot flashes. Also, although tamoxifen is associated with an increase in bone density in postmenopausal women, in whom it helps to counteract osteoporosis, there is some evidence that the drug decreases bone mineral density in premenopausal women.[7] For premenopausal women, there's some concern that tamoxifen may increase ovarian cysts because it stimulates the ovaries and increases estrogen and progesterone levels there while blocking estrogen to the breast.[9] It's also extremely important not to get pregnant while you are on tamoxifen because it can cause damage to the fetus, so if you're heterosexually active, you might want to talk to your doctor about birth control.

Leslie Mouton was diagnosed with estrogen-receptor-positive cancer at age 35. She experienced many different side effects from the tamoxifen treatment she received. "After I finished chemo, my ovaries were not working," she recalls. "But 6 months later they were, and my periods came back. But I was on tamoxifen. Tamoxifen and your ovaries fight each other. They would usually treat what I had with the pill. But, for other health reasons, I can't go on the pill. I'm also afraid of ovarian cancer. And I got all these cysts—four or five on my right and left ovary every month. So 2 months ago I had my ovaries removed, knowing I can still have kids because I still have my uterus." (Leslie and her husband created and froze embryos, which they are planning to implant in Leslie's uterus so that she can bear children after her cancer treatment is over.)

Unfortunately, although tamoxifen is often prescribed for young women, virtually all the data we have on it concern women who have already gone through menopause. In an analysis conducted especially for this book, it appeared that of 14 trials conducted by the National Surgical Adjuvant Breast and Bowel Project (NSABP), less than 1 percent of the participants were under the age of 30, and only 11 percent were aged 40 and under. There is also little information concerning raloxifene, a drug used to prevent osteoporosis in postmenopausal women that is being studied for use in breast cancer patients. While NSABP trial information being gathered on roloxifene applies only to postmenopausal women, one study by researchers at the University of California–San Francisco found that raloxifene acts differently in pre- and postmenopausal women. However, the U.C.–San Francisco study involved only healthy women, not breast cancer patients.[9]

When she was interviewed about tamoxifen for this book, Dr. Susan Love said frankly, "We don't have much safety data on young women. For instance, tamoxifen causes problems in young women, although in postmenopausal women it's effective and lowers estrogen levels. But in pre-menopausal women, it may actually increase estrogen levels," which of course could stimulate the growth of estrogen-receptive tumors. "We don't know the effect of tamoxifen on younger women," Dr. Love concluded.

YSC cofounder Roberta Levy-Schwartz, diagnosed with breast cancer at age 27, is also concerned about the effects of tamoxifen on younger women. "Right now half of our members are on tamoxifen, and yet they've never studied it in our age group," she points out. "I want them to study us while we're on this drug. And they're not doing that—and that's the hard part for me. They need to understand that we're willing to participate, but at the end of the day we want to see the study that says it works in young women or it doesn't work."

Randi Rosenberg worked closely with her oncologist trying to make sense of the data on tamoxifen. "We struggled with whether this was going to be an appropriate treatment for me," she recalls. "What it came down to is that this is the number one drug therapy for estrogen-receptor-positive cancers, so my doctor really thought I should try it." However, says Randi, many questions remain: "I would like to know if the normal time frame for tamoxifen's efficacy, 5 years, holds true for younger women who are premenopausal. Are the benefits equal to the benefits for postmenopausal women? What are the longer-term side effects of tamoxifen? Are 5 years of tamoxifen going to be enough to tide me over for all the estrogen that will be coursing through my body for the remainder of my lifetime? Those are some of the questions for which we don't know the answers—and they're a cause for concern." Randi experienced some initial side effects from tamoxifen, but as her body adjusted to the drug, "those symptoms started to even themselves out."

Although, as discussed previously, tamoxifen may cause uterine cancer, most frequently in postmenopausal overweight women, and ovarian cysts in premenopausal women, it's also showing some exciting possibilities as a preventive drug. The Breast Cancer Prevention Trial (BCPT), a clinical trial funded by the National Cancer Institute (NCI) and conducted by the National Surgical Adjuvant Breast and Bowel Project (NSABP), was designed to see whether tamoxifen could prevent breast cancer in high-risk women. This study involved 13,388 premenopausal and postmenopausal women across the United States and Canada. The results, reported in the September 16, 1998, *Journal of the National Cancer Institute*, stated that women who took tamoxifen had 49 percent fewer diagnoses of invasive breast cancer than women in a control group who took a placebo.[10] Unfortunately, although the study did involve premenopausal women, it included so few women in their twenties and thirties that the findings are not statistically relevant for women in these age groups.

The Study of Tamoxifen and Raloxifene (STAR), one of the largest breast cancer prevention trials ever undertaken, includes 22,000 post-menopausal women. Only women who have stopped menstruating are allowed in the study, since raloxifene has yet to be adequately tested for long-term safety in premenopausal women. However, the National Cancer Institute has launched a separate, though far smaller, study involving 62 premenopausal high-risk women between the ages of 23 and 47. Researchers will monitor raloxifene's effects on bone density, hormone levels, the uterus, and the ovaries.

Aromatase Inhibitors and Inactivators

Another category of drugs, known as aromatase inhibitors and inactivators, has also been found to suppress estrogen production in post-menopausal women. Now researchers are wondering whether these medications might also help premenopausal women, as either a supplement or an alternative to tamoxifen. The inhibitors letrozole and anastrozole and the inactivator exemestane are being investigated as potential replacement drugs that women could switch to after 3 years of tamoxifen. In an overview of aromatase inhibitors published in the *Journal of Clinical Oncology*,[11] Italian researchers concluded that the drugs would be good candidates for future studies of hormonal therapies. An earlier study in the same journal had suggested that aromatase inhibitors and inactivators should not be used in premenopausal women unless the women were also getting oophorectomies or suppressing their ovarian function.[12]

No matter what type of hormonal therapy you choose, doctors seem to agree that shutting down the ovaries for between 2 and 5 years is important for young women with ER-positive breast cancer.

They also seem to agree that more studies are necessary. In an article in the *Journal of the National Cancer Institute*,[13] Dr. Aron Goldhirsch asks: "Is failure to achieve chemotherapy-induced amenorrhea associated with an increased risk of relapse among premenopausal patients with ER-positive tumors?" His answer is yes. "For young patients whose tumors express hormone receptors, endocrine effects of chemotherapy alone are modest, and endocrine therapies appear to be an essential component of an effective adjuvant therapy program. Whether use of 'optimal' endocrine therapy (e.g., ovarian function suppression plus tamoxifen) may be sufficient for these patients is a hypothesis that has not been tested adequately."

Ovarian Ablation

As we've seen, some tumors grow faster under the influence of estrogen or progesterone. If you've got the type of hormonally sensitive cancer that will respond well to hormonal treatments, your doctor will have learned this from your pathology report. He or she may then recommend some type of ovarian ablation, which stops your ovaries from producing estrogen so that more of your tumor cells will die.

Speaking at the Living Well Today for the Promise of Tomorrow Conference, cosponsored by Living Beyond Breast Cancer and the YSC, Angela De Michele, an oncologist at the University of Pennsylvania's Rena Rowen Breast Center, described the process by which some tumors are receptive to estrogen:

> I like to think about the estrogen receptor as a gate, basically a protein sitting on the surface of the cancer cell. It's acting as a gateway for the estrogen to come in and have an effect on the entire cell. And we all know that young women, particularly premenopausal women, have a lot of estrogen floating around.

Young women who undergo ovarian ablation will experience menopause immediately—and the side effects of early menopause may be more bothersome than those of natural menopause.

There are three methods of ovarian ablation: surgery, hormone therapy, and radiation therapy. The choice of treatment is individualized to the patient's preference and her doctor's recommendation.

Ovarian Ablation through Surgery: Oophorectomy

Now that estrogen-blocking drugs are available, oophorectomies are done infrequently, but they remain a very effective option for premenopausal women. Oophorectomies are also performed on postmenopausal women to reduce the risk of ovarian cancer.

As we saw earlier, the 700 women studied in Vietnam and China who were treated with a combination of mastectomy and oophorectomy had relatively high survival rates if their surgeries were properly timed (84 percent lived cancer free for 5 years). According to Dr. Eric Winer, director of breast oncology at Dana Farber's Gillette Centers for Women's Cancer in Boston, "Ovarian cancer risk drops by about 50 percent when the ovaries are surgically removed." As Winer explains, "The risk doesn't go down to zero because ovary-like cells that are normally present in the pelvic area could still form a cancer, even after the ovaries are gone."

Winer believes that in the next few years, doctors will come to prescribe ovarian suppression or removal as an alternative to chemotherapy for some kinds of cancers:

We now have many old studies—and newer ones—that show that in premenopausal women with hormone-receptor-positive cancer, ovarian suppression is a useful strategy and is as good as chemotherapy. Studies do not show it's beneficial in addition to chemotherapy—though it may turn out that way in some patients. But clearly in lieu of chemo, it's a reasonable consideration.

The problem, says Dr. Winer, is that research hasn't determined the ideal relationship among ovarian suppression, chemo, and tamoxifen in the treatment of women with hormone-positive tumors. But recent studies do seem to indicate that some women with breast cancer do better after their ovarian function is suppressed, either through chemotherapy-induced premature menopause or through the actual removal of their ovaries. Particularly for women who have tested positive for the BRCA1 gene mutation, ovary removal is "one of the few effective ways to reduce breast cancer risk," according to Timothy Rebbek, Ph.D., a biostatistician at the University of Pennsylvania School of Medicine, in an article in the *Journal of the National Cancer Institute*.[14]

If you agree to such a treatment, you will be unable to have children, although some women harvest their eggs and have them fertilized and then frozen before undergoing the treatment. (For more on fertility issues, see Chapter 9.)

Chemical Ovarian Ablation through Hormonal Treatments

Other hormonal therapies (also called *endocrine therapies*) cause chemically induced menopause. Hormone therapy drugs that cause ovarian ablation are called *luteinizing hormone–releasing hormone (LHRH) analogues* (meaning that these drugs are similar to chemicals that the body normally produces); they include goserelin (Zoladex). Leuprolide acetate (Lupron is a similar drug), which is called a *gonadotropin-releasing hormone (GnRH) analogue*. Both of these drugs accomplish ovarian ablation through "chemical castration," meaning that they slow or stop estrogen production by the ovaries. Both Lupron and Zoladex are increasingly popular for premenopausal women who are taking tamoxifen. While these therapies can cause permanent menopause in older premenopausal patients, they can preserve fertility in the youngest patients.

Lori Atkinson in Indiana chose Zoladex over Lupron because of the larger body of research surrounding Zoladex.

For the 8 months I was on chemo, I didn't have periods. Later, after I began tamoxifen, my periods started again. My estrogen receptors were positive, and my oncologist told me that in cases like mine, the

Questions to Ask Your Doctor about Hormonal Treatments
- How will these treatments affect my fertility?

- How can I protect either my fertility or my ability to bear children later (through frozen embryos or other fertility procedures)?

- What is the trade-off between preserving my fertility and preserving my safety? How much of a risk am I taking if I choose to protect my fertility?

- What kinds of side effects can I expect? Which are short-term and which are long-term? (*Note:* As previously stated, there is a lack of information on the long-term side effects of any treatment. Find out what your doctor can tell you and where the unanswered questions remain.)

- How do you plan to respond to these side effects, if I do develop them?

studies lean toward shutting down the ovaries for 2 years. Since I already had my kids, both my oncologist and my gynecologist gave me the choice of either a hysterectomy or the Zoladex. I didn't want another surgery, so I opted for the Zoladex. Every 6 weeks I got an injection—although now you can get 3-month doses. You have the same symptoms as going through menopause—at first there's a heavy, heavy week that's like your last period. Then it stops. I went on Zoladex for a year because for the previous 11 months, I'd already gone without having periods. Now, a year later, my periods are back. The studies are saying it's better to get 5 years of ovarian shutdown, so now they're recommending a hysterectomy. I could go on Zoladex again, but it is a drug, and my oncologist thinks the hysterectomy will be better for me. At the time, I didn't want to get rid of all my natural estrogen. I want to stay as natural as I can. And Zoladex bought me another year and a half of staying as natural as possible. I'm going to be setting up my surgery this summer. Zoladex wasn't bad. If I'd had to take it for 5 years, it would've been worth it.

Like Zoladex, Lupron can causes premature menopause; and, also like Zoladex, it can be expensive, but it's most often covered by insurance. Lupron is often used in treating metastatic breast cancer, especially when the patient is premenopausal and the disease has progressed or has recurred after trying at least 3 months of tamoxifen.

Ovarian Ablation through Radiation

Ovarian ablation can also be achieved by treating the ovaries with radiation, which stops them from making estrogen. While this technique *can* work well, doctors often do not recommend it because it produces much slower ovarian ablation than surgery and sometimes does not work. This is especially true for young women who may require higher doses of radiation to shut the ovaries down.

This process involves irradiating the ovaries, usually for a few days on an outpatient basis. Unlike surgery, which will end your periods immediately, radiation causes your menstrual cycle to end slowly. You can expect your periods to stop during the first couple of months following completion of treatment.

If your menstrual cycle continues past that time, or stops and then resumes, it means ablation through radiation has failed. This is a possibility, especially in women under the age of 35. Young women also need to be aware that the higher doses of radiation needed to suppress their ovar-

Questions to Ask Your Doctor about Radiation

- Why do I need radiation?

- How long will each treatment take?

- When do I begin treatment?

- Who will administer the treatments?

- Should I bring someone with me to my treatments?

- What are the possible side effects? How long will they last? Is there any treatment for them?

- Is there anything I can do now or during treatment to minimize side effects and risks?

- Can I continue my normal activities during treatment?

- Is this covered by my insurance?

- What kind of follow-up and monitoring will I need after my radiation treatments have ended?

As recommended by the YSC.

ian function carry the risk of late radiation damage (damage that occurs months or years after treatment) to organs and tissues near the ovaries. Low-dose treatment, which minimizes the risk of late radiation damage, may not be an option for young women, who need the higher doses to achieve ovarian suppression.

Radiation

Radiation is localized rather than systemwide treatment. It is focused on the tissue of your breast and the surrounding area, and it is usually given as follow-up to a lumpectomy, although it may be administered after a mastectomy as well. High-intensity x-rays cut through your cells and damage their DNA structure so that any cancer cells that remain after your surgery will not be able to replicate.

Side effects of radiation include reactions of the irradiated skin, such as itching, redness, dryness, or scaling. This response varies greatly from person to person but is usually gone within 2 weeks after treatment has ended. Fatigue is another common side effect of radiation; this also tends to vanish when treatment ends.

As Dr. Sledge warned us earlier, young women are more likely than older women to have their cancer recur after lumpectomy and radiation. However, Dr. Sledge stresses that this is not necessarily a reason for young women to avoid this treatment.

Another concern about radiation is its effect on genetic mutation. Since younger women are believed to be somewhat more likely to be carrying a genetic predisposition for cancer, some doctors worry that radiation could potentially damage a mutated gene and further increase the risk of recurrence.

The "Breast Cancer Gene"

One of the most publicized aspects of breast cancer research in recent years concerns genetics and the so-called breast cancer gene: the idea that some women, especially those who get breast cancer when relatively young, have a genetic predisposition to the disease.

Researchers believe that some women carry one or two genetic mutations that vastly increase their likelihood of developing breast cancer. The genes known as BRCA1 and BRCA2 are responsible for repairing damaged DNA. Scientists believe that if either or both of these genes are defective, DNA damage will occur in the breast or ovarian cells, increasing the likelihood that cancer will develop. While only 5 percent of all women with breast cancer have genetic mutations, young women with breast cancer are believed to be far more likely to be genetic mutation carriers, which may also be why they have the disease at such early ages.

If you do have mutations in BRCA1 or BRCA2, your chances of getting breast cancer are extremely high. According to Sandya Pruthi, M.D., a breast health specialist at the Mayo Clinic, 20 percent of all women with a mutated BRCA1 gene will develop breast cancer by age 40, 51 percent by age 50, and 87 percent by age 60. (Comparable figures are not yet available for mutations in the BRCA2 gene, which has not been studied as extensively.)

Because there is such a high correlation between mutations in BRCA1 and 2 and breast/ovarian cancer, and because young women with cancer are more likely to carry the mutation, many young women with breast cancer choose to get genetic testing.

The Pros and Cons of Genetic Testing

As a young woman with breast cancer, you may be wondering whether you, too, have the mutation in BRCA1 or 2. You may feel that genetic testing might bring you peace of mind, helping you to answer the question, "Why me?" For some women, it's a relief to know that there is a scientific explanation for their having breast cancer at an unusually young age.

Another reason to get tested is to make decisions about childbearing. If you are carrying a genetic mutation, you have a 50 percent chance of passing it on to your children, vastly increasing the likelihood that your daughters will develop breast and/or ovarian cancer and that your sons may pass the mutation on to their daughters. Both young women and women with a family history of breast cancer have good reason to suspect that they are carrying the genetic mutation; for some women, that's an important factor in deciding whether to bear children of their own.

Finally, learning that you do indeed have the genetic mutation in BRCA1 or BRCA2 may affect your medical decisions. If you tested positive for the gene before being diagnosed with breast cancer, you probably would have had more frequent mammograms and clinical breast exams. You might have been treated with tamoxifen before diagnosis, and you are likely to receive it as part of your treatment.

A more difficult decision is whether to opt for a prophylactic mastectomy or oophorectomy—the removal of breasts or ovaries in an effort to prevent breast or ovarian cancer. According to the National Cancer Institute, "Preventive mastectomy may be an option for women with a strong family history of breast cancer, especially if several close relatives developed the disease before age 50." Yet the NCI adds,

"Although having a preventive mastectomy can reduce the risk [of breast cancer], no one can be certain that this procedure will protect a woman from breast cancer. Because it is impossible for a surgeon to remove all breast tissue, breast cancer can still develop in the small amount of remaining tissue."[15]

The question of prophylactic mastectomy was studied by a high-level task force of doctors, who considered the question for 14 months. As reported by the *Journal of the American Medical Association*, this panel came to no definitive conclusions on the issue of preventive surgery: "These surgeries are an option for women with a high risk of cancer, but evidence of benefits is lacking."[16]

At least one group of scientists does recommend prophylactic mastectomy, especially for women with BRCA1 or BRCA2 genetic mutations. According to a report in the *New England Journal of Medicine*, researchers at the Mayo Clinic concluded that prophylactic mastectomies would reduce the risk of breast cancer by up to 90 percent in women who had strong family histories of breast cancer.[17] A subsequent study by the same researchers found that women with a strong family history—who were also genetic carriers—experienced a "substantial reduction" in breast cancer risk when they underwent prophylactic mastectomy.[18]

Beth Newman, a genetic epidemiologist and professor of public health at Queensland University of Technology in Brisbane, Australia, one of the leading experts in BRCA1 and BRCA2 genes, is disturbed at the prospect that genetic testing might lead to an increase in prophylactic mastectomies. "This drastic intervention doesn't reduce the risk to zero," says Newman. "You can still get breast cancer even if you've had a bilateral prophylactic mastectomy."

Newman argues that genetic information is of only limited value in figuring out who is likely to get breast cancer. Despite—or perhaps because of—her own pioneering role in genetic research, she describes herself as "actually one of the more skeptical people regarding the virtues of genetic testing." Newman was part of the group working with Mary-Claire King at the University of Washington, Seattle, where BRCA1 was first discovered. At the time, Newman says, the group expected to discover a genetic basis for breast cancer that would help scientists understand both how the disease was caused and how to cure it. However, says Newman, "That paradigm didn't pan out. It's not as simple as that." Although researchers did find that some women might be particularly susceptible to breast cancer, genes did not turn out to be the hoped-for "magic bullet" explanation.

Now, says Newman, the BRCA1 and BRCA2 genes have gotten enormous publicity. But she's concerned about the medical consequences of this information. "We don't know how to tell women to prevent breast cancer," she says, "and I fear we're medicalizing their lives decades before it's necessary. If you are diagnosed with breast cancer at a young age and have a strong family history—then yes, I would say that's the best time to have genetic testing—but only if you want to open that Pandora's box. Testing does not give you answers—it just gives you more questions. If you find out that, yes, you are a mutation carrier, what then? Given that there's no concrete advice we can give women about how to prevent the disease, it's hard to know what action to take."

Moreover, getting genetic testing can have a ripple effect throughout your family. If you are indeed carrying a mutation of the gene, what does that mean for your mother, your sisters, and your other female relatives? What does it mean for your children? Finding that the breast cancer mutation runs in your family can have a devastating effect on you and your loved ones.

"There's a history of cancer on both sides of my family," says a woman who prefers to be known as Ann Stone, the alias she used while being genetically tested, in order to protect her ability to get health insurance. "I lost a maternal aunt when she was in her forties. I lost two maternal great-aunts whom I didn't know — one of them to ovarian cancer. And I lost a paternal grandmother to breast cancer." Ann was diagnosed with breast cancer at age 33. When her older sister was diagnosed a year later, the family discussed genetic testing: "But it was so overwhelming to think about that it went on the back burner. We knew we needed to discuss it further—but at that time the most important thing was her prognosis. That's what we dealt with then. It wasn't until the completion of her treatment—almost a year later—that we started talking about it again."

So far, four of Ann's family members have been tested—and all four have been diagnosed with the BRCA1 mutation. But not everyone wanted to be tested: Ann's oldest sister opposed testing from the beginning. She thought the results—regardless of what they were—would be too upsetting for her, and since she had adopted rather than borne children, she felt no responsibility to give her children the genetic information.

Results of a genetic test are never given over the phone, so, nearly three weeks after being tested, Ann met with a genetics counselor who told her that she had tested positive. "I really lost it," Ann recalls. "I was crying really, really hard. And my daughter was sitting on my lap. And

Ellen Feig, Diagnosed at Age 37

Ellen is of Ashkenazi Jewish descent, a population at increased risk for breast and ovarian cancer because of high incidence of BRCA alterations. Ellen has tested positive for the BRCA mutation.

When you're diagnosed with cancer, you feel, rightly or wrongly, that you're being proactive, that there are all these things you can do. Whether they'll work or not is a different story—but there is a pervading sense of hope.

When I found out I had the breast cancer mutation, it was a very different story. I was being told I was going to have cancer again—that I had a 90 percent chance of breast cancer and a 97 percent chance of ovarian cancer. My oncologist went so far as to say that the next time I wouldn't survive it.

I also have a daughter. She's little, but it's terrifying to think I'm giving her that gene potentially. I have a sister, too. The gene mutation didn't just affect me—it affected my family on so many levels. And it really brings up tremendous emotional issues. I'm scared for my daughter. I know my mother feels guilt, and I always try to tell her it's not her fault. The levels of trauma are so great with the gene, it's almost indescribable. I really think finding out about the gene was more devastating than knowing about the cancer.

When the results were in, my oncologist told me that the best thing for me was to have a bilateral mastectomy and an oophorectomy. And so that's what I did —and it was very emotional. But I believe the testing actually saved my life.

that's why I was crying so hard. I couldn't look at her without thinking she might have that mutation, because there's a 50 percent chance she could have it. *Thinking* I was positive was nothing compared to *knowing* that I was. And I really thought that I was ready to handle it. I was so sure I had the mutation—but thinking it and knowing it was like night and day."

Yet despite the emotional turmoil caused by hearing her test results, Ann wished she had had the test done earlier. By the time she was tested, she had been diagnosed with breast cancer 2 years previously and had had a lumpectomy. "If I knew then what I know now—that I was going to be BRCA1 positive—I would have made different decisions," Ann says, suggesting that she might have chosen a more radical surgery. "But then," she adds, "I had never even heard of BRCA1. When I was first diagnosed I had no idea what that was."

By contrast, Jeannine Salamone got her genetic test results early enough to influence her medical decisions. "I decided soon after I tested positive for the mutation that I wanted to get a double mastectomy," Jeannine says. "At that point I had only had a lumpectomy. But with the information I got from the genetic testing, there was no question. I knew what I had to do. I have to do everything I can to keep from getting cancer ever again."

New Prospects for Genetic Research

In June 2002, investigators at Dana Farber Cancer Institute and Children's Hospital, affiliates of Harvard University, announced a major scientific breakthrough: the discovery of six additional genes whose mutations might be related to breast cancer and other types of cancer. The study's senior researcher, pediatrics professor Alan D'Andrea, was actually studying Fanconi's anemia, a rare childhood disease, when he discovered that six genes believed to be implicated in that disease might also be involved in breast cancer. Apparently, the six genes can create a protein that can lead to genetic mutation and, eventually, cancer if BRCA1 and BRCA2 are not effectively doing their job of repairing damaged DNA.

"This has big implications for breast and ovarian cancer screening," says D'Andrea, who believes that this new information will help scientists pinpoint more accurately who is at risk for cancer. "Now that we know about these genes, we will be adding them to the diagnostic screenings that are already being done. As we cast a wider net, we can identify more women and families who are prone to cancer."

D'Andrea can't say when these six new genes will become part of routine testing. But he does hold out the hope that his discovery may lead to more cancer-prevention options than we've had before. "The question is, could drug companies come up with drugs and medicines that potentially strengthen the inherent genetic weakness that exists?" he asks. "Could someone come up with a drug that could enhance or increase DNA repair? If so, then one could delay the onset of cancer, or perhaps do a better job of treating an early cancer." Because of the specific ways in which the six new genes operate, D'Andrea says, they may offer more potential for intervention than BRCA1 and BRCA2 have provided.

D'Andrea points out that despite their names, errors in breast cancer genes 1 and 2 , besides being strongly associated with breast and ovarian cancer, can also cause pancreatic cancer, melanoma, and stomach cancer. He also stresses that women not only can be born with abnormalities in these genes and the six he has discovered but that sometimes

Questions to Ask before Genetic Testing

- Am I prepared to learn that I'm at risk of developing a potentially life-threatening disease?

- What are my medical options if I test positive?

- What emotional support will I need if I test positive?

- If I test positive, should my children also be tested?

- How will my family react if I test positive?

- If I test positive, should the female members of my family be tested too?

- How will the results of my genetic tests be used by physicians?

- What are the long-term effects in terms of insurance coverage if I am carrying the BRCA mutation?

- Who will have access to my test results?

they acquire these mutations later in life. "It's the same culprit gene," he explains, "but it mutates at a different time in your life." If the gene mutates early enough, the person may develop Fanconi's anemia. If the mutation occurs later, another type of cancer may result.

Breast surgeon Dr. Bert Petersen is very much concerned with when genes mutate. "One of the things we notice is that with each new generation, the onset of the cancer is earlier and earlier," he points out, suggesting that perhaps environmental factors are causing genes to mutate earlier, or causing already mutated genes to "misbehave" earlier. Like D'Andrea, Dr. Petersen is hopeful that genetics will offer a new paradigm for understanding and treating cancer, "where we'll treat breast cancer at the molecular, genetic level." He compares this potential leap forward to the discovery of antibiotics, which suddenly made treatments like bloodletting seem outmoded and archaic. Perhaps, he suggests, this new genetic approach to cancer will lead to similar medical advances.

Newman remains skeptical, however, pointing out that the vast majority of women who get breast cancer do not test positive for any genetic problems. In her opinion, the focus on genetic testing gives women a false sense of control, since it isn't clear what kinds of medical responses should follow a positive test. "I realize my view is a minority view," she says. "Most of the people who work in this field see more value for genetic testing. I don't."

If you do test positive for the breast cancer gene, you might consider the following medical responses:

- More frequent screening, ideally with a combination of mammography and ultrasound
- Preventive use of tamoxifen (see the discussion earlier in this chapter)
- Prophylactic mastectomy or oophorectomy

Clinical Trials

A clinical trial is an experiment that's done to develop new treatments for breast cancer. Sometimes trials give you a chance to try out new treatment methods while they're still in the experimental stage, before they become widely available. Sometimes trials compare existing methods, so that we can learn more about which are more effective under various circumstances, or so that scientists can gather more long-range data about their effectiveness, their side effects, and other aspects of treatment.

Dr. Susan Love points out that many young women don't understand how clinical trials work. "Often, women want to pick their treatments and then have someone study them," says Dr. Love. "But that doesn't give us any information, because studying one person is an anecdote. It is their story. What you have to do to answer scientific questions is to get women before their treatment and randomly assign them to one treatment or another, so you don't get biases, and then follow them and see what happens."

Clinical trials fill in some of the gaps in existing research. "We can't complain that there's no data and then not participate in studies," says Randi Rosenberg of the Young Survival Coalition. "The only way anything is going to change is if young women get involved in studies."

Dr. Love echoes these sentiments. "We have to continue to be in studies because it is the only way that we will be able to change things for our sisters behind us," she says.

Kelly Douglas, diagnosed at age 24 with breast cancer, is currently in a major trial on the effectiveness of Herceptin (trastuzumab), a drug used along with several other medications in chemotherapy. Herceptin is not yet widely prescribed and has been used primarily in metastatic cancer patients. It's now going through clinical trials to investigate the possibility of more widespread use. "So many other brave women have gone before me," she says. "I really believe in it, and I think I owe a lot to the women who went through trials before I did. I do feel like I'm on the cutting edge of cancer technology."

Kelly's husband, Mark, shares her commitment to the experimental process. "Because of the advances in scientific research, you expect there's going to be a cure," he says. Therefore, says Mark, he and Kelly agree that she, too, must participate in clinical trials so that the next generation of women can benefit still more. Seeing themselves as part of a chain of people contributing to future generations actually helps Mark and Kelly cope with their experience of cancer, because it enables them to find some meaning in it.

"If I have to be a guinea pig so that others can know more, then so be it," says Joy Simha, YSC cofounder, who was diagnosed with breast cancer at age 26. "But I want a cure. I really want a cure. And the only way we're going to get the answers we need is if people like us volunteer to help find them."

If you're interested in finding out more about participating in clinical trials, ask your doctor about which experiments you might qualify for, or call the National Cancer Institute Information Service at 1-800-4CAN-CER. You can find other resources on clinical trials in the Resources section of this book.

What Happens in a Clinical Trial?

As Dr. Love explained, the essence of the scientific approach is for studies to be *random* and *objective*. Women must be assigned randomly to various groups. Sometimes women know which group they're in. Sometimes their doctors know, but they don't. In *double-blind studies,* neither the women nor the people administering the treatments know who is in which group. That helps keep people's expectations and biases out of the process, so that the results that emerge can be trusted.

Let's say a new drug for chemotherapy is being tested. There might be three groups of women: one group that gets a large dose of this drug, in conjunction with other chemo medications that have already been found to be effective; a second group that gets a smaller dose of the drug, along with the other medications; and a third group, the *control* group, that gets only the other medications. Each group of women would be tracked to see how they do. If the women in the first two groups do better, the drug is probably useful. If they do not, the drug probably isn't effective, at least not in the combinations that were tested. An experiment like this would also keep track of possible side effects resulting from the new medication.

Clinical Trials: Experiments in Three Phases

Actual research trials are more complex and proceed in three phases. *Phase I* clinical trials tend to involve very few patients. Their goal is to test the safety of a new drug. Usually, phase I trials are open only to patients whose disease is furthest advanced.

Phase II trials are primarily designed to test a new drug's effectiveness, as they look at the way individual tumors respond to specific treatments. Sometimes a phase II trial will involve only a single drug, but sometimes it will include a combination regimen—the drug to be tested plus others that are known to be effective. Usually, phase II trials are open only to women with tumors for which there's not yet an effective treatment.

In *phase III* trials, the new treatment is compared to previously accepted treatments to see whether it offers longer-term survival or has fewer or less severe side effects. Phase III trials also measure symptom control. These trials are the largest of the three types and the ones you're most likely to qualify for, particularly if you're newly diagnosed. Only when a drug has done well in a phase III trial does it receive approval from the Food and Drug Administration (FDA) for general use.

"I Feel Like I've Been Dropped out of a Plane": When Treatment Ends

When you complete your treatment, there are probably three words you want to hear above all others: *You are cured*. But be prepared for your doctor *not* to say them. That does not mean that your doctor believes your cancer will come back, or even that he or she believes it is still in your body; it does mean that you may experience increased anxiety about your future. Every ache or pain may make you worry that your cancer has spread. Again, you are not alone. It is common for women to feel anxiety about recurrence for at least 2 to 3 years following a diagnosis. For young women, these anxieties may last even longer because of all their expectations for the future.

For Aquatia Owens, diagnosed at age 32, the posttreatment fears are still strong after 5 cancer-free years. "People always think the worst part of the experience is hearing the words, 'You have cancer.' No, the worst part is after your doctor says, 'Okay, you're fine.' That's when the hard road begins. And when you're walking it, you can't be afraid to talk to other people about your fear issues, because that's part of your recovery also."

According to Roz Kleban, it is "enormously helpful" to connect with other young women who understand what you're experiencing. "It's important posttreatment to be with other people who are feeling like you are. Because your friends and relatives—who may have been enormously supportive while you were going through treatment—are now

Questions to Ask Your Doctor about Clinical Trials

- What's the purpose of the study?
- Why do doctors think the approach may work? (For example, how has it been studied before?)
- Who has reviewed and approved it?
- How are the study results and safety of participants being checked?
- How long will the study last?
- What will I have to do if I join?
- What are the short-term benefits for me?
- What are the long-term benefits for me?
- What are the short-term risks, such as side effects, for me?
- What are the long-term risks for me?
- What other prevention options do people with my risk for cancer have?
- How do the risks and benefits of this trial compare with the risks and benefits of those options?
- How could being in the study affect my daily life?
- Can I talk with other people who are in the study?
- Will I have to pay for any part of the trial, such as tests or the study agent?
- What is my health insurance likely to cover?
- What if I need additional medical treatment as a result of the side effects of the clinical trial?
- Is the study approved by the National Cancer Institute?

Provided by the National Cancer Institute.

finished. They are happy to just put this whole experience behind them and move on. They don't understand what a vulnerable and fragile position you are in."

The key to managing your fears is to understand that you are not alone and that, while fear is normal, you can take control of it, instead of its taking control of you.

Roz Kleban, Social Worker, Memorial Sloan-Kettering

It is true that the posttreatment period is one of increased anxiety. During treatment, you're being taken care of by a whole team of medical personnel and you're being pumped up with lots of drugs. Then, all of a sudden, you hear, "Good-bye, you're finished." And you're not told that there's something you can do to prevent a recurrence. Except maybe taking tamoxifen—and even those who take tamoxifen don't feel like they have the magic rabbit's foot.

The true answer to the question, "How do you deal with the fear of recurrence?" is time. With time, the fear will go away. People roll their eyes at me whenever I say that, never believing that life can ever be the same. But I can tell you for certain, the fear and anxiety will go away. It may not go away for 3 years—but it doesn't stay at the same intensity for all 3 of those years either.

There are people who can't plan a vacation; they are afraid of planning anything. They are afraid that believing in the future will be a sign that they have too much hubris. It's an interesting phenomenon. There's something about this period of time in "cancerland"— they get accustomed to the landscape and feel protected. They're afraid to leave. But you need to keep living. What I tell patients is, when you've finished treatment, you have to recognize the feelings you have but not always act on them.

In addition to her own doctor's visits, bone scans, blood tests, and MRIs making her nervous, Roberta Levy-Schwartz, who was diagnosed at 27, says, "I get a knot in my stomach" about her friends' visits as well. "When I hear someone's running to the doctors, I get scared. First for them, then for myself," Roberta admits. "Rarely do you ever assume something normal is going on, like a hangnail or the flu. You always assume the worst. And in some cases, you get the news that it is." That emotional roller coaster, says Roz Kleban, is normal.

Sometimes, however, the fears get out of hand. They become so intense that they take over your life. According to Roz, if you find yourself afraid or anxious a great deal of the time, feeling hopeless about the future, and being unwilling to reinvest in life, you may want to consider professional counseling to help you remove the "black cancer cloud" that has settled over your life. "If you are unable to go back to your precancer activities," says Roz, "then that's a problem. You should go back to your old life—with fear and with apprehension, yes, but you need to be able to participate in your own life."

Tips for Living with Fears of Recurrence

- Give yourself permission to feel and express your fear of breast cancer. As Roz Kleban advises, "Acknowledge the fear. Do not act on it." The fear of recurrence is a complex issue that includes the fear of death and dying. In our society, it's not always easy to explore these issues, but doing so can be emotionally and spiritually rewarding. If you're interested in this opportunity, but you aren't sure how to get started, you might consider working with a spiritual or religious counselor.

- Understand that your feelings of fear, anxiety, sadness, and anger are normal. It's only when they start to consume you that there's a problem. When negativity takes over, you may feel worse about yourself and your situation, which can interfere with your ability to take good care of yourself.

- Ask yourself the right question. When thoughts of recurrence creep into your mind, you may find yourself repeatedly asking, "What if I die?" Ask yourself another question instead—"What if I live?" It is a subtle but important shift of focus that substitutes the best possible outcome for the worst.

- A sense of connection—to friends, to family, to community, to life— is the single thing that young women say helps them most in getting through the breast cancer experience.

- Put your mind at ease by realizing that your fears are generally worse than the reality. Roz Kleban suggests getting worrisome aches and pains checked out within a week or two— "not because it is something, but because the anxiety is too much."

- Be good to yourself. Staying well rested is critical to your emotional and physical healing and well-being. Even the smallest fears can take on gigantic proportions when you're tired. This is why many women say that nighttime is the most difficult time of the day. If that's true for you, you may want to consider sleeping in another room or redecorating your own room as a way of creating a new safe area.

- Give yourself credit for all you've already accomplished. Remember, the postsurgery treatments you've been through are designed to destroy any lingering cancer cells. Remind yourself that you've done and are doing everything you can to beat breast cancer.

- You are strong. You've faced breast cancer before. And if you have to, you can do it again. Recurrence is not a death sentence. No matter what happens, there is always something that can be done to help you. Local recurrence can be curable. Metastatic disease may be put into long-term remission.

Dr. Bert Petersen, Surgical Oncologist and Director of the Family Risk Program at Beth Israel Cancer Center

From the time of diagnosis through the first 2 years, I see a woman once every 3 months. And during these visits I really want to make sure she's getting the support she needs during this very difficult time. In the 3 to 5 years after diagnosis, I see patients once every 6 months. Now it's more about celebrating each day. With each visit, I really make a point of saying, "Okay, we've gotten this far. This is great. This is your 3-year anniversary. This is your 4-year anniversary." And really celebrating the moment. I want women to be aware of this accomplishment, and to really focus on the good. It's important not to spend a lot of time focusing on what ifs.

After the 5-year anniversary, I'll see my patients once a year. Usually people are sailing at this point. They're so happy they've made it through 5 years. After 5 years, the anxiety level tends to really drop. But there's always that little voice in the back of the head. My patients always say there are two things they dread doing every year: going for a mammogram, and having to come and see me. I can understand that.

Aquatia has found that redirecting anxiety about recurrence into energy for taking action helps her cope. She keeps herself busy with new challenges like African dance, yoga, group knitting classes, and meditation. She also focuses on having a positive attitude and surrounding herself with others who feed that positive energy. "The idea of death doesn't scare me like it used to. I've learned to deal with my emotions and the anxiety. But do I have fear? Oh, yes. I fear recurrence. I fear more treatment. But I'm dealing with that. I've learned that it's okay to be afraid. I'm not letting the fear slow me down. I'm out there enjoying life, getting the most out of every single day. The demons are still talking in the back of my head, but I'm not listening."

CHAPTER 4

"Can I Still Run the Marathon?"

Fitness, Diet, and Taking Care of Your Body

When Joy Simha finished her chemo, her first thought was, "How soon can I get back out on the river?" Joy had recently taken up whitewater kayaking, and she had come to love it more than anything else in the world. The sooner she got back into a kayak, she thought, the sooner she would regain faith in her body. "When I first heard my diagnosis, I felt my body had betrayed me," Joy explains. "Here I was enjoying my body so much—going to the gym, swimming, kayaking. I thought I had a strong body, and yet a little piece of my body was betraying me." Setting out with her kayaking buddies to challenge the rapids helped Joy restore her sense that her body was her ally, that her life was larger than her disease. "I tried to have fun while beating breast cancer," she says. "It wasn't all about chemo and surgery—it was about the little gifts God gives us. The blue sky—the sunshine—a day with great friends. The precious moments."

Three weeks after she had finished her chemo, Tracy Pleva Hill took up kickboxing. The following year, she took part in a 60-mile walk for breast cancer. "I felt great right then," Tracy recalls. "I had a great time. And I felt strong. It was one of those things that I did to prove to myself that I was strong—that my body was strong. My body was healthy. It was my way of saying, 'I can deal with this.'" For Tracy, kickboxing wasn't just a fabulous form of exercise, it was a source of emotional strength.

When Lanita Hausman was diagnosed with breast cancer at age 32, she was well on her way to her long-time goal of running the New York City Marathon. Because her cancer had been caught at such an early stage, Lanita was told that she wouldn't need chemo after her double mastectomy, which was scheduled for March 18, 1996—just 7 months *before the big race. To Lanita, running the marathon was her chance to show that she, not cancer, was victorious, and she was determined to make the most of that chance. "From the time I was diagnosed, one of my first questions was, 'Can I still run a marathon after cancer?'" Lanita recalls. "Every doctor answered, 'I don't know why you'd want to, but there is no medical reason why you can't.'"*

What We Know about the Benefits of Diet and Exercise

For Joy, Tracy, and Lanita, exercise was far more than a way to achieve an ideal body image, or even to regain their health. It was a way to reconnect to their bodies, to restore their physical sense of self after the trauma of breast cancer and mastectomy. It would be nice to add that, in addition to the pleasure it brings, exercise has been shown to have specific beneficial effects for breast cancer survivors, that it will help you recuperate from your illness and your surgery and maybe even prevent a recurrence of the disease. Unfortunately, that's a claim that so far we can't make. Although the general health benefits of exercise are well known, there is no scientific consensus about the specific relationship between exercise and breast cancer, particularly for young women. Two of the few significant studies that did include large numbers of young women, the well-publicized Nurses' Health Study (NHS)[1] and Nurses' Health Study II (NHSII),[2] were inconclusive on the relationship between exercise and breast cancer, according to Beverly Rockhill, Ph.D., assistant professor of epidemiology at the University of North Carolina, Chapel Hill, who conducted analyses of those studies' data.

"Exercise is so important to women's health in general," says Dr. Rockhill. "But with respect to overselling it as a breast cancer benefit—and a survival benefit—that's where you have to be careful. Exercise has a lot of physical and mental benefits. But if we're making women feel guilty about not exercising without having a strong scientific consensus, that certainly isn't helpful. There are so many women who could be described as 'pictures of health'—they eat right and exercise regularly—and they still have gotten breast cancer."

Because exercise *is* so important to women's health in general, and because there are so many misconceptions about its relationship to breast cancer, let's look a little more closely at what we do and don't know about exercise.

Analyzing the Data

Everyone who considers the question of exercise, young women, and breast cancer agrees that we just don't know enough. Anne McTiernan,

M.D., Ph.D., a scientist at the Fred Hutchinson Cancer Research Center in Seattle and the author of *Breast Fitness: An Optimal Exercise and Health Plan for Reducing Your Risk of Breast Cancer,* is an international leader in research on exercise as a method of preventing the occurrence and recurrence of breast cancer. She's a strong proponent of the idea that exercise is beneficial to breast cancer survivors, and she sees exercise as a possible means of preventing breast cancer in the first place. Yet even she acknowledges that little research into how exercise affects breast cancer survivors has been done. "There is an absolute dearth of studies," she says. "There is a big hole in the research."

The few studies that do exist, Dr. McTiernan says, are short-term research projects that looked at exercise for 3 months or less and dealt mostly with quality-of-life issues, such as whether exercise reduced anxiety or depression. And in this regard, Dr. McTiernan says, exercise is indeed helpful: "Exercise, at least for this amount of time, did seem to reduce anxiety and improve the quality of life." But, she adds quickly, the research does not tell us what effect exercise has upon a woman's survival.

Kathy Burgau, Diagnosed at Age 26

I've always loved softball. It started in elementary school.

I finished chemo in May of 1997, and in August I was playing coed softball. They put me right back in the outfield. It felt so good to do something normal again.

I remember one time, I hit a triple, and as I slid into third base, my friend Myrna said, "Kathy, adjust yourself." I said, "Myrna, I'm not a boy!" She said, "No, your breast." And I look down, and there's my boob in the middle of my stomach. So I took out my fake breast and threw it at her.

I didn't plan on having reconstruction until after I'd had kids, but I just wanted to be rid of that thing in my bra. It was always in my way. So in November 1997, I had the expander put in, and then 3 weeks after the expander was in, I was back playing volleyball. I usually schedule my surgeries around volleyball and softball. With the implant in, because I lift weights and have muscle, I can move my boob. I've got pecs like a man.

In September of 2000, I ran my first race—one I won't soon forget. I was so happy, even though I was crying. It was such an accomplishment for me to think I was back to the old me!

"We need studies in the future, to show what women are doing after their diagnosis and how it relates to survival," Dr. McTiernan says. "That's where the advocacy comes in. We need to get the word out about what needs to be done."

Exercise before and after Diagnosis

Leslie Bernstein, Ph.D., an epidemiologist and researcher at the University of Southern California, has also looked into the question of how exercise might affect young women's chances of getting breast cancer. Dr. Bernstein explains that there are actually three separate questions:

1. Does exercise reduce the risk of breast cancer in young women?

2. Does it reduce the risk of breast cancer in postmenopausal women?

3. Does it reduce the risk of recurrence in women of any age who have already been diagnosed with breast cancer?

In Dr. Bernstein's view, the answer to the first question is an emphatic *yes*. In her studies, for healthy women aged 40 and under who exercise 4 or more hours a week during their childbearing years, the risk of developing breast cancer is reduced by 50 percent.[3] With regard to postmenopausal women, Bernstein believes that exercise can also help prevent breast cancer, especially if the women have been active for most of their lifetimes.

For women who already have breast cancer, however, it isn't clear what role exercise plays. "No one has ever even created an exercise program whose goal was to reduce recurrence and increase survival," says Dr. Bernstein. "Most of the exercise programs that have been studied have been designed to increase the quality of life during treatment." She adds that it would be difficult to study the effects of exercise on women after diagnosis because there are so many factors that might affect a survivor's ability to exercise, including the fact that women who have had mastectomies or have been treated with radiation therapy often have limited upper limb mobility.

However, Dr. Bernstein says, it is possible to speculate that if exercise helps to prevent breast cancer in healthy women, it might also be helpful for women who already have breast cancer. In both cases, she says, exercise might have the same beneficial effect: the reduction of estrogen.

Exercise and Estrogen

In Dr. Bernstein's view, the reason she found such dramatic evidence of the usefulness of exercise in preventing breast cancer is that exercise lowers women's estrogen levels. Breast tissue, of course, is responsive to estrogen, which is why young girls grow breasts during puberty, as their female hormones kick in. And while the relationship between estrogen and breast cancer is not yet fully understood, many doctors and researchers believe that, at least in some cases, estrogen may accelerate tumor growth. (Dr. McTiernan points out that one-third of young women with breast cancer have estrogen-receptor tumors, which grow more quickly when a woman's hormone levels are higher.) "So," concludes Dr. Bernstein, "anything that reduces a woman's cumulative exposure to estrogen is something we're interested in, because it might help reduce breast cancer risk."

Dr. Bernstein also studied how exercise affects menstrual cycle patterns in adolescents. She believes that when teenagers exercise even as little as 2 to 3 hours a week, their estrogen levels are reduced, setting up a pattern in which their cumulative lifetime exposure to estrogen would be lower than that of women who were sedentary. Likewise, she thinks, when the women under 40 whom she studied exercised at least 4 hours a week during their childbearing years, they were lowering their exposure to estrogen. Therefore, she concludes, exercise helps reduce the risk of breast cancer because it lowers women's estrogen levels. And perhaps this beneficial effect might also extend to women after diagnosis.

Dr. Rockhill is more skeptical about this line of reasoning. In her own analysis of the Nurses' Health Study II, which included a population of over 100,000 premenopausal women and 370 cases of breast cancer, she found no relationship at all between exercise and breast cancer risk in premenopausal women.[4] In older women in the original Nurses' Health Study who exercised 7 hours or more a week, Dr. Rockhill says, there was a 20 percent lower risk.[5] "That's not the magic bullet," she points out. "*If* the lower risk is caused by the higher activity, something which isn't proven yet, *and if* we could get *all* women in this country to do 7 hours of exercise, then the 180,000 cases of breast cancer that occur each year would be reduced to 144,000. I would say that's a modest reduction."

It is important to recognize that both Dr. Rockhill and Dr. Bernstein are committed to finding answers about the effects of physical activity on breast cancer and that they regard their different findings as evidence that further study is needed. As the chair of the Scientific Advisory Committee for the Nurses' Health Study, Dr. Bernstein has worked with those investigators to initiate a case-control study within the population of nurses (similar to the approach in her study) to determine if there are different results regarding physical activity. "One of the difficulties with cohort studies like the NHS is that they do not have information on life-time exercise activity—the key to assessing activity," says Dr. Bernstein.

Both scientists also agree that the relationship between estrogen and breast cancer is a crucial one. The problem is that estrogen is produced differently in pre- and postmenopausal women, so that studies of older women don't necessarily apply to women who are still menstruating. In young women, estrogen is produced mainly by the ovaries. In women who have stopped menstruating, estrogen is produced mainly by body fat. That's how exercise may help reduce breast cancer among older women—by reducing body fat.

For younger women, though, body fat has far less impact on the hormones. "A young woman must be either extremely thin or very obese before her weight has much effect on the functioning of her ovaries," says Dr. Rockhill. While exercise may indeed lower estrogen levels in young women to some extent, Dr. Rockhill isn't sure how much exercise would be required to lower those levels to the point where breast cancer risk would also be reduced.

Dr. Rockhill points out that women in countries where the breast cancer rate is relatively low go through puberty at far older ages than women in the United States. Thus they have several more estrogen-free years than their U.S. counterparts. "In China, in the past, the average age of menarche was close to 17," she says. "In America, it's getting earlier and earlier—11 and 12—and even in China it's starting earlier. Maybe we can reduce breast cancer by delaying puberty. But I think there are a lot of ethical problems associated with that."

Perhaps, adds Dr. Bernstein, "you don't have to delay puberty if you encourage girls and young women to be physically active." A study she conducted of a racially diverse population of high school girls in the United States showed that physical activity after menarche dramatically reduced the frequency of ovulatory menstrual cycles and therefore affected the cumulative exposure to estrogen and progesterone during adolescence.[6] "Menarche is not simply a chronological marker of the onset of estrogen exposure," argues Dr. Bernstein. "It is also a marker of the amount of early exposure to estrogen once menstrual cycles begin."

Researchers also agree that early childbearing can help reduce the risk of breast cancer.[7] "Breast cancer rates are very low in societies where women have their first child very soon after puberty," says Dr. Rockhill. "Obviously, in America, this is not a solution." While her goal is not to advocate a particular medical or social policy, this example illuminates the difficulty of understanding the relationship between estrogen and breast cancer in young women.

Body Weight and Breast Cancer

What about the relationship between breast cancer and body weight? If exercise helps you lower your weight and reduce your body fat, can we assume that it will help to prevent the onset or recurrence of breast cancer?

Joy Simha, Diagnosed at Age 26

After breast cancer, I could no longer stay in smoky bars. I couldn't be around smokers, or around people who just wanted to drink to get drunk. Breast cancer just changed me that way, made me feel like, "Yuk, that's a useless life. I'm going to make every moment count."

And there was that recurring fear that I would die, and die alone, or have a recurrence of breast cancer alone. I felt that I could do it, but I didn't want to. I decided I needed to take every opportunity that I could to try to get out there and live life. I realized that kayaking was the best way to meet guys. I was out there on the river, one of the only girls, and there were all these men running around. And so I just kept up with kayaking and figured that one day my little kayaker would float on by. And that's where I focused my energy from May through October.

Really, I didn't care if I met the man of my dreams—I was having fun. And that went along with my desire to keep biting, chewing on life, taking in every second.

Then I moved to an apartment building where there was a gym in the basement, and I started to go to the gym on a daily basis, and I started to build up my body. I could run on the treadmill, spend half an hour on the Stairmaster. And I realized that my body was growing more and more beautiful every day. And you know what? It's just a shell. My soul is really beautiful. I'm a good friend. I have other things to offer the world. And I started to see myself as this beautiful person.

I probably wouldn't be back whitewater kayaking if they had told me when I first got breast cancer that they'd be removing my lymph nodes and that my arm would be in jeopardy for lymphedema, and maybe I wouldn't want to cut my arm in the river. If I had taken that to heart, I wouldn't be a whitewater kayaker. I wouldn't have been back on the river. I wouldn't have met Vasu and gotten married. And I wouldn't have my beautiful baby boy.

Once again, the experts disagree. Dr. McTiernan says flatly, "For a woman of any age with breast cancer, being overweight decreases your chances of survival and increases your chances of recurrence. We know that. Being overweight is not healthy for women who have already gotten breast cancer at any age."

Dr. Leslie Bernstein says the data are strongest for older women. "Obesity is a major factor for breast cancer in older women." In a study of postmenopausal women aged 50 to 64 that was published in the *British Journal of Cancer,* Bernstein and her colleagues found the most evidence for decreased risk of breast cancer in those who gained the least weight over their lifetime, starting at age 18.[8] However, she points out that once again there are simply not enough data on the relationship between obesity and breast cancer in young women.

What Dr. Rockhill stresses is that exercise is generally beneficial to all women of all ages, including young women with breast cancer. "Women who exercise more do have a lower risk of dying from any disease," Dr. Rockhill says. "It seems like common sense. Physical activity is associated with a lower total risk of mortality—it lowers the risks of nearly all the major diseases that women face." But then she adds, "Sadly, breast cancer appears to have only a modest association with exercise. Based on what we know of physical activity, if women think that by exercising and eating right they won't get breast cancer, they may be disappointed."

Drawing Your Own Conclusions

If even the experts can't get together and recommend something as apparently simple as exercise, you may wonder how you are supposed to know what to do. The first thing to keep in mind is that the experts themselves don't believe that their studies are necessarily the best means of making recommendations for individual women. The statistics that they gather on the large groups of women in their studies give them overall probabilities. But how the statistics affect any individual woman is far more difficult to calculate.

"We personalize these things that are very gross averages for the population," says Dr. Beverly Rockhill. "I give the analogy of flipping a coin. We could have a model of how many times we'll get heads if we flip a coin one thousand times. We have a really good statistical model for that. But with every individual flip, we still will be wrong half the time."

The good news for you in all this is that your destiny as a breast cancer survivor is not ruled by statistics. While there are general patterns that can be followed throughout an entire population, you as an individual are unique. In that context, you may find it helpful to know that

Lanita Hausman, Diagnosed at Age 32

Before I was diagnosed with breast cancer, I had been running for a couple of years, averaging 20 miles a week, and I'd completed a half marathon. I had promised myself that one day I would run a marathon and had started working on a training strategy, when my life took a temporary detour.

Those 26.2 marathon miles became very important to me. The first thing I did was get my doctor's assurance that when I recovered, I could continue training with no risk to my health or well-being. With his reassurance, those miles became my focus when the pain threatened to overtake me and depression lurked in the corner of my hospital room, ready to pounce at the first inkling that I was wavering in my resolve to beat breast cancer. The first time my mother held me up as we shuffled down the hospital corridor, I said, "These are my first steps toward the marathon finish line."

As my treatment progressed, so did my training. One day, several weeks after my mastectomy and reconstructive surgery, I had to meet the plastic surgeon, who was taking fluid out of my breast implants because they were too big. My appointment was for 10 a.m. She said, "I'm sorry I'm making you miss running." I said, "You didn't." I'd gotten up at 5 a.m. and done my 10 miles, in the rain.

My friends told me that this was my way of delaying dealing with the breast cancer—my way of saying, "No, this disease is not so devastating." They might have been right. But I think what the marathon really did was take me out of that "Why me, poor me" syndrome. I ran the marathon to prove to myself that cancer didn't beat me—that I won. My sanity probably was in question! But I finished it and made a personal record—5 hours and 25 minutes.

I have my medal and number and picture framed at home, and I look at it whenever I need inspiration as to whether I can do the things I've chosen to do. Every goal I meet brings many more to conquer.

exercise is extremely beneficial in all sorts of ways—it combats anxiety and depression, it raises your general level of health, and, as the women in this chapter have related, it simply helps you feel alive and energized in your own body. If it turns out down the road that exercise has also had a specific impact on your breast cancer, so much the better. But even without that particular benefit, there are still many good reasons to exercise.

So far, we've considered only how ordinary exercise might affect your breast cancer. There is one type of exercise, however, about which there is absolutely no doubt: specific exercises that you can do after surgery to help you regain strength and range of motion in your arms and shoulders. When done correctly and at the pace that is appropriate for you, these exercises are definitely beneficial for every young woman with breast cancer.

Postsurgery Exercises

Sad to say, there are still some old-fashioned doctors out there who advise their breast cancer patients to avoid all activity after surgery and during chemo. Of course, as Lanita found, there may be a period when it's a struggle simply to take a few steps down the hall or raise your arms over your head. But inactivity promotes muscle wasting, which makes it even harder for you to regain normal functioning. So whether or not you were exercising before, you might seriously consider becoming active as soon as you can.

Obviously, you should always consult your physician before starting any exercise plan. Just be sure you've found a doctor who understands the importance of exercise.

Getting Started

It can be a bit scary to start exercising after surgery, especially if you've never exercised before. You may experience some discomfort in your upper arm and shoulder after surgery, which can be disconcerting if you don't expect it. That's because during surgery, some of your nerves may have been injured, which creates numbness. In some cases, the injury is permanent and you regain only limited feeling or no feeling at all in the affected areas. In other cases, as the nerves grow back, you feel a kind of pins-and-needles sensation. According to Diana Stumm, a physical therapist and the author of *Recovering from Breast Surgery*, the pins and needles usually go away. Meanwhile, though, the sensation may make you reluctant to move your shoulder. In Stumm's words:

> The natural inclination is not to move your arm when it's in pain, so many women find themselves walking around looking like Napoleon. You hold your arm away from your side with your hand across your stomach. But if you do this for a while, the surgical scar tissue tightens and the tense muscles shorten. This is particularly true if the surgery was done on your nondominant side [your left side, if you're right-handed, and vice versa], so you're not forced to use it. The joint stiffens without use, and this can take several months of intense physical therapy to resolve.

You Shouldn't Exercise If . . .

- Your pulse is irregular.

- Your resting pulse is higher than 100 beats per minute.

- You have recurring leg pain or cramps.

- You have chest pain.

- You feel intensely nauseous when you exercise.

- Exercise makes you feel disoriented, confused, or dizzy, or it gives you blurred vision or causes you to faint.

- You've got new pains in your bones, back, or neck.

- You're extremely pale or anemic.

- You're ill and/or have a fever.

- You experience sudden shortness of breath, muscular weakness, or unusual fatigue.

During cancer treatment, it's hard to know how to read your body's signals, since you will naturally be feeling more tired and achy than usual. That's why it is essential that you work with a physician, and perhaps also with a physical therapist, so that you can learn when you should push yourself a bit and when you need to stop and rest.

Rather than falling into a vicious cycle—surgery makes you reluctant to move, which in turn causes further problems for your muscles and joints—try to do at least these simple muscle-strengthening exercises. They'll take only a few minutes a day, and you can even do them while watching television! Talk to your doctor about what kinds of slightly uncomfortable sensations you should exercise through, as opposed to feeling actual pain, which should cause you to stop. You might also find a physical therapist who can help you design your own back-to-health exercise program.

Recommended Postoperative Exercises

The following exercises, based on recommendations of the University of Washington Breast Cancer Specialty Center,[9] can help you regain your full range of motion in your arm and shoulder while building up muscle strength and flexibility. If you have been fitted with a surgical drain, your surgeon may recommend that you wait to exercise until it is removed. In any case, either your surgeon or your physical therapist should monitor your exercise for the first several weeks after the operation. Usually, it takes only 4 to 12 weeks to get back your full range of motion, but some women have trouble with ongoing tightness and restricted motion.

Try all four of these exercises on the floor or on a firm bed, from one to three times a day.

For each of these exercises, be patient with yourself and take it slow. Each day you can do a little more—though sometimes you may hit a plateau or even feel as though you're going backward. Don't worry; that's just part of the process. Doctors agree: Quality is better than quantity. Think of yourself as gently coaxing your muscles awake, rather than rudely shaking them out of sleep.

Hand Leaning

For this exercise, your goal is to feel tension—a pleasant stretching of your muscles—but not pain. Keep your shoulders loose and relaxed. Avoid putting them in a "hiked" or raised position, as this will actually shut down muscle activity and bring on spasms and pain in your shoulders and neck. "Slow, steady, and gentle" should be your watchwords.

- Sit on a bed or couch with your hand resting by your side.
- Lean on your hand. Start with just a little pressure. Each day, lean a little harder.
- As you build up strength, try moving your hand farther away, out to the side and behind you. Again, gradually lean a bit harder on your hand in each new position.
- When you can easily lean on your hand, graduate to crawling on your hands and knees.

Start the next three exercises lying on your back with your knees bent and your feet flat. If you like, put a pillow under your head and/or your lower back.

Daydream

- Clasp your hands behind your head. If you like, support yourself with a pillow under each elbow.

98

- Let your elbows drop down as far as you can.
- Hold your elbows down for 1 minute. Gradually, build up the amount of time you can hold them down until you can do it for 10 minutes.

Snow Angel

- Extend your arms out to the sides, palms up if possible, with your elbows and wrists on the floor (or bed). If you can't rest your elbow on the floor, put a pillow underneath it to support it.
- Keeping your arms on the floor, gradually move your arms up over your head. Stay there as long as you can, working up from 1 minute to 10 minutes. Your goal is to feel a pleasant stretch in the arm or side where you had the operation. If you feel pain, stop.
- Start by repeating this exercise three times, and do it three times a day. As you become more comfortable, you can increase the number of times you do it until you feel that you've recovered your full range of motion.

Hand Clasp

- Clasp your hands together and lift your arms up over your head, keeping your elbows slightly bent.
- Raise your arms as high as you can, but stop when you feel tight. Very gently, let the weight of your arms stretch your tissue just a little bit more.
- Relax for 1 minute with your arms in their upright position. Work your way up to 10 minutes in that position. That may sound like a long time, but it is what doctors recommend. Take your time and work your way up gradually to that time. Standing, place your left hand behind your neck and your right hand behind your back. Then put your right hand behind your neck and your left hand behind your back. When your affected arm is in the upper position, press a little to stretch the area. Again, your goal is tension, not pain.
- It's also helpful if you use your arms as much as possible after surgery: reaching, eating, washing yourself, combing your hair. If you can, move your arms back and forth in a swinging motion from the shoulder as you walk, perhaps while bending your elbows. Swinging your arms will help increase your shoulders' range of motion.

Tips for Starting an Exercise Plan

- *Take it slow.* This goes for potential marathon runners as well as for women who have never been physically active—and for everyone in between. You and your body have been through a lot, and you've got a long way to go. So pace yourself. Take some time to discover what you can and can't do, even as you build up your strength, endurance, and range of motion.

- *Ask your doctor to refer you to a physical therapy program at your clinic or hospital.* A physical therapist can help you strengthen your arm and shoulder after surgery, and can work with you on regaining the range of motion you need for your daily routine. A physical therapist can also tell you about ways to prevent and manage lymphedema.

- *Start with low-impact exercise that develops whole-body strength and includes at least some aerobic components.* Aerobic exercise like walking, swimming, and yoga helps you breathe deeply, and the therapeutic effects of deep breathing are too numerous to mention. Once you have restored your range of motion, a physical therapist can advise you on strength-building exercises with light weights to help you regain your strength and endurance. Especially if you've never been active before, these forms of activity are good "starter" choices.

- *Pick activities you like.* Are you a do-it-yourselfer or someone who likes groups? Do you like variety or routine? Can you combine exercise with something else that you like, such as walking through different city neighborhoods or cycling down a country road? Or would you rather just go to the gym, work out, and get it over with? Try to develop a workout plan that allows you to enjoy yourself—and do consider some creative choices, just for fun. Things like t'ai chi, martial arts, salsa lessons, kayaking, water ballet, and African dance may be available in your community, offering you many kinds of pleasure besides the obvious health benefits.

- *Don't forget to rebuild muscle.* It's hard to stay active during much of the diagnosis and treatment process, so when you're ready to get active again, you may have lost muscle. Increased muscle can add to your store of energy, lessen your fatigue, and help you to manage pain, so it's definitely worth going for. Building up your muscle can also help you with daily activities, such as playing with your kids, doing yard work, or engaging in other physically demanding chores.

- *Start your weight training with machines rather than free weights.* Your abdominal, back, and shoulder muscles don't have to work as hard with machines—and that might be the head start you need, especially if you've never trained with weights before. However, if the surgery has left your muscles relatively intact, using very light free weights (as little as 1 or 2 pounds) can help restore abdominal tone and improve your muscle balance.

- *Try not to slouch.* Women who have had mastectomies sometimes have a tendency to slump forward, either in response to their new shape or because of the chest tightness that can result from the surgery. Stretching your chest and shoulder muscles and strengthening your back muscles will be good for your whole body—and your whole outlook. It's also helpful to occasionally walk with your hands clasped behind your back while pulling your shoulder blades together.

Nutrition and Breast Cancer

Just as there has been a lot of confusion over the usefulness of exercise in breast cancer, so has there been a similar confusion over the usefulness of diet. Apart from the relationship between breast cancer and weight, how does the food you eat affect your chances of surviving breast cancer?

The answer, once again, isn't clear. The American Cancer Society has issued a set of guidelines for a healthy diet and a physically active lifestyle that provide general recommendations for good health. But the specific relationship between breast cancer and diet is not yet known.

For a while, says Dr. Beverly Rockhill, the idea that a high-fat diet led to breast cancer was "very popular." But, she says, when researchers have interviewed women with and without breast cancer about their diets, they've found that "women with breast cancer overreported the amount of fat they were eating. They were looking for the cause of their getting breast cancer." That may be human nature, says Dr. Rockhill, but it's not hard science. "I'm amazed that people aren't more cautious about this issue," she says. "The idea that there is a breast fitness diet or exercise plan is flawed. I'd rather see a health plan."

Dr. Rockhill acknowledges that some evidence seems to suggest that a diet that is high in plant foods "binds" more estrogen than a diet that is high in animal protein. Once estrogen is bound, it may become less active in the body, and some is expelled in the urine. And, as we've seen,

Tips for Finding a Nutritionist Who Knows about Breast Cancer

- *Ask your doctor for a recommendation.* Although some doctors are skeptical about the role of nutrition in health, many work closely with nutritionists or may have colleagues who do.

- *Check out the nearest center for complementary or integrated medicine.* Complementary and integrated approaches to medicine draw on alternative traditions to complement the contributions of Western medicine, seeking to create an integrated approach. Many prestigious cancer centers, such as Memorial Sloan-Kettering, have established departments of complementary and/or alternative medicine, and these may employ or consult with nutritionists of all types. (For more information on complementary and integrated medicine, see Chapter 5. For contact information on particular medical centers, see the Resources section.)

- Look at the bulletin boards of the local health food store, yoga center, or t'ai chi/martial arts center.

- Find a women's clinic or health center.

- Ask people who get or give alternative health treatments—massage, acupuncture, Ayurvedic medicine, and the like—if they can recommend a nutritionist.

having less estrogen active in the body may be a good idea for women with breast cancer, especially young women whose ovaries are still functioning. But Dr. Rockhill is still cautious about drawing straightforward conclusions about nutrition.

"There is a lot about breast cancer that we don't understand," she says. "Portraying it as simple is misleading. The mentality of 'More estrogen bound, more estrogen out, equals less breast cancer' simply doesn't hold up. I think women need to know that there are no simple answers."

With or without hard scientific data, there are many people, holding a wide range of nutritional philosophies, who believe that breast cancer can be greatly affected by diet. You can read about some of those approaches, including a soy-rich diet and macrobiotics, in Chapter 5, which concerns alternative and complementary medicine. You might also look for a nutritionist who has a particular interest in breast cancer and/or women's nutrition. Many nutritionists point to studies that they feel offer a good basis for making dietary choices, even if the evidence is not yet conclusive.

Breast Cancer and Smoking

Given what you've already learned about exercise and nutrition, it may not surprise you to discover that scientists cannot even say conclusively that smoking is bad for breast cancer. Dr. Beverly Rockhill, who wrote the chapter on smoking in the Surgeon General's Report on Breast Cancer, says that although smoking increases the risk of lung cancer dramatically, finding a link between smoking and breast cancer is not so simple. "Women who smoke go through menopause earlier," she points out. "So some would argue that smoking would be good for breast cancer. And there's a report in the *Journal of the National Cancer Institute* saying that women with the BRCA1 gene [believed to increase the risk of breast cancer] who smoked, actually lowered their risk of breast cancer by 50 percent.[10] Of course, I haven't seen that study replicated. But you can't scare women about smoking by saying that it's related to breast cancer."

Rockhill wants to emphasize that there is a strong scientific consensus that the negative effects of smoking are so overwhelming that women should simply avoid or quit smoking. However, she says, there is no consistent link to breast cancer that has been demonstrated at this time.

The American Cancer Society's Nutrition and Physical Activity Guidelines: Points to Remember

Note: These guidelines are not specific to the prevention or treatment of breast cancer.

Eat a variety of healthful foods, with an emphasis on plant sources.

Eat five or more servings of a variety of vegetables and fruits each day.

- Include vegetables and fruits at every meal and for snacks.
- Eat a variety of vegetables and fruits.
- Limit French fries, snack chips, and other fried vegetable products.
- Choose 100 percent juice if you drink fruit or vegetable juices.

Choose whole grains in preference to processed (refined) grains and sugars.

- Choose whole-grain rice, bread, pasta, and cereals.
- Limit consumption of refined carbohydrates, including pastries, sweetened cereals, soft drinks, and sugars.

Limit consumption of red meats, especially those high in fat, and of processed meats.

- Choose fish, poultry, or beans as an alternative to beef, pork, and lamb.
- When you eat meat, select lean cuts and smaller portions.
- Prepare meat by baking, broiling, or poaching, rather than by frying or charbroiling.

Choose foods that help maintain a healthful weight.

- When you eat away from home, choose food low in fat, calories, and sugar and avoid large portions.
- Eat smaller portions of high-calorie foods. Be aware that "low fat" or "fat free" does not mean "low calorie" (and that low-fat cakes, cookies, and similar foods are often high in calories).
- Substitute vegetables, fruits, and other low-calorie foods for calorie-dense foods such as French fries, cheeseburgers, pizza, ice cream, doughnuts, and other sweets.

Adopt a physically active lifestyle.

- Engage in at least moderate activity for 30 minutes or more on 5 or more days of the week; 45 minutes or more of moderate to vigorous activity on 5 or more days per week may further reduce the risk of breast and colon cancer.

Examples of Moderate and Vigorous Physical Activities

Exercise and Leisure

- *Moderate activities:* Walking, dancing, leisurely bicycling, ice-skating or roller-skating, horseback riding, canoeing, yoga
- *Vigorous activities:* Jogging or running, fast bicycling, circuit weight training, aerobic dance, martial arts, jump rope, swimming

Sports

- *Moderate exercise:* Volleyball, golfing, softball, baseball, badminton, doubles tennis, downhill skiing
- *Vigorous exercise:* Soccer, field hockey or ice hockey, lacrosse, singles tennis, racquetball, basketball, cross-country skiing

Helpful ways to be more active

- Use stairs rather than an elevator.
- If you can, walk or bike to your destination.
- Exercise at lunch with your workmates, family, or friends.

- Take a 10-minute exercise break at work to stretch or take a quick walk.
- Walk to visit coworkers instead of sending an email.
- Go dancing with your spouse or friends.
- Plan active vacations rather than only driving trips.
- Wear a pedometer every day and watch your daily steps increase.
- Join a sports team.
- Use a stationary bicycle while watching TV.
- Plan your exercise routine to gradually increase the days per week and minutes per session.

Maintain a healthful weight throughout life.
- Balance caloric intake with physical activity.
- Lose weight if currently overweight or obese.
- Being overweight or obese is associated with an increased risk of developing several types of cancer.

ACS advice specific to reducing the risk of breast cancer:
- Engage in vigorous physical activity at least 4 hours a week.
- Avoid alcohol or limit your intake to no more than one drink per day.
- Reduce lifetime weight gain by limiting your calories and exercising regularly.

Reproduced by permission of the American Cancer Society

Eating Your Way to Health

When you see the American Cancer Society dietary recommendations for general health and suppressing breast cancer, you probably won't be surprised. For general health, experts recommend a low-fat, high-fiber diet rich in fruits and vegetables and no smoking; as regards breast cancer, they also recommend limiting alcohol intake to one drink per day.

Unfortunately, a lot more research is needed in order to better understand the relationship between nutrition and breast cancer, and no study is really conclusive on any point. But here's some of what we do know:

Countries where the standard diet is high in fruits, vegetables, and fiber and low in fat tend to have far lower rates of breast cancer than countries with high-fat diets that are low in fruits, vegetables, and fiber.[11]

And when women from low-fat countries come to high-fat countries like the United States, their breast cancer rates skyrocket, suggesting that environment and not genetics is involved.[12] Whether diet is the most important piece of this puzzle is a matter of much debate. After all, women in the United States have little in common with women in rural China, and what they eat is just one of many differences.

Lab animals that are given high-fat diets have significantly higher rates of breast cancer than those on low-fat diets.[13] However, experts aren't sure how to translate those results to people. Some experts recommend a diet in which less than 20 percent of the calories come from fat. Others say that reducing fat is not enough—you need to adopt the whole package, including a high intake of fiber, fruits, and veggies.

Women who have two or more alcoholic drinks a day are more than twice as likely to get breast cancer as nondrinkers. That's probably because alcohol seems to increase the levels of estrogen in the blood, perhaps because of alcohol's toxic effects on the liver, which interfere with that organ's ability to cleanse the blood of excess estrogen.[14] Alcohol can also make it harder for your immune system to function. A report from the Nurses' Health Study suggests that taking folic acid can help counteract the increased risk from alcohol.[15]

The New Science of Phytohormonals

Recently, a whole new branch of nutritional science has been attracting attention: the science of phytohormonals. Nutritionists have discovered that certain plant foods can affect women's estrogen levels—and perhaps also affect their risk of breast cancer. Soy is the most famous source of these phytoestrogens, although many other foods, including garbanzos, black beans, and some other legumes, have the same key ingredients, known as isoflavones. (For more information on soy, see Chapter 5.)

Reconnecting to Your Body

When all is said and done, the reasons to consider fitness and dietary changes may have as much to do with your mental health as with your physical health. Tracy Pleva Hill feels that being physically active is almost a spiritual way of connecting to her life:

> I took up kickboxing. I signed up for the Avon Three Day 60-mile walk. I just don't want to stop. I guess there's something in the back of my head that tells me that if I don't stop, it can't catch me. So by being active, I'm telling myself that I'm one step ahead of it. I'm beating it.

Cindy Kim also believes that the choices she makes allow her to cope with breast cancer better. "I'm the first to tell people that I was diagnosed at age 26. And every day of my life I feel like I am renegotiating with my body." She describes her new approach to her body as:

Complicated. And yet somehow very simple at the same time. I want the best for my body. Every time I sit down to a meal, or think about having a glass of wine, the question crosses my mind: Is this good for me? I try not to obsess over it, but I know I want to make the best decisions I can to be the healthiest person I can be. In so many ways I've felt like the unhealthiest person because of this— and anything I can do to change that, I want to do. It's not so much about control as it is about balance. It's about finding that inner balance emotionally and mentally.

CHAPTER 5

"This Empowers Me"

Alternative, Complementary, and Integrative Approaches to Healing

Juanita Lyle was first diagnosed with breast cancer when she was 32. Today she is a 58-year-old survivor who has endured three recurrences of her cancer, even as she raised her two children, continued to work, and became active in the breast cancer community. Juanita credits such practices as meditation, visualization, and affirmations with helping her with her often painful but ultimately triumphant journey through breast cancer. "Going back to chemo after I thought I had finished with it was the worst," she recalls. "It took a whole lot of self-talk to get me through it. I said things to myself like, 'Okay, your veins are going to work today. You're not going to smell the chemo today. You're not going to get real sick today.' I'd say to myself, 'You've been down this road before; you can do this.'" Juanita believes that her use of affirmations helped her both to manage her pain and to recover her health.

✦

"Eastern medicine saved my life," Cindy Kim says bluntly. "Lots of people in my family are Chinese acupuncturists—they're running around doing yoga and martial arts and acupuncture and acupressure, and they are so at peace with themselves. And their bodies are functioning." So when Cindy was diagnosed with breast cancer at the age of 28, she turned to her father, a licensed doctor in Chinese medicine, for help in handling her debilitating responses to chemotherapy and radiation treatment.

"During radiation I was going through full-blown menopause," Cindy recalls. "I called my father, crying, and within 2 weeks of taking what he gave me, I started my period. It's all about an imbalance of hormones, which an herbal remedy can help rebalance. I believe there is a cure for every ailment; we just need to find it."

✑

"When you're a cancer patient, everyone wants to send you books about alternatives, along with their favorite supplements," says Beth Brokaw, who was first diagnosed with breast cancer at age 37 and diagnosed with metastatic breast cancer at age 44. "I've felt terribly overwhelmed, and I don't want a crash course on alternative medicine, but you have to be informed. I've tried to sort through the supplements and advice, and to follow through on those that I find have some credibility. As a cancer patient, I don't have the energy to go walking through the library. So I appreciate that my friends have done some research for me."

Understanding Alternative, Complementary, and Integrative Medicine

Over the past few decades, the mind/body connection has become an increasingly popular approach to health. "There is a close working relationship between the body and the mind," explains Barrie Cassileth, Ph.D., director of the Integrative Medicine Service at Memorial Sloan-Kettering Cancer Center in New York City and author of *The Alternative Medicine Handbook*. "If you can relax one, the other will benefit. It doesn't matter whether you come at it through the body, as with massage, or through the mind, as with meditation. If you relax the muscles, then you will become emotionally more relaxed. So you've got the same effect as if you had an intravenous dose of Valium, but this is noninvasive and nonpharmacologic."

In addition to mind/body approaches, a growing number of people, particularly young people, have developed an interest in so-called alternative treatments—approaches to healing that come from traditions and philosophies that are different from standard medical practice. Such disciplines as Chinese medicine, Ayurvedic medicine, macrobiotics, and nutritional approaches are not grounded in the scientific method that is the foundation of Western medicine, in which a hypothesis is tested and then proven by means of a controlled, randomized experiment. Rather, these forms of healing have developed out of tradition, intuition, trial and error, and experience, although many of them are now beginning to be studied by scientists who see them as having some potential for helping patients.

Initially, alternative healing was strongly resisted by most physicians, who considered it harmless at best and dangerous "quackery" at worst. But as the popularity of these techniques grew, at least some portions of the medical community have gradually begun to accept them. When Memorial Sloan-Kettering, one of the nation's premier sites for cancer treatment and research, established its Integrative Medicine Service, it sent

Defining CAM Approaches

As you consider CAM approaches, it might be useful to break them down into categories:

- *Approaches that focus on the mind and spirit.* This category would include psychotherapy, counseling, and support groups, as well as your own attempts to find meaning in your illness by drawing upon your philosophy and/or your faith.

- *Alternative approaches to medicine.* In this category are medical traditions that aspire to be complete in themselves, although doctors recommend that you use them to complement, not replace, your standard medical care. Chinese medicine, the Ayurvedic medicine of India, homeopathy, and naturopathy are such autonomous medical systems.

- *Nutritional, herbal, and dietary approaches.* Many people believe that what you eat can have an enormous impact on your health, and that particular foods, herbs, or supplements can help to combat breast cancer and/or the side effects of breast cancer treatment by building up the immune system. Again, these systems vary and so do their proponents' claims for them, but the doctors who are most sympathetic to these nutritional approaches recommend integrating them with standard medical care.

- *Mind/body approaches.* Disciplines like meditation, yoga, Qigong, and t'ai chi have been shown to help create a sense of calm and serenity, as well as potentially reinforcing the body's own healing energies. These approaches are not considered self-contained healing systems, but people who advocate them believe that they can have an enormous effect on your health. Visualization and affirmations are also considered effective in many circumstances.

a powerful signal to the cancer community that these once-reviled approaches had some measure of credibility. Likewise, the National Cancer Institute, one of the major sponsors of cancer-related research, now includes the National Center for Complementary and Alternative Medicine. Indeed, the very word *complementary* suggests that alternative approaches can complement standard medicine, and the term *integrative* indicates that alternative treatments can be integrated into standard medical practice.

According to David Rosenthal, M.D., formerly head of the American Cancer Society and currently director of Harvard University Health

Services, complementary and alternative medicine (CAM) approaches are particularly popular among young people. "The younger people are, the more interested they are in complementary care," he says. "We've found that only 3 in 10 pre-Baby Boomers use some form of CAM. In the Baby Boom era, 5 in 10 people had used some form of CAM by age 33. And for the post-Baby Boom generation, 7 in 10 people have used CAM by age 33. So the young ones are using it more."

However, says Dr. Rosenthal, doctors still resist this approach, and as a result, "Fewer than 40 percent of CAM therapies are disclosed to physicians. Patients simply aren't telling them. Research shows that 61 percent say it's not important for the doctor to know, 60 percent say the doctor never asked, 31 percent say it's none of the doctor's business, and 20 percent say the doctor just wouldn't understand."[1]

Dr. Rosenthal understands that many patients fear that "If I tell my physician, he or she will no longer *be* my physician." But, he adds, "It's so important that the doctor knows what's going on," particularly since some CAM approaches, such as herbs or nutritional supplements, can interact with drugs and medications. Indeed, educating doctors about CAM approaches while subjecting those approaches to rigorous scientific scrutiny is part of the mission of the Sloan-Kettering division.

CAM and Standard Medical Care: A Growing Relationship

As CAM approaches have become more popular, the medical community has begun conducting research on various alternative treatments. Currently, the National Center for Complementary and Alternative Medicine is funding clinical trials to study the healing effects of prayer, the impact of hypnosis and guided imagery, and the conscious effort to find meaning in one's illness. The center is also studying the interaction of tamoxifen with dietary soy and herbs, as well as carefully exploring the role of phytohormonals, the plant-based sources of estrogen that many nutritionists claim can have a profound effect on a woman's hormonal balance. In addition, the center is exploring the use of massage and acupuncture and studying various nutritional issues, such as the ability of the phytochemicals in red wine to prevent breast cancer, the protective powers of grape seed extract, and the possible effectiveness of shark cartilage powder in treating colorectal cancer.

Moreover, many leading medical schools and research institutions are creating programs or divisions focusing on CAM approaches. In addition to Sloan-Kettering and Harvard's Dana Farber, the University of California at San Francisco is developing an integrative therapy program, funded by a $10 million grant to the UCSF medical school for research and education in CAM techniques. Dana Farber received a similar grant to create a new institute to explore complementary care.

Dr. Debu Tripathy, an oncologist at UCSF's Mount Zion Medical Center, is currently studying Chinese and Tibetan herbs and medicines in clinical trials. Dr. Tripathy explains that the impetus for this research came from the discovery that 80 percent of the center's patients were using some form of integrative medicine. "And young women under 50 tended to be the most common users," he notes. "We had an overwhelming number of questions from our patients, so we realized that we needed to set up research to come up with scientific answers to their questions."

Dr. Tripathy also developed a personal interest in herbal and Eastern medicines when his mentor, the director of the cancer research program at the California-Pacific Medical Center in San Francisco, developed breast cancer. Although Dr. Tripathy's mentor was an internationally known figure in the world of medicine, "she was being treated by a Tibetan doctor with herbs—and that physician, who used to be the personal physician to the Dalai Lama, agreed to do a trial with me," he says. Because Tibetan medicine is highly individualized, it does not lend itself to the standardized practices of Western medicine, and as a result there were research difficulties. Yet the experience left him with a strong commitment to find out more.

While some current doctors may be opposed to CAM, future doctors may be more sympathetic to CAM approaches, according to Dr. Rosenthal, who notes that medical schools are now training future doctors in at least some alternative approaches. "We're seeing that about one-third of medical institutions have programs teaching about integrative medicine," he says. "For the first time, students are studying herbs and nutrition. A lot of the classes are still electives. But at least it's getting into the coursework."

Dr. Rosenthal suggests that part of the impetus for the study of CAM techniques is coming from patients themselves, who are expressing an enormous desire for information. "The industry is already generating $30 to $40 billion a year in the United States alone," Dr. Rosenthal says. Support for this industry, he speculates, comes partly because there are so many diseases for which there is no cure—including breast cancer, but also including other forms of cancer, AIDS, and Alzheimer's. "As a result, there are twice as many visits to alternative practitioners as there are to primary care physicians."

According to two major studies on the subject conducted by David Eisenberg, Ph.D., Director of The Center for Alternative Medicine

Research at Beth Israel Deaconess in Boston, there was a dramatic increase in the public's use of CAM approaches between 1990 and 1997. The total number of visits to CAM providers in 1997 was 629 million (up from 427 million in 1990), thereby exceeding total visits to all U.S. primary care physicians (386 million). Dr. Eisenberg also found that Americans were spending 45 percent more on alternative therapies and professional services in 1997 than in 1990. He conservatively estimated expenditures at $21 billion in 1997, with more than half of that paid out of pocket.[2]

Yet another reason for the growing popularity of CAM approaches is simply that so many people have found them helpful. "Complementary therapies allow patients to have a major role in their own care," says Dr. Cassileth. "It gives them a very important sense of control." Complementary therapies that are available at Sloan-Kettering include massage, acupuncture, relaxation techniques, reflexology, music therapies, yoga, and t'ai chi. "These strengthen the body and relax the muscles and mind," says Dr. Cassileth. "This is not just about pain reduction. Complementary approaches also reduce other major symptoms, such as fatigue, shortness of breath, depression, and anxiety. These types of therapies can reduce the amount of pain medication that a patient needs. And in some cases, they can even relieve the pain completely."

Dr. Cassileth is especially enthusiastic about acupuncture, particularly for helping women to cope with the premature menopause that often results from various cancer treatments. "We don't have solid data yet," she says, "but I can tell you that women with breast cancer who have horrible hot flashes are finding tremendous relief through acupuncture. So far, we've had a lot of success. We have one staff member who was going through normal menopause, and after she had one acupuncture treatment, the problem was gone. This is amazing. As you know, you can't treat menopause very well in breast cancer patients, because it's dangerous to give them estrogen and standard hormone replacement therapies." (Doctors are concerned that estrogen supplements might encourage tumor growth and awaken dormant breast cancer cells elsewhere in the body. For more information, see Chapters 3 and 9.) Dr. Cassileth reports that researchers at Sloan-Kettering are in the process of conducting several studies into the efficacy of acupuncture.

Dr. Cassileth also feels strongly that CAM approaches can vastly ease women's passage through the sometimes harrowing symptoms and side effects of radiation and chemotherapy. "Many patients tell us they couldn't have gotten through treatment without access to complementary care," she says. "Sometimes we will do reflexology or use some mind/body relaxation technique during chemotherapy itself."

Dr. Cassileth explains that a hallmark of complementary therapies is that "they are not diagnosis-specific; they are good under many different circumstances." In standard medical practice, a particular ailment calls for a particular medication. But in CAM approaches, the same approach might benefit many different people with a wide variety of complaints. Consequently, Dr. Cassileth encourages women with breast cancer to explore their options and find the form of CAM that helps them the most. "These therapies are all helpful," she says. "It depends what an individual is drawn to. Some love music. Others don't find that helpful and would prefer to do t'ai chi." Whichever technique you choose, Dr. Cassileth says, you are likely to be struck by its powerful and

Questions to Ask a CAM Practitioner

- What exactly does this treatment involve?

- Are there are known side effects or dangers?

- What is the rate of success with this treatment?

- What factors—such as age, general health, or type of cancer—affect the rate of success?

- Have any scientific studies been done on this type of treatment?

- Can you refer me to anyone you've helped who might be willing to talk about her experience?

- Do you work in partnership with medical doctors? Can I talk to them?

- How would you integrate your treatment with the medical regime I'm currently following?

- •Do you know of any interactions between your treatment and my current medical regime? Are there any scientific studies about how the two types of treatment interact?

- How will I know if your treatment is working? How will I know if it's not working? How long before I can see signs of success? How long before we achieve "total" success?

- How do you define success for this treatment?

- What is required from me for this treatment to be as successful as possible?

lasting results. "We do follow-up calls," she says, "and we know that the benefits endure for at least 48 hours. That's pretty impressive."

Mary A. Tagliaferri agrees that an integrated approach to medicine can often benefit women in profound ways. Tagliaferri was a licensed acupuncturist whose own diagnosis with breast cancer at age 30 prompted her to go to medical school and obtain an M.D. to supplement her knowledge of Chinese medicine. With Isaac Cohen, L.Ac. (licensed acupuncturist) and O.M.D. (Doctor of Oriental Medicine), and Dr. Tripathy, she founded the Breast Cancer Center Complementary and Alternative Medicine Program (BCC-CAMP) at the University of California–San Francisco, in order to conduct clinical trials of herbs used in Asian medicine. Her work at BCC-CAMP exemplifies the notion of integrative treatment, which she defines as "combining many forms of medicine to achieve the best possible outcome for women going through breast cancer."

Tagliaferri sees integrative medicine as a way to "optimize treatment by utilizing more than just Western medicine," because, she says, "There are several unmet needs in Western medicine." Tagliaferri contends that an integrative approach using herbs and acupuncture can boost red and white blood cell counts, support the immune system, and help women resist infection. After all, she points out, "If you get an infection and are too weak to go on to the next cycle of chemotherapy, then you've delayed treatment." A complementary approach to treatment, on the other hand, can enable women to benefit from the best in both Western and Asian medical approaches.

Finding Meaning in Your Illness

The concept of "meaning" as a cornerstone of healing comes from the work of Viktor Frankl, author of *Man's Search for Meaning*. Frankl was a Jewish psychoanalyst imprisoned in Auschwitz during World War II. As he observed both his own and others' efforts to survive under horrific conditions, he discovered that an inner sense of meaning was far more important than physical strength. Some prisoners found their sense of meaning in religion, believing that they were somehow part of God's plan. Some found meaning in their political ideals, while others drew on relationships with fellow prisoners. In a similar vein, the writer Elie Wiesel, also imprisoned in a camp, felt that he survived by taking care of his father.

Clearly, the prisoners observed by Frankl and Wiesel had very little control over their circumstances—and, indeed, many died or were killed. But those who were able to find meaning in their experience were more likely to survive and, in Frankl's observation, were also better able to face death "with a smile on their lips and a prayer in their hearts."[3]

Roberta Levy-Schwartz, Diagnosed at Age 27

I never bothered to ask the question, "Why me?" The question was more, "Why not me?" Why breast cancer? What does this mean? I still don't understand it.

My friends view the world as if they're going to live until they're 80 or 90. And I'm jealous that they don't have to think about the things that I do. I want to live that carefree life, and I don't have that any more.

On the other hand, I enjoy things more than they do. Every year when the flowers bloom, I get all excited. And every year when there's the first snowfall, I've got to go out and play, and I've got to enjoy it, because who knows? Who knows what's going to happen? For them, they just go, "Oh, it's cold today." We look at things differently.

After cancer, you feel everything. Everything is intensified. You almost go back to that childlike state where you're more honest about everything. Everything's more vivid.

I'm proud because I took an experience that could have been negative, and I've made it one of the most positive things in my life.

Frankl's insights are echoed in the work of Lawrence LeShan, Ph.D., a researcher and clinical therapist and the author of *You Can Fight for Your Life* and *Cancer as a Turning Point*. In working with thousands of people with cancer, LeShan found that those who did best were those who could find what he called "their own unique song," using cancer as a turning point or as a source of meaning. It seems to matter little whether you view that meaning as something that is somehow intended for you in the experience or as something that you make yourself by the power of your choice and your response. Whether you find it or make it, seeing meaning in your illness (or in any of life's hardships) can prove to be a powerful therapy.

A Spiritual Response

For many young women with breast cancer, spirituality becomes a crucial part of their response to the illness. In some cases, the spiritual response comes through the expression of a particular religion or an explicit belief in God. In other cases, the spirituality is more personally defined: the sense of being connected to the universe or a feeling for what matters most in life.

For most of human history, spirituality has been an integral part of the healing process, with shamans, priests, and medicine men/women serving as both spiritual leaders and community healers. Now, science is returning to a study of faith and spirituality, with many new studies revealing a close connection between spirituality and healing. For example, an analysis of 42 published studies on death and dying, involving some 126,000 participants, revealed that people who reported frequent religious involvement were significantly more likely to live longer than people who were less involved.[4] Whether the religion itself was the healing force, or whether the healing came from being involved in a supportive community and engaged in a meaningful exploration of life's big questions, it seems clear that some kind of spiritual involvement promotes longer life and greater health. Likewise, in a study of 1600 cancer patients, many patients reported that spiritual well-being was as important to their quality of life as physical well-being. And among patients who experienced significant fatigue, pain, and other debilitating symptoms, those who reported higher degrees of spiritual well-being also enjoyed a significantly higher quality of life.[5]

A particularly intriguing study published in the *British Medical Journal* noted that both prayer (in this case the Hail Mary said 150 times during the rosary) and the recitation of a mantra (a combination of syllables used in Buddhist and Hindu meditation) could improve heart health by slowing breathing to a level where it was optimally synchronized with heart rhythms.[6] Dr. Luciano Bernardi, associate professor at the University of Pavia in Italy and lead author of the study, found that reciting a repeated prayer could help slow breathing to six breaths per minute, which leads to improved blood oxygen levels and perhaps better mobilization of the heart muscles.

While Bernardi's study involved only 23 patients, it is part of a growing body of research on the health benefits of meditation and prayer, including work done by Herbert Benson, M.D., president of the Mind/Body Medical Institute and chief of the Division of Behavioral Medicine at Beth Israel Deaconess Medical Center in Boston. Benson points out that prayer and meditation can induce a "relaxation response" marked by slower breathing, lower metabolism, reduced blood pressure, and lower heart rate. Slower brain waves are also associated with this response, which can be induced by many different kinds of repetition, including words, sounds, or moving a particular muscle. Benson has further noted that the "relaxation response" is deepened when the word or movement has some deep personal significance to the individual, such as during prayer.

In response to such studies, and with the growing interest in CAM approaches, many cancer treatment centers are reintroducing a spiritual

Aquatia Owens, Diagnosed at Age 32

I'm a spiritual person to begin with. My family is Baptist. I'm a Catholic. You go through routines of religion. Following the rules. But when you're down and out, that's what you're going to come back to. Thank God, I had a foundation of knowing God and not having to find Him. And I had the faith to believe I was going to get better. I can't imagine not having that faith. I had people praying for me—priests and reverends. It might sound sappy, but I believe in God, and it makes a big difference in my life.

I read the Bible every day. I like knowing I am not here without God. I don't mean God in the religious "rule" aspect of God—but that I know Someone loves me. My husband comes from a religious family—his brother is a priest—and that helps. His brother never said, "You're going to be okay." He said, "Whatever God's plan is for you, that's what it'll be."

My husband and I pray. I remember when I was in treatment, we were dating, and I remember seeing him pray for me for the first time. It was so powerful. It takes away all the macho man stuff—there he was just asking God to help his girlfriend. He was sitting next to my hospital bed praying, "Help us get through this." I prayed, too. And I wasn't praying for God to help me live—I asked God to give me the strength to get through whatever He had in store for me.

People ask, "How often do you pray?" I don't have formal prayer—but things will happen during the day that will make me prayerful. I talk to God every day about everything that happens good or bad—no matter what. Whatever's going on at work, or with the breast cancer, I'll say, "What am I going to do?"

Sometimes people are afraid to ask God for help. It gives me strength and courage. It brings me peace.

component to the healing process. According to the Rev. Percy W. McCray, Jr., director of pastoral care and social services of the Cancer Treatment Centers of America, "Spirituality is a part of the human being that transcends the basic aspects of what a patient is in the health care environment—it speaks directly to that part of us that cannot be treated by science or medicine." And for young women with breast cancer, spirituality is especially important "because it's a part of your being that can't be extracted."

Although McCray is himself a Christian minister, he sees the spiritual dimension as available to all people, regardless of their religion. "Spirituality is about getting to the center of your very being and feeling a one-ness with the Creator and creation," he says. "When you're dealing with your own mortality, your priorities shift. Forgiveness, reconciliation, clo-sure—these catapult to a primary level of importance. Spirituality be-comes the best place to deal with these questions: What if I'm not here tomorrow? Was I the best mother I could have been? Am I the best daughter or sister I can be? What kind of legacy would I leave? What kind of relationships do I genuinely have? And the only thing that helps to answer these questions is spirituality. It's the only thing that can give you closure."

In McCray's experience, connecting with your own spirituality can help you move to new levels of healing. "It's a magical thing," he says. "When people connect with their spirituality, it helps them move away from the negativity of a situation and fight back emotionally and spiri-tually in a positive way. Relationships are healed, and families are re-united. There is enormous healing that goes on—not necessarily being rid of the disease entirely, but healing that happens on so many different lev-els within yourself and with the other people in your life."

Childhood cancer survivor Susan Nessim offers a similar perspective on healing as an emotional journey rather than as simply being rid of a disease. In her book, *Cancervive,* she writes,

> Cancer has taken us on an amazing journey. When we look in the mirror, we may see our lives as unchanged, but the person they be-long to has undergone a spiritual metamorphosis. We have shed our old skins. Now we must assess who we've become and where we're headed. . . . We've gained new insights into the depths of our spiri-tual strength, physical resiliency and courage. . . . *For those fortu-nate enough to have gained a new perspective, the lessons learned are as precious as life itself.*"[7]

Creativity and Meaning

One way of making meaning is to create something: a poem, a journal, a painting, a sculpture, a song. Giving a shape to your feelings, your ex-periences, and your ideas about life, whether through words, music, or images, creates a kind of meaning of its own. A number of healers ad-vocate creativity as one response to serious illness, including Michael Lerner, Ph.D., president and cofounder of Commonweal, a health and environmental research institute in Bolinas, California. Dr. Cassileth has also instituted creative programs at Sloan-Kettering. She is particularly impressed with the power of music therapy.

Music seems to hit a very primitive part of the brain, and the calming effects that can result are simply amazing. Music reduces heart rate and blood pressure, relaxes muscles, and just generally relieves tension. It has effects on the brain that can be measured with MRI. It raises endorphin levels and relaxes the muscles.

Art therapy can also be a powerful gateway to self-expression. Some art therapists work with sand trays, a large wooden box full of sand that is accompanied by hundreds of little toys and objects. An art therapist may ask you to select some objects and arrange them in the tray. When you feel that your image is complete, you're invited to talk about it. People working with sand trays often discover that they've told a story or created an image that has great significance to them.

Another way of working with imagery is to write down your dreams. People who do dream work often report that the very process of paying attention to their dreams has a profound healing effect. They feel calmer and more in touch with themselves, simply by virtue of acknowledging this part of their inner reality. They also discover that when they write down their dreams, they dream more, and that the dreams are often more elaborate, interesting, and provocative. It's almost as though dreams were one-half of a conversation with your inner self. When you start listening to that self, it responds the way most of us do when we're being listened to and respected: It speaks more often, more clearly, and more profoundly.

If working with imagery and creativity appeals to you, explore the following options:

- *Just begin.* There's no wrong way to be creative or to work with the images that matter to you. Start keeping a journal, writing down your dreams, creating poems, or drawing pictures. Pick up a nice notebook, a watercolor set, a musical instrument, or some modeling clay. Follow your instincts, trusting that your creativity has "a mind of its own" and will lead you wherever you need to go on your healing journey.

- *Take a class.* You don't necessarily have to link this activity with having cancer. There are plenty of adult-education and community-center classes in the arts, as well as dream workshops, journal workshops, and other creative programs offered by various groups.

- *Find a CAM program.* There are some cancer-related programs that offer art therapy, music therapy, or other creative activities. In some cases, you work individually with a therapist, counselor, or specialist. In other cases, you join a support group, which can be good both for your creative production and for overcoming the isolation that sometimes goes with having cancer.

Therapy, Counseling, and Support Groups

Many women find that having breast cancer raises profound questions about their life choices, their relationships, and their identities. Part of their search for meaning involves exploring who they are and what they really want to be doing with their lives. Although therapy, counseling, and support groups do not claim to help you treat your cancer, they can be helpful resources for considering the "big questions," or simply for enduring the difficulties of a life-threatening disease. There are a wide range of therapeutic approaches, some of which are listed here.

- *Psychoanalysis.* Psychoanalysis may be practiced by a psychiatrist (M.D.), a psychologist (Ph.D., M.A., or M.Ed.), or a social worker (M.S.W. or C.S.W.) with training in psychoanalytic therapy. Analysts working in the Freudian tradition (also known as modern analysts) tend to focus on childhood issues, sexuality, and anger; they often view life as a struggle between the need for love and connection and the will to power and control. Jungian analysis works more with archetypal images that express universal human concerns, such as love, death, family, and religion. Other types of analysis may borrow elements from Freud and Jung, or they may draw on different philosophies. Whatever its philosophic basis, an analytic approach generally involves talking with the therapist on a regular basis (once or twice a week) over a period of time, with the goal being to resolve both immediate concerns and long-term issues.

- *Cognitive-behavioral therapy.* This therapeutic approach holds that many of our problems spring from incorrect understandings, or "cognitions." For example, if someone criticizes us, we may think, "If this person is critical of me, he hates me; if he hates me, so does everyone else; if everyone hates me, I'll always be alone and I'll never find anyone to love me." To the extent that this chain of negative thoughts affects our emotions, it can make even a minor criticism seem far more significant than it actually is. A cognitive-behavioral approach works on identifying negative thoughts and replacing them with more realistic perceptions, while also changing behavior patterns that don't work for us. The focus is less on analyzing where these thoughts and behaviors come from and more on helping to overcome them. Generally, cognitive-behavioral therapists treat people for a few weeks or months, rather than the lengthy time period associated with analysis. Like analysis, this type of therapy can be practiced by a psychologist, psychiatrist, or social worker.

Juanita Lyle, Diagnosed at Age 32

When I was diagnosed in the 1970s, it was much harder to talk openly about breast cancer. So, I turned inward. I turned to my faith. My husband really had a hard time dealing with the diagnosis, and treated me like I'd already died and had a funeral. When the cancer came back, he asked me, "How can you believe in God?" I asked the chaplain to counsel us, to help everyone in the family understand that it was okay to be angry with the cancer, but that didn't mean we had to be angry with God. Talking to the chaplain was great therapy for me. I would've loved to talk with other young women, too, but that just wasn't possible then.

I also found a lot of healing from doing visualizations. I would put my hand on the area with pain, and I would visualize light going there. It was a very peaceful feeling. Some people think that it can't work, that you're just fooling yourself. But I can tell you, the mind is a powerful tool.

- *Hypnotherapy.* There are many different schools of hypnotherapy, but all of them are based on working with people in a hypnotic trance, an extremely relaxed state in which a person is generally more receptive, open, and vulnerable than in his or her normal state. Hypnotherapy can be used for short-term goals, like quitting smoking or overcoming anxiety attacks. It can also be part of longer-term therapy, in which the hypnotherapist helps the patient revisit the scene of a traumatic event, often from childhood, and re-experience the emotions that were repressed at the time, bringing new adult strength to bear on an incident that was too much for the child to handle. This approach may also be useful for people who feel out of touch with their emotions, or who are experiencing strong feelings—including panic attacks, ongoing anxiety, or overwhelming grief—that they need help in managing.

- *Treatment with medication.* In the past 2 decades, conditions like depression and anxiety have increasingly been treated with medications, including antidepressants, anti-anxiety medications, tranquilizers, and the like. Only a doctor or a psychiatrist can prescribe medication, but therapists without M.D.s often refer patients to a psychiatrist for medical treatment while other types of therapy are continuing. If you are seeking medication to cope with your responses to cancer, make sure that both your prescribing psychiatrist and all doctors involved in your cancer treatment know about all the medications you are taking, both cancer-related and psychiatric.

- *Treatment with herbal remedies.* St. John's Wort and kava are two herbal remedies that are now frequently used to treat certain forms of anxiety and depression. There are also herbal remedies for insomnia and other conditions. While herbal remedies can be obtained without a prescription, herbalists and medical doctors agree: *Do not treat yourself with herbal remedies!* Find a practitioner you trust, either an herbal specialist or a medical doctor, and take the herbal remedies under his or her supervision. Herbs have a powerful effect on your body (if they didn't, why would you take them?), and you need to approach them with the same respect that you'd give to any other type of medication. Make sure that all your doctors, herbal and medical, know about any herbs you're taking, so that you can be monitored for possible side effects or interactions with your other treatments.

- *Support groups.* Many women with cancer find that being in a support group is extremely helpful. Support groups take many forms, but they are usually short-term groups that meet once a week for a few weeks or months, offering people a space in which to share their experiences and concerns, and to ask for advice on specific issues. Some support groups are relatively unstructured; others choose specific topics for each weekly meeting. Some support groups are self-governing, while others are led by therapists, counselors, or people who have experience with the issue involved. Support groups for breast cancer survivors allow women to talk about dating, relationships, body image,

Joy Simha

Breast cancer puts it all into perspective. I was in therapy for 3 years before being diagnosed with cancer. And during the last 3 weeks in August, when this was really coming to a head, my therapist went away on vacation and was nowhere to be found. And I had to make the decision about the mastectomy all on my own. And that was empowering. After the mastectomy was over and I was home, when I was scheduled to go back in for therapy, I left her a message: "I don't think I need you any more." They say breast cancer cures all other neuroses, and it's true. I'm here to tell you it's true.

Dr. Kathryn Kash, Psycho-Oncologist, Beth Israel Hospital, New York City

The disease is terribly unfair. We don't know why it happens to younger women, and when it does, there's a lot of anger and fear. There's a fear of dying. There's a fear of not moving forward in your life. Sometimes women get really angry. And they have a right to be angry. They didn't bring the cancer on themselves.

Those reactions are real, they don't come in any order, and they don't last for any particular period of time. When a woman is first diagnosed, she usually feels shock and anger: "Why me?" And no one can really answer that question. Women are entitled to feel self-pity and anger, but at some point they need to move on and say, "This is unfair, but what am I going to do about it?"

Sometimes people say that having breast cancer is a good thing, because it makes them think about their lives and where they are going. They see that there are far bigger issues, and they can let the little things slide. When women are faced with a life-threatening disease, being proactive is excellent. They can really make choices and move on.

families, children, and work, as well as to share their fear of cancer, treatments, and death. Many young women report difficulty in finding support groups in which they can talk to other young women with breast cancer, saying that the groups tend to be dominated by women in their fifties and sixties. Although the YSC is not a support group, YSC chapters have sometimes provided the nucleus for support groups that operate independently.

Alternative Forms of Medicine

In addition to the Western medical allopathic tradition, there are a number of other medical traditions available to women in many parts of the United States. Chinese medicine, the Ayurvedic medicine of India, homeopathy, and naturopathy are all self-contained medical systems that operate from different premises and with different techniques from those used by allopathic medicine. Most medical doctors—and many alternative practitioners—agree that these systems are not necessarily a substitute for surgery and/or chemotherapy. Because these systems have been studied so sparingly, even though many have existed for centuries, there are no scientific data comparing their effectiveness with that of surgery and chemo, but there are also no scientific studies saying that they are *not* equally effective. From a purely scientific point of view, while we know the effectiveness rate for allopathic treatments, we simply don't know how well these other systems work.

For that reason, many women choose to have surgery and chemo but to combine that approach with these other traditions. While many medical doctors support this integrated approach, others are indifferent to it, and still others are actively hostile. As always, it is important to work with your doctor to find the integrated approach that is right for you.

Traditional Chinese Medicine

Traditional Chinese medicine has two components: acupuncture and herbs. In the United States, there are a range of people with widely varying levels of training who practice traditional Chinese medicine. Some acupuncturists are not qualified to prescribe herbal treatments or choose not to do so. If you are interested in traditional Chinese medicine, do what you can to find out the qualifications and track record of the practitioner you approach, and bear in mind that, just as Western doctors have varying levels of skill and specialization, so do practitioners of Chinese medicine.

In the Chinese medical view, breast cancer is seen as a result of the lengthy and gradual accumulation of many apparently trivial factors, which together gradually undermine the body's ability to protect itself. Environmental pollution, exposure to harsh climates, infectious diseases, the quality and quantity of food available, diet, water balance and metabolism, mental and emotional attitudes, balance between work and rest, sexual life, and psychological issues may each play a part. In the Chinese view, each woman's breast cancer is unique, representing a particular chain of events and set of interactions; thus, each woman's breast cancer will behave in its own way, with its own prognosis and requirements for treatment.

Isaac Cohen, O.M.D. (Doctor in Oriental Medicine) and L.Ac. (licensed acupuncturist), has pioneered efforts to translate traditional Chinese medicine into scientific terms. In his view, "There is not enough scientific evidence to justify the use of Chinese medicine to replace any of the current Western medical treatments: surgery, radiation, chemotherapy, and hormonal therapy."[8] However, Cohen asserts, "There is no doubt . . . that Chinese medicine is useful in all stages of the disease to augment the benefits of conventional treatments, to prevent recurrence and metastasis in early stages of breast cancer, and to promote health, improve quality of life, and prolong life in advanced stages."[9]

Aquatia Owens

There are some people who don't believe in complementary medicine and some who swear by it. Do those approaches work? Or are they just psychological? They make me feel better mentally, and that translates to physically. I'm going to try anything that helps my energy level go up. If someone said skydiving would make you feel good about yourself, I'd be skydiving. With the strains of work, marriage, and family, everyone needs to do something.

I started acupuncture when I was diagnosed, and I love it. One of the ladies from my support group (who doesn't use any drugs) recommended it. I was going through chemo and had some side effects, but I felt great. Was it because I was doing all these alternative things? It wasn't hurting me.

The acupuncture empowers me because I'm doing something for myself. While I'm there, I'm meditating. Acupuncture puts me in another place and makes me feel like I'm not being passive.

I starting reading up on meditation, and while I'm not sure I'm good at it, I'm having fun with it. Breast cancer has opened so many doors. First I got these tapes, just to relax. Most people don't know how to relax. It allows you to come down from where you are and takes you away from what you're thinking. I'd love to get away from all the anxiety and issues of the day to day. Am I there yet? No, but I'm trying.

That's why a lot of people do yoga. You're trying to get connected to your body. It takes you away. And I need that. Something to see if my body still functions. Even though I wasn't the most limber person, I've always worked out. Now, I'm learning to do things I probably wouldn't have done before. I'm using my brain and my body, and I have the strength to do these things. I walk out feeling like, "I'm alive." When you're going through chemo, you think, "I won't be able to rollerblade again." Now, it's like, "Hey, let's do this."

Acupuncture is based on the Chinese medical theory that *qi* (pronounced "chee"; energy or the life force) circulates through the body within the blood and through a network of channels known as meridians. Therefore, a needle inserted, say, between the thumb and the index finger is tapping into the large intestine meridian and may help cure a headache. Both scientific evidence and clinical trials have affirmed that acupuncture does indeed produce particular physiological responses, including pain control, changes in hormonal activity, and stimulation of the bone marrow to produce more blood cells.[10] Moreover, acupuncture seems to affect the central nervous system, and thus a person's entire body and sense of well-being, by stimulating production of neurotransmitters, chemicals involved in many mental and emotional functions.

A skilled acupuncturist will usually diagnose a patient by listening to the pulse, looking closely at the tongue, and observing other signs that reveal the body's condition, level of energy, and state of balance (or imbalance). He or she will then insert several needles at various points and leave them there for 30 to 45 minutes. The needles are about the thickness of a piece of thread. While they sometimes cause discomfort upon entry, it is at most very minor discomfort, and they are supposed to cause no discomfort at all once they are inserted (if the acupuncturist you go to causes you ongoing discomfort, you might consider switching practitioners). Most people experience profound relaxation during the treatment, often falling asleep or "spacing out." At the end of the treatment, the acupuncturist removes the needles, reexamines your body's signs, and suggests a time to return for the next treatment. He or she may also prescribe herbal treatments. Some acupuncturists sell their own herbs; others will send you to an herbal pharmacy with a prescription.

According to Cohen, Chinese herbal medicine works well to complement Western therapy by

- Reducing such side effects as nausea, vomiting, fatigue, insomnia, and pain
- Reducing potential toxicities resulting from the chemo, such as bone marrow inhibition, immune suppression, cardiac toxicity, and hepatotoxicity (toxic liver)
- Enhancing the effectiveness of the chemotherapy by lowering drug resistance and increasing the body's blood flow
- Supporting the immune system by preventing immune suppression and protecting the organs and glands that produce immune cells[11]

Unfortunately, at least in Cohen's view, Chinese medicine is unlikely to help prevent hair loss. However, he believes that its ability to combat numerous side effects of surgery, chemo, and/or radiation therapy makes it an ideal supplement to Western medical treatment.

Ayurveda

Ayurvedic medicine is an ancient system founded in India that focuses on the harmony among mind, body, and nature. Like other systems of Asian medicine, it incorporates diet, exercise, meditation, and herbal

---

Cindy Kim, Diagnosed at Age 28

When I was diagnosed, everyone was devastated. I contemplated not going through chemo. My father said, "Take advantage of both Eastern and Western medicine." Which I did—against all the doctors' advice. The first 3 months I was given herbal chemotherapy, to make sure the cancer was contained. And I took different types of roots. My father formed an herbal cocktail according to my body type. The goal was to get my immune system stronger. That's the whole point of Eastern medicine: it's to build up your immune system.

I used Chinese medicine to detox. I was doing chemo every other Friday. I'd let the chemo do its thing for 5 days. Then I'd start on herbal tonics for 4 days. Then I'd rest. The herbal tonic detoxed my liver. It helped me have a healthy system, so I wouldn't be affected as negatively by the chemo.

---

remedies. Ayurvedic treatments may also involve intestinal cleansing, yoga, massage, breathing exercises, and visualization.

Although Chinese medicine has been vastly more popular in the United States in the past few decades, interest in Ayurveda is growing. A 1994 report by a National Institutes of Health panel cited a study showing that 79 percent of patients with various chronic diseases had improved health after Ayurvedic treatment. [12] Some laboratory and clinical studies suggest that Ayurvedic herbal treatments may be useful in the treatment of breast, lung, and colon cancers, although randomized clinical trials have yet to be carried out. Meanwhile, however, the National Cancer Institute has added several Ayurvedic herbal compounds to its list of potential anticancer agents.

Ayurvedic medicine is based on the notion that there are three *doshas*, or basic metabolic types: a heavy, calm type, known as *Kapha*; a medium-sized, ruddy, fair-haired type, known as *Pitta*; and a slender, nervous, energetic type, known as *Vata*. Each person is affected by all three *doshas*, but is generally categorized by a single predominant one, which indicates the person's physical, metabolic, and emotional type, as well as his or her habits. If a person is unhealthy, his or her *doshas* need to be brought back into balance.

An Ayurvedic practitioner will inspect a patient's tongue, nails, lips, eyes, ears, nostrils, mouth, genitalia, and anus; examine his or her secretions; and listen to the lungs, pulse, and various parts of the body. The practitioner will also take a detailed life history of the patient, asking about the past, present, and intended future. He or she will then rec-ommend a course of action designed to rebalance the *doshas*. Many pa-tients describe their experience with Ayurveda—including meditation, yoga, and breathing exercises—as bringing about a sense of serenity and well-being.

Like Chinese doctors, Ayurvedic practitioners in the United States can have vastly different levels of training, experience, and skill, so use some care in choosing a healer from this tradition. The American Cancer Society warns against certain Ayurvedic practices, such as bloodletting and inducing vomiting, which can be potentially debilitating for people with cancer. And, as with all treatments involving herbal preparations, patients should watch out for possible interactions with conventional medications.[13] However, as with Chinese medicine, there seem to be many indications that Ayurveda may be a useful supplement to Western treatments, especially to combat the symptoms of chemo and radiation therapy.

Homeopathy

Homeopathy works on the principle that "like cures like." In this tradi-tion, you are exposed to minute quantities of a particular substance that is causing you trouble, so that your body will be stimulated to marshal its own ability to overcome that illness. Unlike acupuncture, which has found quite a bit of support in the medical community, at least as a sup-plement to standard treatment, homeopathy is still viewed with enor-mous skepticism by most doctors and scientists. Nor is homeopathy supported by a growing body of scientific studies, as acupuncture and some other alternatives are. Nevertheless, many individuals swear by ho-meopathy and believe that they have been helped by it.

Naturopathy

Naturopathic medicine works to prevent and treat disease by support-ing the body's own healing ability. It relies on natural medicines and on people taking personal responsibility for their own health. It draws on a wide variety of natural therapies, including herbs, nutrition, hydro-therapy (treatment with water), homeopathy, yoga, movement, and psy-chological counseling, in an effort to achieve optimal, total health.

As with homeopathy, there is little enthusiasm for this approach among doctors and scientists, and there is little scientific evidence to sup-port it. However, many individuals report great success with it, particu-larly in overcoming some of the more distressing symptoms of chemotherapy and radiation.

Laurie Goldstein, M.D., Obstetrician/Gynecologist, Diagnosed at Age 39

I think when you first hear a diagnosis of cancer, particularly breast cancer, you think immediately, "I'm going to die," and you start making deals with the devil to just get to your next birthday. I was 39—I was just approaching my fortieth birthday—and I promised myself that I'd never complain about my birthday again. But after a while, you start to realize, "I'm not going to die." And if you're not going to die, what are you going to do with the rest of your life? You're entitled to have a life even if you've been diagnosed with breast cancer. And so you go on and you need to contemplate what's next.

Nutritional and Herbal Approaches

Like other CAM approaches, dietary and herbal treatments have been supported by a wealth of anecdotal evidence but virtually no scientific studies. And as with many other approaches, this is largely because few scientific studies have been conducted. It's fairer to say that the results are not yet in than to claim that the benefits attributed to these approaches have been disproved.

If you are considering a nutritional approach, you should keep in mind that different people have vastly different nutritional needs. While some people may benefit from a macrobiotic approach, a diet rich in complex carbohydrates, or a low-fat diet, other people may find that these approaches are not only not beneficial but are actively harmful. Even a woman who needs to lower her intake of certain types of fats may at the same time be suffering from a shortage of essential fatty acids, and a woman whose best friend flourished on a vegetarian diet might find that she herself needs a daily intake of red meat, at least for awhile. Nutritional approaches can be dramatically effective in boosting energy and supporting the immune system, but the approach you use has to be right for you and your own unique biochemistry. Moreover, cancer, surgery, and chemo/radiation, along with the lifestyle and emotional changes that your illness has caused, may have changed your biochemistry significantly, requiring new dietary choices on your part.

Herbal remedies must also be treated with the same respect you'd give any powerful prescription medication. Just because a remedy is "natural" doesn't mean that it can't have negative effects, either by itself or in combination with other herbs, dietary supplements, or medications.

So if a nutritional or herbal approach appeals to you, be sure to work closely with a dietitian, nutritionist, herbalist, or other qualified, experienced practitioner—and be sure to keep your doctor up to date on what you're doing.

Macrobiotics

The word *macrobiotic* has been used in many contexts, but today it primarily refers to the work of Japanese philosopher George Ohsawa and his student Michio Kushi. Kushi wrote several books explaining both the philosophical basis for the macrobiotic diet and its potential for creating health and overcoming disease. The standard macrobiotic diet emphasizes whole plant foods. High in complex carbohydrates and low in fat, it calls for organically grown foods whenever possible. Over the course of a week, the person on a macrobiotic diet will eat

- 50 to 60 percent whole cereal grains
- 25 to 30 percent vegetables, preferably organically grown
- 5 to 10 percent soups—about two bowls a day—ideally made from sea vegetables
- 5 to 10 percent beans[14]

Macrobiotic eaters who are concerned about cancer are also advised to avoid aluminum pots and microwaves and to walk outside at least half an hour a day.

Much of this diet is echoed in less stringent recommendations by the American Cancer Society and the American Institute of Cancer Research/World Cancer Research Fund, which emphasize plant foods over animal foods. More dietary research on low-fat and high-fiber diets is currently being conducted in a number of places.

It's useful to note that many nutritionists and other healers believe that this diet is ideal for some people but harmful for others, while many others believe that the diet is generally useful but needs to be modified in many individual cases. Because of the recent popularity of low-fat diets, a macrobiotic approach—either pure or modified—may appeal to many women and may indeed be helpful to many. Women should remember, however, that their bodies need omega-3 fatty acids (found in fatty fish and flaxseed oil), along with some other essential fats. Women also need calcium in their diets, so a woman who cuts out dairy products should be sure to consume lots of dark green leafy vegetables and seaweed. Again, if you are considering "going macrobiotic," work with a qualified nutritionist who can help to ensure that all your dietary needs are being met.

Soy

A lot of recent attention has gone to the role of soy in preventing women's hormonal problems and in preventing or treating breast cancer. Researchers first caught on to the relationship between soy and breast cancer when they realized that Asian women have a far lower incidence of breast cancer than most U.S. women—and they also eat far more soy.

Whole soy foods are rich in nutrients called isoflavones, which are also found in garbanzos, black beans, and other legumes. These isoflavones seem to be the key ingredient in soy's relationship to cancer. Indeed, some studies have shown that soy consumption or the ingestion of isoflavones in other forms can lower estradiol levels in women by 20 percent or more. (Estradiol is a form of estrogen.) In theory, the lower estrogen levels can help reduce the risk of breast cancer. More research is being done all the time on this issue, and new findings may have made their way into the public eye by the time this book appears. However, one of the most persuasive studies that have been done is a meta-analysis of nine different studies conducted by Dr. Bruce Trock and his colleagues at Georgetown University, including five studies completed in Asia, one study of women of Asian ancestry living in the United States, and two studies of nonAsian U.S. women. Trock and workers found that there did indeed seem to be a correlation between a high soy intake and a decreased risk of breast cancer.[15] Further analysis of the data, however, showed that the beneficial effects of soy intake on breast cancer risk were limited to premenopausal women.

However, says Tagliaferri, who used soy as part of her own anticancer diet after she was diagnosed, Trock's data leave some key questions unanswered: Does it help to start taking soy later in life? And if you do start, is it dangerous?

"No one knows these answers," Tagliaferri explains. "When you look at Asian women, they've been eating soy since they were very young, and that affects the way the breast tissue is laid down during puberty." Still, Tagliaferri is excited about the potential for soy to help women with breast cancer, and she believes that eating a moderate amount of traditional Asian foods containing soy helped her combat her own cancer.

Two other recent studies seem to support the notion that higher levels of soy isoflavones in the body—a result of eating whole soy foods—lead to a lower risk of breast cancer.[16] These findings—all involving studies done on humans—are further supported by animal studies and laboratory studies. For example, in January 2000, U.S. researchers announced the results of a U.S. Department of Agriculture study showing that rats were less likely to develop mammary tumors when fed a soy protein diet.[17] And a 1998 study found that soy isoflavones seem to be able to block the proliferation of breast cancer cells caused by environmental estrogens.[18]

Soy and Female Hormones

Why do isoflavones seem to have such a powerful impact on breast cancer risk? The answer lies in their relationship to female hormones. Isoflavones convert to a weak form of estrogen inside our digestive tracts. Under some circumstances, particularly when the body's estrogen levels are already high, isoflavones bind with the body's estrogen receptors—the chemical compounds that hold on to estrogen. The remaining unbound estrogen in the bloodstream can then be cleansed from the bloodstream by the liver and eliminated through the urine. Thus, isoflavones act to reduce excess estrogen among women who have not yet reached menopause—women whose estrogen levels tend to be high. As we saw in Chapter 4, lower estrogen levels in young women—what scientists refer to as "decreased lifetime exposure to estrogen"—may help prevent breast cancer.

But there's a catch. Since isoflavones are actually a form of estrogen, however weak, they can also boost the body's estrogen levels rather than reducing them. This is particularly true in postmenopausal women and in other women whose estrogen levels are low. Paradoxically, isoflavones seem to boost estrogen levels when they're low and lower them when they're high.

That would be fine, if it weren't for the other catch. In test-tube and animal studies, isoflavones have been shown both to retard the growth of breast cancer cells—and to increase it. Scientists don't yet understand the reasons for these contradictory results. Moreover, some animal studies have suggested that soy and other isoflavones might encourage estrogen-dependent tumors to grow.

Tagliaferri stresses that the effects of soy are extremely paradoxical. Estrogen levels in the body are determined by a number of different factors, and the ways that soy interacts with the body's estrogen levels are highly complex. Researchers are learning more all the time about how estrogen acts within a woman's body and how soy and other factors can affect estrogen's behavior.

Certainly, many women with estrogen-receptor tumors are extremely skeptical about soy and other legumes, actively avoiding these foods for fear that the isoflavones that benefit other women will cause their tumors to grow. Most doctors likewise advise caution about soy for young women with breast cancer, especially for women with estrogen-receptor tumors.

Yet Tagliaferri continues to believe that soy is "good medicine" for young women with breast cancer. Based on her study of the available medical and nutritional evidence, Tagliaferri recommends that U.S. women—with or without breast cancer—should consume the FDA recommendation of four servings of at least 6.25 grams of soy protein per day, or 25 grams total per day. This, she says, is the rough equivalent of the daily amount of soy that Japanese women have consumed for centuries, and Japanese women have only one-sixth the breast cancer rate of U.S. women and are one-third as likely to die of the disease. She stresses that these four servings should be consumed in the form of traditional Asian foods—tofu, tempeh, edamame (green soybeans), miso, and perhaps also soy milk—and that women should definitely avoid isolated soy protein powders. Likewise, soy products— soy franks, soy ice cream, soy bars, and other foods containing isolated soy proteins— are problematic: They contain nonsoy ingredients, they have fewer isoflavones, and some nutritionists believe they can create food sensitivities and digestive problems for women.

"Women need to consume soy in a way that their dosages aren't more than they would be in traditional Asian practice," Tagliaferri explains. "But often people are looking for a magic bullet, and will take larger quantities of soy than were ever used traditionally. People tend to say, soy is good. I'm just going to, say, eat soy. Yes, soy is good, but it's just one of the many things we can do. And soy was never supposed to be taken as a protein powder, where everything is taken out of the soy. There may be some other part of the tofu or soy product that is beneficial."

Tagliaferri is also frank about the possible limits to soy's effectiveness. "We don't know if you need to begin eating soy at a young age—if that's the only way for it to have a protective effect," she explains. "It's unclear at what age you need to begin eating soy to have that protection."

If you are intrigued by Tagliaferri's approach, you can find out more in *Breast Cancer: Beyond Convention*, an anthology of CAM approaches written by leading doctors and researchers. And if you yourself are interested in using soy as a nutritional response to your breast cancer, *be sure to check with your doctor first,* particularly if you have an estrogen-recepor tumor.

Nutrients and Supplements

As Dr. Tripathy has noted, many patients (as well as some nutritionists) have faith in micronutrients and nutritional supplements as a way of treating cancer symptoms and the unpleasant side effects of chemo and radiation therapy, as well as boosting general health. Because this field is so complicated and so controversial, your best bet is to find a qualified nutritionist who can help you make the specific choices that are right for your body and your condition. Many people make the mistake of self-medicating with vitamins and other supplements, casually following the advice of a friend or suggestions made in a news story. But if you believe in the power of nutrition, you should give it the respect it deserves, realizing that nutritional supplements can have profound effects on you and can sometimes have disturbing interactions with your medical treatment. Just as you wouldn't give yourself chemotherapy without a physician's guidance, you should *avoid being your own nutritional specialist.* If this approach interests you, find a qualified practitioner you trust to guide you through it.

Mind/Body Approaches

As Dr. Cassileth pointed out, mind/body approaches have proved to be enormously helpful in relieving the side effects of cancer treatment, as well as in helping women achieve a sense of control over their health. Meditation, yoga, Qigong (a Chinese form of exercise), and t'ai chi all focus on achieving physical relaxation and flexibility, mental clarity, and a total focus on the "now." Each of these activities is suitable for someone who is recuperating from cancer treatment, and you can progress to more vigorous forms of yoga, Qigong, and t'ai chi as you regain your strength.

For many young women, the traditional female pastime of knitting has actually become "the new yoga." In New York City, Los Angeles, and other metropolitan centers, young women gather in daily or weekly "knitting circles," knitting and chatting over their lunch hour in an effort to find relief from the stress of the workday. According to Bernadette Murphy, author of *Zen and the Art of Knitting,*[19] knitting helps lower the heart rate and blood pressure, creating the classic relaxation response described by Harvard University professor Dr. Herbert Benson, founding president of the Mind/Body Institute. Indeed, Murphy says, Benson himself has referred to knitting as one of the recognized forms of meditation and a good way to induce relaxation.

"Knitting, and its meditative power, has the ability to center you," says Murphy, who took up knitting when she became injured and couldn't walk. "It was one of the few things I could do that would let me sit still enough to heal," she recalls. But the knitting itself, she now believes, helped the healing process as well.

"When you're dealing with a physical problem like fighting a disease, your mind starts running with all the what ifs," she explains. "You start to think there's this huge list of things you need to take care of now. I talked to a breast cancer patient while writing my book. She said she started to feel like she had to exert this enormous will to change things. But knitting brings you back into your body and calms you down. You let go of all those other things you think you should be doing. By taking the time to do that, the other things reprioritize themselves. You have a better sense of how to spend the energy you do have."

Aquatia Owens found that knitting helped her calm and center herself in ways that she hadn't expected. "It's relaxing because I'm creating something," she says. "It's repetitive, but not monotonous. It's very calming. You get into somewhat of a meditative state. There's the clicking of the needles, it soothes you." Paradoxically, Aquatia says, while knitting relaxes her, it has also intensified her appreciation of life. "Before, I would look at sweaters and not see their beauty, their intricacy," she says. "Now I walk around stores, and I'm amazed at the small details that I would have completely overlooked before. I definitely have a better sense of the world around me. And breast cancer opened up that world to me."

Visualization

One mind/body approach that many women have found especially effective is visualization, using the power of the mind and the imagination to overcome pain, manage symptoms, and, ultimately, create health. In its most general sense, visualization involves seeing yourself as you want to be. If you're undergoing a painful medical procedure, for example, you might visualize yourself in a peaceful meadow—or you might see yourself exactly where you are, but without pain.

To use visualization for specific situations, like painful procedures, you might experiment with a number of different techniques. Some women find it helpful to picture a safe or magical place and put themselves there. Other women bring imaginary helpers into the treatment room: a favorite animal, a beloved relative, or a religious figure that you can feel nurturing and protecting you. For some women, abstract images work best: seeing themselves as a shaft of light or as a wave serenely breaking on the shore, indifferent to the sharp rocks and vicious sharks.

You can also use visualization for longer-term goals, such as defeating the cancer within your body and regaining a state of glowing health. Formerly, advocates of visualization suggested that women imagine themselves fighting and subduing the cancer, using such images as a vacuum sucking up the cancer cells or a knight in shining armor slaying them with her sword. Now people who work in this field recommend eliminating all negative imagery from your thoughts entirely and simply seeing yourself as healthy and strong. Again, you might create literal images (you as you used to be, moving happily through your day), or you might come up with symbols (you as a bird soaring over a field). The images that you create express your deepest understanding of yourself and the world, so any positive, meaningful personal image that works for you can be helpful.

Affirmations

As Juanita Lyle found, affirmations can also be a powerful way to draw upon your own strength and overcome pain. Affirmations are short, positive statements about yourself, always said in the present tense, such as

I am healthy and safe in the world.

Every day, I grow toward health.

I love my body, and my body loves me.

You can repeat affirmations whenever you need to, although people who practice the technique recommend saying a single affirmation at least three or four times, either aloud, in a whisper or as a mental statement. It's important to avoid negative affirmations—do not say, "I am no longer sick," but rather say, "I am supremely healthy." The theory is that by affirming this particular idea you will make it true. Certainly, Juanita found that by affirming her belief in her own ability to transcend the pain of her treatment, she created a situation in which she actually felt less pain.

Designing Your Own Approach

As you can see, the beauty of CAM approaches is that they are so flexible and adaptable. Only you can decide which approach will work for you, and you are the best person to design your treatment.

Precisely because there are no predetermined answers, developing your own approach may take awhile. You may need to experiment a bit, following your instincts to see where they lead you. You may want to start small, beginning with one new activity or treatment, rather than either trying to do everything at once or feeling so overwhelmed that you don't do anything. Find a way to start at a place that is comfortable for you, and work from there.

The good news, according to Dr. Barrie Cassileth, is that you can expect your CAM approach to grow in effectiveness as your treatment continues. "Complementary techniques can help women go through the initial diagnosis and treatment in a fair degree of comfort," she says. "And that, in turn, enables you to feel better as time goes on. Whichever approach you choose, it's a tool that you can carry with you wherever you wish."

CHAPTER 6

"I See the Pain in Their Eyes"

Getting Support from Family, Friends, and Community

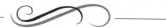

Lisa Muccilo was only 27 when she was diagnosed with breast cancer, but her family was well aware of the disease: Lisa's mother had also been diagnosed with breast cancer and had had a mastectomy at age 48, just a few years before Lisa's condition was discovered. Lisa's mother's cancer, however, was caught at stage 0, whereas Lisa's cancer had metastasized and has since recurred five times. "I always feel like, 'Oh, God, how could I do this to my family?'" Lisa says. "And that feels really sad, because I don't want to be a burden to anybody. I don't even want them to worry about it. That bothers me, that they have to deal with it all the time, too. That's the worst part of it for me. I don't want them to worry or be upset, because I think it's all because of me, my fault. It's tough."

"You think maybe down the road you'll have to deal with something," says Mark Douglas. But Mark and Kelly never expected to be facing a life-threatening illness only 2 years into their marriage. "In some ways it's kind of good," says Kelly, who was diagnosed with breast cancer at the age of 24. "It sounds weird to say that, but you always hear that something that's distressing or a hard event in people's lives either draws them closer or pushes them apart. I think this has been one of those points for us. It just happened a lot earlier in our marriage than most people have to deal with."

Roberta Levy-Schwartz says that one of the hardest parts of having had a mastectomy was the sense of being "one big cancer gene, and it's written all over your T-shirt, all over your forehead. You feel like you're

139

broadcasting it." But, she says, "With your really good friends, most of them don't let that stop you. Even if you feel that way, they say, 'Get over it, let's go out, let's do things.'" Roberta, diagnosed at age 27, met the love of her life, the man she eventually married, while she was recovering from breast cancer. But, she says, it was really her friends who enabled her to survive the experience.

Getting Support: Another Part of the Challenge

Young women who have survived breast cancer agree: Getting support from family and friends is a crucial part of making it through. Knowing that some combination of parents, siblings, friends, partner, and in-laws is there for you is an essential part of the journey through diagnosis, treatment, and recovery.

But getting support can be a challenging process in itself. Even couples who have been married for 20 years have difficulty coping with a life-threatening illness. Think how much greater the challenge will be for a new marriage. Our twenties and thirties are often a time when we are moving away from our families of origin, so having to lean heavily on Mom, Dad, and siblings can seem like a loss of hard-won independence. Building friendships is like building a marriage—it takes time to develop trust and communication, that precarious balance between healthy boundaries and happy intimacy. But under the pressure of a breast cancer diagnosis, young women have to find ways of working through these issues far more quickly, with far higher stakes.

This chapter will introduce you to some of the hardships you may face and help you get support from family, friends, and loved ones—which can bring a whole set of additional challenges at a time when you're already facing an enormous one. The good news is that as you meet these

---

Lee Schwartz, Husband of Roberta Levy-Schwartz

Roberta has this amazing network of friends. I think it's self-selecting. I think the people who are attracted to Roberta are people who are attracted to someone who is very capable and very positive. They often have a similar personality

Cancer weeded out a lot of her friends. The friends who were not strong and positive were the ones who didn't contact her. And that's an experience that very few of us ever go through—finding out, as the saying goes, who your friends really are.

new challenges, you get to find out what an incredible support network you have—or you have the chance to build one. Many young women report that surviving breast cancer has led them to relate to friends, family, and community in a whole new way, with a vulnerability and an openness that has actually enriched their lives.

Support for Medical Procedures

One of the most useful times to draw on your support network is during the period of diagnosis and decision making. Having a friend or family member accompany you to appointments with your doctor means that he or she can help you to do several things:

- *Ask questions.* Talking to a doctor about your breast cancer diagnosis and treatment can be an upsetting experience. It can be hard to remember all the questions you want to ask or to stay focused on the doctor's explanation long enough to ask follow-up questions. Of course, it helps to go into these meetings with a list of questions in hand. But a friend or relative can be an excellent backup.

- *Remember.* Lots of women like to have their backup person take notes while they themselves simply listen. (Some women also bring a tape recorder.) Afterward, it can be helpful to discuss the interview with someone else who was actually there. If you need to vent about the doctor's attitude or behavior, you'll have someone who knows exactly what you mean. And if you need help figuring out how all the nuances went (what the doctor seemed to be recommending, how optimistic he or she was about a particular course of treatment), a support person can help you talk it through.

- *Advocate for yourself.* If you feel that the doctor isn't listening to you or isn't taking your wishes into account, a friend or family member can help you stand up for yourself, or even speak directly to the doctor on your behalf. In the wake of a breast cancer diagnosis, dealing with doctors can be an overwhelming experience. Even if you never need to use your backup, it can be nice to know that it's there.

- *Cope.* Visits to the doctor can be emotional experiences under the best of circumstances. Having someone accompany you means that you don't have to be alone afterward: Someone is there to comfort and support you. You may not need that type of emotional support, or you might prefer to be alone. But you may not know ahead of time what you're going to need, so bringing someone with you at least gives you the option of companionship.

Joy Simha

After my biopsy, I went to my parents' house on Long Island to recover. I'll never forget the night before I got the diagnosis. I was in total fright mode.

My sister went out and rented videos for us to watch. I don't remember what. I think comedies. I didn't pay attention to it. The TV was on, and I was awake, but I didn't pay attention. No one was sleeping. The next day, my mom and I traveled to the doctor together. It was comforting having her there, but I wasn't thinking about that. I was worried about troubling her. I would look into her face and see a very worried person. I was worried that I was aging my mother, making it more difficult for her. It was a huge responsibility—that all this heartache was because of my sickness. I wished I could have done it alone, but I'm glad someone else was there.

In hindsight, if I had known the doctor was going to give the diagnosis, I would've brought a third person who wouldn't have been as upset as we both were, and who could've taken notes.

We left the office, my mother and I, and walked through Central Park, heading downtown, toward my house. My mother was really confused and talking a lot, trying to cover the silence, peppering me with questions. I said, "Mom, I need you with me, but I need you to be quiet." She thanked me for being honest. We held hands, and walked the rest of the way in silence.

Although she was married when she was diagnosed with breast cancer, Lisa Muccilo chose to have her mother come with her, first to her initial mammogram after she'd felt a lump, and then to her subsequent visits. "We were upset," she recalls. "We were crying. I didn't want to go back to work. I didn't want to go home. I went to my grandmother's. We started calling everyone. I just remember hearing, 'Don't worry about this, you're gonna be fine.' All these phone calls were happening. It was like rallying the troops. It was very emotional. Everyone was just really shocked. My mom has been with me for every appointment. It's great support that's gone a long way in helping me."

Although most young women who bring loved ones to the doctor are glad they did, some find that there are also painful aspects to the experience. Having a friend or family member accompany you may mean coping with their feelings as well as your own. You may have to speak up and tell your support person what you need: silence or speech, to be hugged or to be left alone for a while. For most women, though, the initial company is definitely worth the mixed feelings—even if there comes a time when they need to be alone.

Being Open to Support: Negotiation and Communication

As other young women's experiences reveal, finding and accepting support may be important, but it's not always easy. Roberta found herself turning to friends for support, but then was struck by how different their lives had become:

"I remember having a total meltdown one Fourth of July. We were watching the fireworks with a whole group of friends, and I was quietly sobbing in the back. Because it was like, 'Is this my last Fourth of July?' And from what I knew about the facts, I knew I was going to live. But the idea in my head didn't always match the feeling in my heart. And it's hard to get your mind to overshadow your heart, which doesn't know how to act."

Roberta also found that she lost some friends who couldn't deal with her having breast cancer. "I don't know anybody who hasn't had one or two experiences with having to write off people because those people couldn't handle the illness," she says. "There's one story that I'll never forget: This woman called her friend and said, 'I have breast cancer,' and the friend said, 'Oh, my, what's your husband going to do without you?'"

Susan Kolevsohn also found that her friends' support was something of a mixed bag. Susan was diagnosed at age 22, when she was a senior at the University of Georgia in Athens. "I was surprised by the support I got," she recalls. "A lot of people came out of the woodwork who had no obligation to be there. I was also hurt and disappointed by a couple of my best friends, who kind of ignored it. I called them to tell them, and that was the last time I spoke to a couple of them. Overall, even those who were there for me didn't know what to say. I think it was because we were so young."

One of the hardest parts of being a young woman with breast cancer can be the loneliness. Of course, having breast cancer isn't easy at any age. And friends from any generation might turn away from someone who's sick because of fears about their own mortality. But older women who get breast cancer are more likely to be facing aging and death alongside a cohort of friends who are concerned about the same issues. For a younger woman, being struck with a potentially fatal illness can often seem completely outside the natural order of things.

"I read an article the other day, which I was crying over, about a woman who had just had a child," says Roberta. "She was hoping that she lived until the child was four so that the child would remember her. And that was terrifying for me, that I should even think those things. That I should even think about hoping to live until my child is 4 years old.

"My friends don't think like that—they don't view the world that way. My friends view the world as if they're going to live long, full lives. I have as much chance of getting hit by a car as I do of getting breast cancer again, but I still think about the fact that I might not be here past my child's bat mitzvah or wedding. There's definitely a disconnect with the other people my age. It's like overnight you go from being young to feeling old."

Susan Kolevsohn had a similar sense of being isolated from her friends, who were all graduating from college the spring she was diagnosed. "My biggest fear was that they'd forget about me," she recalls. "Graduation is a transition time—some of them were going on to grad school or getting married. So just the fact that they took the time not to forget me made a huge difference."

In the midst of dealing with the cancer, Susan relied on her friends for a sense of normalcy. "Everything is so serious all the time when you're sick," she says. "It's nice to hear what nail polish is in fashion, or who's dating whom. I don't think my friends even realized all the little things that helped."

Susan is also aware of how hard her illness was on her friends: "They'd apologize for not knowing what to say. They'd send cards and try to relate. But the reality was that they were going to frat parties while I was in chemo. It's such a lonely thing. No matter how many people are around, it's lonely being a young woman with breast cancer."

Susan's surgeon put her in touch with two breast cancer survivors, both older women. "One of them called me," she explains, "but I wasn't ready to talk to anyone. And I definitely wasn't comfortable talking to someone my mom's age about it. It took me well into chemo before I was ready to talk about it at all. So then I asked a lot of my doctors, and none of them had any young women to put me in touch with. I looked on the Internet, and one day, by accident, the Young Survival Coalition came up. That's how I started connecting with young women."

Susan finds it hard to meet new people who don't have breast cancer. "It's just too frustrating to explain yourself all the time," she says. "When I talk about a fear of recurrence, people will try to be rational about why it can't happen. They'll say, 'You can't think that way. You have to be positive.' I *am* positive. My prognosis is very good. But it's frustrating. Sometimes I need to talk about my fears."

Leslie Mouton, Diagnosed at Age 35

I didn't want anyone saying, "Poor Leslie." That would've driven me nuts. That's what was so great about my support system, from work to friends: Everyone just accepted me bald. It wasn't a topic of conversation every time I walked into a room. They treated me like the same person, and that was exactly what I needed. I remember sitting at the table with my best friends at our house two nights before my first chemo treatment. My nickname is Blondie, and they said, "Blondie, I just can't see you bald." Then they saw me bald, and they didn't make an issue of it. My best friend said, "It seems normal. Now Leslie doesn't have hair, big deal."

My family and friends gave me the space I needed, but when I called, they were right there for me. And it was the little things they did that meant so much. Once when my white blood cell count plummeted and I was quarantined in the house, I wanted Popsicles so bad. My friend Ginger knew she couldn't come inside because I was susceptible to any little thing, so she left the Popsicles outside on the front porch. It's something thoughtful like that that made it possible to get through this.

I think it's harder for the spouse. You're going through it; you deal with it every minute of every day. And your spouse can do nothing but sit by and watch. Which for a man is very difficult. Tony just wanted to protect me, to fix the problem. But he couldn't fix it. That was so hard for him. He's a fighter pilot—he's used to going to war and being shot at. Now, here he is, looking at his wife, and there's this war going on inside my body, and he can do nothing to defend me. He had me and my cancer, a full-time job, and a 2-year-old to take care of. There were probably days when he wanted to quit—but he never let me know it.

"Still," says Susan, "It helps not to carry the weight of the world on your shoulders, and to get help from other people. I'm still working on that."

Working Things Out with Your Partner

Married women turn to their spouses for support—and find a variety of responses. Some women learn that they can count on their husbands or life partners absolutely. Others discover that their marriages or partnerships end under the strain of the cancer diagnosis. Still others find that their relationships are transformed, with issues that had been buried before rising insistently to the surface. These transformations can cause a relationship to dissolve—or help it to reform on a whole new basis.

When 32-year-old Lanita Hausman heard her diagnosis, she was far from her husband and her home. In a hotel room on a business trip, she got the news by phone. "I called Tom at work, and I dropped this bombshell on him," she recalls. "An amazing thing happened. Mountains started to move." Somehow, Lanita arranged to switch her flight, check out of the hotel room, call the car service, and contact her parents. "All through this, I would call Tom," she explains. She used the hotel phone for her business calls, while staying in touch with Tom through her cell phone.

"Tom was there for every painful, scary moment. He may not have had a road map of scars across his chest, but he carried them hidden deep inside where no one sees. Tom survived this ordeal just as much as I did. If people call me courageous and inspirational, so was Tom. Our motto was, 'We'll get through this with humor and hard liquor.' We even created our David Letterman–style list of the top 10 reasons for having breast implants. Number one? How else can you carry around the price of a BMW on your chest?"

Kelly Douglas also vividly remembers calling her husband, Mark, to give him the news. "The phone call I made to Mark was the most difficult," she says. "It's just so hard to tell your spouse you have cancer. I think it's hard to tell your spouse you have any serious disease or sickness. And I really felt bad. It's not what you want for your spouse. When you marry someone, you want them to have this wonderful life. You want to be bringing something to their life, you don't want to be taking something out of it."

For Mark and Kelly, the cancer meant facing the possibility that they might not be able to have children—a possibility that few couples have to face when the wife is only 24. "I think you start bargaining," Mark says. "Because Kelly said, 'I don't care about losing my breast or my hair, but having kids is important to me.' Well, it's important to me, too. But what it boils down to is, to me, she's the most important thing. We've got to take care of her first. If it's meant to be that we're parents, God will take care of that."

Both Mark and Kelly felt a sense of uncertainty at having to deal with a life-threatening disease as such a young couple. "Being diagnosed at a younger age," says Mark, "you don't have the wisdom that comes from having seen close family or friends go through that experience." Mark is a nurse practitioner, so he's seen more of illness and death than most people his age. But he still feels the inappropriateness of having his first personal encounter with a serious disease involve his wife rather than a parent or an older relative.

Both Lanita and Kelly were deeply in love with their husbands and considered themselves blessed to have their support. But both also felt the tragic side of that life-giving link. Kelly feels the anguish of bringing pain to her husband. Lanita underwent the sorrow of losing her soulmate. Five years after her cancer treatment was over, Tom was killed in a plane crash.

"One day, you're a normal person," Lanita says, "and the next day you get a phone call that you have cancer. So you pull yourself up by your bootstraps . . . and we weathered that storm. We were in the process of adopting a baby girl from Russia. . . . The day he died, we even talked about that in the morning on the way to work, how we were so excited, we were going to get a picture of her. Twelve hours later, he's dead. Again, you're a normal person one day. . . . And then 12 hours later, I'm watching the floating plane footage on the water." Lanita refers to fighting breast cancer as a "dress rehearsal" that prepared her for the greater ordeal of enduring Tom's death.

Women who feel secure in their spouses' support talk about the sense that the two of them are facing their challenges together. Roberta says that this sense of shared struggle was what convinced her to marry Lee, whom she met while she was undergoing chemo. "We had faced everything," she says. "We had faced, I think, the hardest things a couple can face. Once you get through the breast cancer and the scares of having tests come back, you feel like there's nothing you can't handle together. Obviously he's going to be there through anything life could throw at us."

Joy believes that her marriage to Vasu, whom she met soon after she had finished chemotherapy, is strengthened by Vasu's sense of her as a survivor. Both Joy and Vasu are devoted kayakers, so, Joy says, "I think Vasu has had the good fortune to see me on the river—and that's one of the places I'm a strong, strong person. I think I'm very focused. I have a survival instinct." Vasu agrees. "She'll be upside down for 2 or 3 minutes, and then finally she'll come up. Most other people in that situation would have swum out of the boat and swum to the next rapid, but she'll still be in there. And finally she'll come up. She'll be upright—"

"—And usually it's without my paddle!" Joy says, finishing his sentence. "I'm hand-paddling, going 'Where's my paddle, where's my paddle?' So I think he's seen me as a true survivor."

Kelly says that as she goes through the treatment process, "Mark is my source of strength. He's so steady, and I was actually like a couple of

Tips for Working Things Out with Your Partner

- *Communicate.* One of the hardest parts of having a disease like breast cancer is that your experience and that of your spouse are so different. Negotiating differences and similarities—and establishing good communication across the differences—is one of the biggest challenges in a relationship. For women with breast cancer who are in new marriages, the challenge can seem overwhelming. Romantic visions of "the perfect lover" may feed the fantasy that a "good" partner will automatically know what you need or that your spouse will leap to do whatever you ask. Having a potentially fatal disease may magnify these expectations, encouraging women to feel even more entitled to have their needs recognized intuitively and their requests met. Finding ways to really talk and really listen to your spouse can help cut through the unrealistic expectations, allowing the two of you to connect in more authentic ways.

- *Consider counseling and support groups.* As we've seen, one of the hardest things about undergoing breast cancer, especially for young women, is feeling isolated and lonely. Young men who suddenly find themselves married to breast cancer survivors also feel lonely, out of place, and even invisible—and with even less social support than their wives. Female partners of women with cancer may feel doubly invisible: If their relationship wasn't fully acknowledged before, it's now even harder for their needs to be recognized. Working with a counselor or talking with other young couples who are going through the same thing can help break through that isolation and give both partners more space for their feelings.

- *Cast a wide net for meeting your needs.* Don't expect your partner to be everything to you. Of course, he or she is your life partner, and you're entitled to lean on him or her. But friends and family can also offer support. Whether or not you have breast cancer, it's unrealistic to expect one person to meet all your needs. Because our culture places such a high premium on romance, it's easy to have fantasies of a partner whose love will "save" you or "make everything okay." The more you can see yourself as being at the center of your life, with a wide network of supportive loved ones, the easier it will be for all your friends and family—including your life partner—to give you the support you need.

- *Remember that it's OK to want things to be normal—and it's OK to accept the fact that they're not normal.* Sometimes, all you want is to forget that you have cancer and to be treated like a "regular person." Sometimes, you need your partner to remember how sick you are and respond accordingly. If you're like most young women with cancer, you'll probably have both feelings—and your partner may have a hard time responding to them. The more you can accept your own contradictory wishes, the easier it will be for your partner to respond. And, of course, the more clearly you communicate what's going on with you, the more likely it is that your partner will be helpful and supportive.

- *Remember that your partner has needs, too.* There's no question that it's harder for you to have cancer than it is for your partner to watch you have cancer. Still, your partner is also going through a life-shaking experience that he or she never expected and needs time to recharge, people to complain to, and ways to be self-nurturing. Encourage your partner to take care of him- or herself—or, at least, be understanding of the need to do so!

times, 'Are you okay? Are you doing all right?' Because he's just provided me with so much strength, it's helped me stay in a good mood and stay happy and be okay with it all. He's been a wonderful nurse—he really has. Starting with my throwing up on his feet! After the first time I threw up, my eyes were all bugged out, and he's like, 'It's okay.' And my head is all shaved, and he still tells me I'm beautiful—it's just so reassuring. And I think he's really been helpful with our friends and family, filling them in on what's going on. I couldn't ask for anything more, I really couldn't. He's been absolutely wonderful."

For some women, however, the strain of a breast cancer diagnosis can be too great a burden on a relationship. Dr. Robert Taub, Lisa Muccilo's physician, recalls a moving story about Lisa and her husband. "When Lisa developed the breast cancer, she had just been married," Dr. Taub recalls. "And at first, I wondered how the husband was going to deal with this. Her first visits, I remember, she came with her mother, and her husband would stay outside the room. It seemed like the illness automatically brought her closer to her mother and her father than to her husband, because she hadn't been married to him very long.

"I knew she was starting Adriamycin, and she was going to lose her hair. The very next visit, she came in with her husband, and he had shaved his head—smooth down to the scalp to show his support for her. I was very taken with that."

Mark Douglas, Husband of Kelly Douglas

It was hard seeing Kelly lose her hair. But the hair's gone; okay, let's move forward. We've tried to keep a sense of humor about it. And I love my wife regardless of how much hair she has—or doesn't have, in this case! And that's part of the deal when you take those vows to get married, you make that commitment. So I was happy to shave her head and be part of that, and to be part of the process of going through this together.

There's one thing this has done: It's kept us focused in the moment. I think too often you get lost in the future and all those other things. That's good—but I think that too often we're so worried about what's happening next week that we can't live our life right now. And that's one thing this diagnosis of cancer has done; it's helped us to appreciate the moment. That's been a blessing for sure.

We're a young couple, and clearly there have been some changes in some of the things we'd wanted to do career-wise. We've had to refocus our priorities—looking at other options for becoming parents, like adoption. We have definitely not given up hope that she'll be able to get pregnant naturally, but we've also accepted the fact that some of the drugs she's taking could make her sterile and we may not be able to.

But when I look at Kelly, I see my soulmate, my life, my true love. I see that inside her head, there are so many amazing things going on. I wish I could crawl in there and see what's going on. She's such an incredible artist—she's so creative, she has such an amazing voice. She's a beautiful woman and a beautiful person, but her soul is unbelievable—it radiates the most amazing energy.

I didn't marry the hair or any other part of the body. I married the person. Kelly's the person I fell in love with, the deep-inside person, so it's pretty easy to say all these things because it's truly how I feel. And she brings it out in me, and she brings it out in other people all the time. I hear it all the time: "You have such a wonderful wife." And I do. I'm not sure how she ended up with me. I'm lucky.

Despite this moving gesture of solidarity, Lisa and her husband grew apart emotionally, and eventually decided to separate. "I had to focus all my attention on fighting cancer, and I didn't want any negative influence in my life. I couldn't worry about fixing the relationship when I was focused on staying alive," says Lisa about the reason for the split.

Sometimes a spouse has difficulty being supportive right from the beginning. "I had problems with Joseph, brought on by my cancer," Cindy

Tips for Partners of Women with Breast Cancer

- *Focus on being there, not on "fixing" anything.* One of the hardest parts of watching someone you love struggle with cancer is knowing that you can't really help her with her biggest problem. You can't cure the disease for her or bear the pain on her behalf. Accepting this can be a struggle, but if you can accept it, that acceptance can be your greatest source of strength. Knowing what you can't do means that you'll have more energy and clarity to focus on what you can do—provide comfort, practical help, and love.

- *Accept the fact that you and your spouse have different experiences.* One of the exciting parts of a life partnership is sharing experiences with your partner. But unless you've also had a bout with cancer or a potentially fatal illness, you probably won't fully understand what your partner is going through. The more fully you can accept this, the more genuinely supportive you'll be able to be. Accepting the fact that your experiences are different will make it easier for you to ask your partner to explain when you don't understand what she's going through. It will also give her the space to find support from other cancer survivors. Knowing that you can't fully understand some parts of your partner's experience can be sorrowful, even painful. But if you can get through that pain, you can actually be more supportive in the long run.

- *Accept that things are not "normal."* Sometimes, in an effort to reassure a beloved person with cancer, the partner is tempted to insist that "everything's fine." The woman with cancer may herself be sending mixed signals, asking to be treated "like a normal person" even as she's making new demands or setting new limits. Of course, if it's possible to continue "life as usual" to some extent, that can be helpful to both of you. But sometimes, the cancer is simply going to disrupt your lives—and the stress will often seem to change your personalities, too. There's no way for the process to be easy. But the more you accept the fact that things are not normal, the more gracefully you'll be able to cope.

- *Remember that support is both practical and emotional.* Sometimes you can help your spouse by doing practical things for her, like pitching in on the child care or making sure that the kitchen is stocked with the few foods she can tolerate during chemo. Sometimes what she needs is emotional support—knowing that you still find her beautiful or that you care about what happens to her. You won't always be able to provide both kinds of support, and sometimes you may not be able to provide either kind. But knowing that your spouse needs both practical and emotional nurturing can help you come through for her in a range of ways.

- *Make sure you're getting the help and support that you need.* Having a partner with cancer is almost as difficult as having cancer yourself. Although it's appropriate to focus on her most of the time, it's important that you take care of yourself, too. Find people to whom you can vent, people who will listen supportively as you complain, blow off steam, and express the feelings that you choose not to share with your spouse. As Mark suggests, don't let your support network become a reason for shutting your partner out, but don't deprive yourself, either. We all need to be the ones whose problems are most important, at least some of the time. The more support you get, the more supportive you can be.

Kim says frankly. "We had been together 2 years and had been engaged for less than a year. And once I started treatment, I had no sexual appetite. I didn't feel good about myself, and I definitely didn't feel like having sex. He was starting a new business, and it wasn't going well, and I was scared about my career, too. But I was also scared that I was going to die."

"Right before I started radiation, I just couldn't take it any more. I told Joseph, 'No more, get out.' I was having a midlife crisis right then and there."

One month later, Cindy and Joseph were reunited, and they eventually eloped. They went to couples therapy, which Cindy believes helped her to express her feelings and to develop what she now considers more realistic expectations for Joseph—and for men in general. "I know that Joseph was exhausted from hearing me say that I was sick, that I felt sick, that I felt fat and ugly, that I was going to die, that I was scared this was going to come back. He was exhausted. And in a way I think he felt let down. I let him down because I was sick. And in a way he knew he was letting me down too, but there was nothing more he could give. He's really a good man, and he has a great heart. He just didn't know what to do or how to do it. I think it can be really hard for men to give of themselves emotionally."

Tony Mattox, Husband of Leslie Mouton

If it had been me who got cancer, it would've been so much easier for me. It should've been me.

When I saw the expression on her face after she received the diagnosis, I felt my heart sink. The word cancer *conjures up so many images—so many people think that death is near. That it's all downhill from here. My heart sank, and my stomach turned. And I relate that feeling back to being in a war. I've been in two different wars—and I have to say, it's easier to be shot at than to sit there and watch her go through this. I wanted it to be me going through the whole ordeal of losing my hair and feeling the body aches. It didn't seem like there was enough I could do to take away the pain—physically, mentally, or emotionally. I wanted to do more.*

There's definitely a feeling of complete helplessness. I went to every consultation, every treatment, every everything with her— so I could hear from the doctors directly and see how she was reacting. Especially when she started chemo—I would take her to treatment and then come home and be in the house with her. Me and our 2-year-old daughter, Nicole, would check in on her. I would look at her sleeping and think about all the things happening inside her body at that moment—and I would feel so helpless.

I tried to be the mom. I tried to be the dad. I tried to be the husband, the cook, the cleaner. Everything. I knew it'd be tough. And not just physically—it's especially tiring emotionally, when you can't know exactly what's in her mind and what her body is feeling. Even when you want to be by yourself, you can't get away. There's nowhere to go. But I knew I couldn't lose the positive attitude, as hard as it was. On some days that attitude was a façade—it takes every ounce of everything you have to stay positive. And there were times when I'd think, "Okay, it's time to cry now." And we did. There were nights when we held each other and cried. We kept telling each other, "We'll get through this. We'll get through this together."

Generally for me the hardest time was the day of the treatment, when she would sleep for 24 hours at a time. Nicole and I would go into the bedroom and check on her to see if she needed anything. But when we would leave the bedroom and come down those stairs, it would just be me and Nicole, and we'd snuggle. Nicole would ask me, "How's Mommy? Is she okay?" It was hard to explain things to her without crying. It was an outlet for me to

*have Nicole there and to hold her and tell her, "Mommy is fine."
But when the tears were coming out of my eyes as I was saying it,
Nicole understood that something was not right. Nicole and I
would just hold each other and cry to each other. It's amazing how
little ones can tell you, "It'll be okay." And it does make you feel
better. It made me feel better.*

*There were so many times during the treatment that Leslie
didn't even want to be touched. Sometimes I thought she might
want me to touch her hair or her head, or rub her back or her
arm, and she would say, "Please leave me alone." She'd say, "It's
not you. It's just I can't be touched right now." And not touching her was so hard for me—but it was the best thing I could do
for her at times.*

*It wasn't that I ever wanted to quit, but you're just so tired.
You're worn out. You feel like you're not doing any good. I didn't
want to quit—I just wanted more hours in every day or more
strength. That was my one promise to myself going into this: I said
to myself, "I don't want Leslie to ever see any expression on my
face or hear any words from my mouth that gave her the impression that I didn't believe we could make it through this." And I
never believed it was bigger than we could handle. I always knew
in the bottom of my heart that we could get through this.*

Support for Your Spouse or Partner

Husbands of breast cancer survivors often stress the need for spouses to
develop their own sources of support. "It's not always easy to express
your emotions," says Mark Douglas. "And this is a very emotional thing.
You are watching your wife go through something so quick, so traumatic—it's body-image-changing, it's attitude-changing—there's so much
change going on. And you are many times put in that caregiving role, acting as the cheerleader, the supporter."

"I've told Kelly that I've had to take care of myself. I've had to make
sure I'm doing some things for myself, to make sure I have people I can
talk to openly. Clearly, the most important person for me to be talking
with is Kelly, and we do, we talk about it all the time—but you need to
be able to step away from it a little bit and be honest about when you've
reached a limit. And Kelly'll say, 'Let's not talk about this—let's go out
and go to a movie, hang out,' and it's like, Cool."

"So I would encourage men to seek a friend, a sibling, a spiritual advisor, in addition to building that support network. They need to under-

stand that it's okay to be angry and frustrated. It's okay to cry, to be un-certain—to have fear. Those things are going to happen. Find a way to try to express it. Talk to your wife, if nothing else. But also understand that some aspects of it may be better expressed to someone else."

Tony Mattox, Leslie Mouton's husband, found that it helped him to remember what was most important to him about his marriage. When asked what advice he'd give to other young spouses, he says, "I'd tell them to realize there are going to be some really tough days ahead, and if you know that going in, it's better. You just have to be who you were before this happened. Don't let this change your feelings about the per-son you love. There are weird outward issues that you're going to have to deal with: the paleness and the hair loss. You just have to love that per-son the same way you loved her before. And you have to keep your fam-ily together with a positive attitude."

"Men should know that tucking in and giving one last kiss can make a big difference. Most likely, you fell in love with the person you mar-ried for a reason, and that's all still there. All those reasons are still there. You can't let the cancer get in the way of that love.

"Men have to realize, what they're going through is nowhere near what she's going through. No matter what I was feeling, I always tried to think of what she was going through, and I tried to put myself in her place. I tried to understand. But no matter how hard I tried, ultimately there was no way I could ever physically feel what she felt."

Getting Support from Families

Even at the best of times, families can be both a blessing and a curse. When a young woman has breast cancer, she's likely to find that both the nurturing and the painful aspects of family life are magnified. Fami-lies provide support and encouragement, and many young women rely on this. The connections can also be difficult, however, if only because women are sorry that they are causing pain to their parents.

Parents and Daughters

As you heard earlier in this chapter, Roberta, Joy, and Lisa all relied on their mothers for support and comfort during and after diagnosis. They discovered that this crisis transformed their close relationships with their mothers into even closer ones. As Joy found, however, the relationship can also be made more complex because of the guilt that both you and your mother may be feeling. "I know she was thinking, 'Why my daugh-ter, why not me?' And that was really hard for me. And I know it was really hard for her too."

Mothers and daughters typically have complex relationships. The mother's role as a nurturer and caregiver is often assumed. But if you have a strained relationship with your mother, this time period can be a particularly difficult reminder of the emotional distance that already separates you. Still, where a relationship does exist, mothers both want and are expected to be there every step of the way.

In fact, there's even a national organization called Mothers Supporting Daughters with Breast Cancer (MSDBC) that focuses on helping mothers deal psychologically and emotionally with their daughters' diagnosis and treatment.

Where does this leave your father?

Your father's reaction upon learning that his daughter has breast cancer is likely to be to try to protect you. Your natural instinct is to let him. Just as he did throughout your changing relationship with him as you grew up, he may now be looking for cues from you about how to act and what to say.

Parents like to fix things. Your father can't fix cancer, but he may be searching for a concrete problem that he can solve. For James Muccilo, taking responsibility for the mounds of insurance paperwork that followed his daughter Lisa's diagnosis at 27 was his way of overcoming his sense of helplessness. "Just dealing with the doctor's bills and insurance is a monumental problem. I took that on. I don't want Lisa worrying about the bills. I don't know how anyone in her position could handle the volumes of paperwork that need to be dealt with, and fight cancer. You almost have to be a paralegal to get through the maze. It's an unbelievable task."

When dealing with your father, it may be worthwhile to try to figure out when your relationship with him is working the best. Is it, as with Lisa and her dad, when he's taking responsibility for details like insurance and visits to the doctor? Is it when he can take you in his arms and just *be* there as a source of comfort? Can he do certain research tasks that you don't feel up to, that he may have some special skills in, or is there someone he knows who can help you?

If you've always seen your father as a source of loving strength, it may be hard for you to understand how vulnerable he may be feeling right now. As a man, it may be difficult for him to even talk about his daughter's breasts. If he initially distances himself from you because he's embarrassed or uncomfortable, he may unwittingly send you a message that he's not going to be there for you. And he might make an assumption of his own: that you're more comfortable sharing this experience with your mother, or your husband, or your friends.

James and Theresa Muccilo, Parents of Lisa Muccilo

Theresa: *We're a very close family. We do everything together. That started with my parents always having us over for Sunday dinner, and we just continued that, even when I had my children.*

James: *When we found out, it was 1997. And my wife had just been through breast cancer 2 years prior to that. Lisa was 27 when she was diagnosed. We always said, "We gotta worry about this, because of the genetics," because my mother had it, too—but not at 27. When we got the call, it was devastating.*

Theresa: *When they found out it was cancer, we thought it would be like what I had: "OK, she'll have the lump removed, and everything's going to be fine." But then they called, and it was not like what I had. It had spread to her lymph nodes.*

James: *I mean, just the initial word* cancer—*27 years old, breast cancer, how can that be? It was just devastating for all of us, the whole family. And you get over the shock, and you get over the anger, and you start dealing with it. Then you focus on fixing it and curing her, and since then, that's what we've been trying to do. We try to keep her spirits up, and do everything we can to keep a positive attitude for ourselves and for everybody else in the family, which isn't easy, because you get a lot of depressing news. For a while it was one thing after another. And then she went through various treatments, some of which at this point I would categorize as not working. And every time a bad test result comes back, you get smacked down.*

Theresa: *Well, every time you get the bad news, you're disappointed, of course, because with each new treatment is the hope that everything is going to get better.*

James: *The initial feeling is the same. You get depressed.*

Theresa: *From my own experience, I had both breasts removed. I didn't want that for her. I didn't want her to go through that. I was 48 when I had my breasts removed. I had lived my life. But she was only 27 and just married. She hadn't had a chance to live her life yet. I felt worse for her than I did for myself.*

I keep thinking it's going to be fine—but it's not going to be fine. She's fighting really hard. And she's going to continue to fight. She's a fighter.

James: *The only reason I can deal with it is that Lisa deals with it. She makes it easier. After the initial depression, she snaps back, puts a smile on her face, and keeps everyone else upbeat.*

157

You may also have an expectation that your father will always be emotionally strong. In our society, being emotionally strong may be equated with showing no emotion at all. However, as James Muccilo learned, sharing emotions can become an important part of strengthening the family—especially, in his case, in the face of a disease that seemed intent on striking the women he loved. First his mother was diagnosed with breast cancer, then his wife, and finally his daughter. "You get the news, and it's devastating," he says. "And you cry. The family has a lot of tears. But then we say, 'Okay, what are we going to do about it?' And you dry the tears and go into action. And Lisa makes it easy. She's always been so positive and so upbeat that she keeps the family moving forward, always focused on the future."

For most families, holidays are special times, though they can also be fraught with emotion. When a young woman has breast cancer, family holidays may take on a special resonance, or they may diminish in importance. "Every time I'm with my family is a special occasion," Lisa says. "I feel that way a lot because I'm with them so much. So I don't feel like a birthday or Christmas is 'very, very special.' I feel like one more day that I get to spend time with them is very special."

On the other hand, Lisa's sister-in-law, Lise Muccilo, thinks of each holiday with Lisa as a kind of milestone. "I won't voice my opinion to the family," says Lise, "but I'm grateful that Lisa is here this Thanksgiving." When Lise heard the previous October that Lisa's cancer had metastasized, it was the holidays that she thought about. "You're like, 'Oh, my gosh. Let's savor this Christmas, let's savor this Thanksgiving.' You should do that on a daily basis, but it makes you really think: What if Lisa's not here with us next year? I think it—I never say it to Lisa, I never say it to the family. But it eats me up inside. It makes me crazy sometimes."

For Kelly and Mark, breast cancer has shifted their sense of the holidays, particularly since Kelly had chemo treatments scheduled right before Christmas. "I think in some ways it's allowing us to enjoy the holiday a little more," she says, "since we're not going to be running around to different places as much. This is usually such a busy time of year, where you're running off to parents and running off to see siblings. I think that since this year we're going to do it day by day, it's allowing us to enjoy the time more, and to enjoy each other and take it easy—which is what you're supposed to be doing during the holidays."

Mark points out that the breast cancer has moved him and Kelly to do something they've been talking about doing for a while, which is to celebrate Christmas in their own house. "We'll get off to see some family," he says, "but the most important thing for me is just being with my wife. I look at this as being one of many Christmases we'll spend together. But clearly this Christmas is different, and it's affected us differently. I think it's just special in the way that we've slowed down and focused on the now."

Getting Support from Friends

Friends often occupy an ambiguous place in our culture. On the one hand, we rely on our friends, especially before we get married and have children. On the other hand, though, there's often a sense that friends are secondary to our spouses, children, and families of origin. There can be a kind of invisibility surrounding friendship that downplays the significance of these ties.

As a result, it can be hard to know what we can expect from our friends. A great deal of romance surrounds the idea of husbands and life partners, and many of us have the idea that our families of origin should always be there for us. But how central can friends be in our lives?

Likewise, we expect to have to work at marriage, and by the time we're in our twenties, we understand that families can be full of conflict as well as love. It can be harder to grasp that even the most wonderful friendships also take work and might even be marked by conflict.

When a woman is diagnosed with breast cancer, a strain may be put on any friendship. Friends struggle with their own fears and anxieties about their own mortality. They worry about not being able to say the right thing, not being able to come through—or they simply may not want to deal with such a demanding challenge. The woman with breast cancer has to reevaluate whom she can count on and for what—at a time when she naturally wants to focus on herself and her own needs, not on reworking her relationships.

These issues are magnified for young women with breast cancer. Friends in their twenties and thirties are less likely than older women to have thought about their own mortality or to have gone through the loss of other loved ones. There can be a vivid sense of contrast between the friends who are just starting their lives and the cancer survivor who is worrying about facing the end of hers. Women in their forties, fifties, and beyond may have friendships that have already weathered a few hard knocks over the past 10 or 20 years. Younger women's friendships are more likely to be newer, and perhaps more fragile.

Sometimes there's a conflict between friendship and romance. If you're unmarried when you're diagnosed with breast cancer, you may wish that your friends could take the place of a spouse. It can be easy for single

Tips for Getting Support from Friends

- *Take your friendships seriously.* Expect them to require the same kind of work and commitment that you'd devote to a romantic relationship or to your family ties. Certainly your friendships are different from your love and family relationships. But they require a similar focus—and they may have similar conflicts.

- *Communicate and negotiate.* Just as with a spouse, you need to tell your friends what's going on with you. This can be hard at such an overwhelming time—and sometimes even you don't know how you feel or what you want. But to the extent that you can, let your friends in on your experience, and tell them what they can do to help. Even the most sensitive friend fails at being a mind reader some of the time, and even the most generous friend may go through periods of feeling overwhelmed. The more you and your friends can be clear with each other, the more support you'll be able to receive.

- *Share your feelings with your friends—but remember that they have feelings, too.* It's hardest to be the person with the cancer, but it's also hard to be the person whose friend has cancer. Your friends will need to set limits, cope with their emotions, and develop their own networks of support. That's not your problem, of course—but just making space somewhere in your consciousness to be aware of your friends' needs can help them make the space they need to take care of themselves while taking care of you.

women to build up a picture in their minds of how helpful and supportive the "ideal spouse" could be, and then to judge every other relationship as wanting in comparison to this ideal. Since you know that you're *not* married to your friends, you may underestimate how much support they can provide for you.

If you're married or in a life partnership when you're diagnosed, it may seem natural for you to focus entirely on your spouse, ignoring the important role that friends can potentially play in your life. Some women feel drawn to their friends but experience a certain amount of guilt, as though they should be finding all that they need in their marriages. Married or partnered women, especially those with children, may feel that they simply don't have time to extend themselves beyond the immediate family circle.

Mark and Kelly Douglas are a married couple who have relied heavily on their network of friends during Kelly's bout with breast cancer. Mark has found that maintaining that network also required a certain amount of work—and called for setting some limits.

"I know I have good friends, and I've been able to talk about all this," he says. "Kelly and I have done it together—talked to friends who have no idea what we're going through, but who are there to listen and support. And I think sometimes we need to have faith in our friends and family. It's OK to say, 'I'm having a bad day.' Or to take the phone off the hook. We were having these marathon conversations night after night. We wanted to try to get information to people, but at some point, I was like, 'Turn off the phone, I'm not talking to anyone any more.'"

As a single mother living with her own mother during her treatment, Robyn Mitchell felt that her close friends were "a godsend." During the chemo, one friend dropped her son off at day care every day and then picked him up. "Walking into day care was like walking into a germ dungeon," explains Robyn, "especially when my white count was down so low. She offered to do it."

Roberta Levy-Schwartz depended heavily on her network of friends, who often found creative ways to be thoughtful. "My friend Abbey sent me a card that arrived the night before every chemo treatment. There were people who showed up in the hospital with things that just made me smile. They'd take me out and wouldn't let me wallow."

Roberta's friends really operated as a group, which Roberta thinks made it easier for them to offer support—both to her and to one another. "A lot of my friends had a network around me," she explains. "I would only have to call two or three of them, and then they would handle calling all the rest of my friends, so they would tackle the problems of people who were upset or people who were crying. They'd say, 'OK, get over it before you call Roberta.' They'd say, 'OK, this test didn't look good—you have to be OK with that before you talk to her.'"

While Roberta leaned on her existing network of friends, she found that she wasn't interested in making any new friends while she was being treated. "You do build a pretty strong wall at that point," she says. "You can only handle the people you already know. You don't know how to talk to new people. Even people I meet now whom I didn't talk to during that time period—people I've fallen out of touch with—I almost don't know what to say to them. Because I'm a different person now than I was then, and that new person was almost in the embryonic stage of forming when I was in cancer treatment. It was like, 'I'm a normal person—no, I'm a cancer patient—no, I'm a normal person again.' You don't

Tips for Friends of Women with Breast Cancer

- *If you don't know what to do, ask.* It's hard enough to have a friend who's got breast cancer. Don't add to your burdens by expecting yourself to be a mind reader. Your friend can help you help her by telling you what she needs.

- *Be creative in offering support.* It may be easier for your friend to accept help if you give her a "menu" or make some concrete offers. Women with breast cancer most often need help with the practical things—stocking the fridge with food, getting the housework done, taking care of other work and household chores. Is there anything you can help with, on a one-shot or an ongoing basis? Women with children may appreciate your making a regular child-care date. Are there special treats that your friend can enjoy while she's going through treatment—an escapist video, a joke book, some scented lotion, a pretty scarf or turban? Try picturing yourself in her place and think about what might make you feel loved and supported—and what might help you to make it through the day.

- *Try to stay involved.* Often, friends rally round during the initial diagnosis and operation, and then fall away during the chemo or just after treatment. Your friend's needs will change as time goes on, and she'll look to you for different things. But even when the emergency is over, your support is still important.

- *Accept that you may not understand what she's going through.* If you haven't had breast cancer or another life-threatening disease yourself, there probably will be limits to how much you can empathize with your friend, however close you feel to her. At the best of times, it can be hard for women friends to accept their differences and to realize that there are limits to what each can know of the other. When one of you has a major illness, accepting your differences can be especially challenging. Do what you can to accept the fact that on some level, you really don't know what your friend is going through—and that she may need to be close to people who do.

- *Remember that you have needs, too!* It can be tempting to think that if you simply suppress your own needs, you can help your friend, but the fact is that no matter what you do, you're not going to be able to cure her cancer. While you probably will want to put out more for her and cut her more slack than usual, that doesn't mean that you have to passively accept bad treatment or let her take her frustrations out on you. Nor does it mean that you can't set limits or focus on your own life's priorities. There are no right or wrong answers as to how much one should sacrifice for a friend, but it's always important to remember that there are two people in a relationship. After all, how can you be there for her if you're not there for yourself?

- *Make sure that you're getting the support you need.* Having a friend face a life-threatening illness is one of the hardest things there is. Your friend with breast cancer probably can't offer you support for what you're going through, but your other friends probably can. Develop your own support network of friends, family, mentors, and/or spiritual advisors to help you through this difficult time.

know how to be. So when someone asks, 'Hi, how are you?' even those normal things are incredibly difficult. You don't know what to say to answer that simple question. On the one hand, you want to say, 'Oh, I'm fine.' And on the other hand, you want to say, 'Chemo last week really sucked, and I'm throwing up, and the drugs really aren't working.' You can't say that to someone new. You can say it to your friends. It's a confusing stage of life."

CHAPTER 7

"I Was Just Starting to Like My Body"

Coping with Body Image, Dating, Sex, and Intimacy

"I never even hoped for marriage—I just wanted to live," says Joy Simha, who was 26 years old and single when she was diagnosed with breast cancer. "*I didn't know if I would ever really fall in love with anyone. The mastectomy was what initially made me feel like no one would ever look at me the same way again. Then going through chemo reinforced the idea that I would need to come to terms with myself in a way that I could never have imagined before. There I was with my thinning hair and dark circles under my eyes—even my fingernails, which were once really long, weren't growing the way they used to. There were times when I couldn't even look in the mirror because I didn't recognize myself. I thought, 'Who is this person staring back at me?'*

"You never look at breasts the same way any more," says Aquatia Owens, who had her mastectomy at age 32. *"You see Baywatch, and you're like, 'Those are just breasts.' The mastectomy didn't bother me— I just wanted to live. And I'm alive. But you have scars. Is it ever going to be perfect? No, but it beats dying. People are in love with breasts. But I'm happy with my new breasts. I'm okay."*

"That's when I cried—when I found out I was going to lose my hair," says Leslie Mouton. Leslie was 35 and working as an anchorwoman on a San Antonio news station when she was diagnosed with breast cancer. Her bright blond hair was part of her job, but more important, it was

*part of her self-image; it was even the basis for her nickname, "Blondie."
Leslie managed to maintain a certain amount of calm about her cancer
diagnosis and surgery, despite her fears for her 2-year-old daughter,
Nicole, and concern for her husband, Tony Mattox. But she broke down
when she realized that having chemotherapy for breast cancer meant that
she was going to lose her hair: "I said, 'I can't lose my hair, that's part
of who I am.'"*

Coping with Body Issues

If you're still in your twenties, you may still be making friends with your
body—exploring your sexuality, discovering your physical abilities, trying out different looks, hairstyles, and body images. You may be dating,
just beginning a serious relationship, or newly married. If you're in your
thirties, you may also feel as though you're still finding out what you're
capable of—physically, sexually, and socially. You may also be dating or
involved in a relatively new relationship.

And if you're like most young U.S. women, your breasts have a central
place in your body image, your sexuality, and your sense of yourself as
a woman. Whether you think your breasts are too small, too big, or just
right, you probably have a strong sense of where they fit into the image
you project, your sense of your own social power, your attractiveness,
and your femininity. It's hard for women of any age to cope with the idea
of losing a breast, but it's a special challenge for young women. Likewise,
it's upsetting for women of all ages to think of their breasts as a source
of danger, but such a view can be especially trying for young women,
who are still coming to terms with their bodies.

Single young women who are diagnosed with breast cancer worry
about having the courage to expose their new, postcancer bodies to new
sexual partners, while women who are already in relationships are concerned about their partners' losing desire for them. Women in all situations often notice their own loss of sexual desire, along with occasional
symptoms of fatigue, vaginal dryness, hot flashes, and other aspects of
premature menopause brought on by their treatments. (For more on cancer treatments and premature menopause, see Chapters 3 and 9.)

"If you're over 35, the chance of premature menopause after chemotherapy is very high," says Leslie Schover, Ph.D., an associate professor
in M. D. Anderson's Department of Behavioral Science. "Going through
the sudden change of chemically induced menopause seems to be much
harder on women than going through menopause naturally. You get hot
flashes, vaginal dryness—and it goes beyond the loss of estrogen in the
vagina. Women simply lose interest in sex." While this loss of sexual

desire is usually temporary, says Schover, it can be devastating to the woman—or the couple—who encounters it, especially if, as is often the case, oncologists and gynecologists have failed to warn you of what might be coming.

Cindy Kim, who was diagnosed at age 26, felt that her breast cancer almost ended her relationship with her fiancé, Joseph, whom she'd been with for 2 years. "I just had no thoughts about sex," she says frankly. "He didn't repulse me, but I didn't have the strength to do anything. And it made him feel like he had cancer as well. He thought that I didn't care about his needs any more. He thought that he wasn't good enough for me any more. And I was like, 'How could you think that way? I'm the one with cancer. How did this all of a sudden become about you?'" As a result of Cindy's cancer and the conflicts it generated, the couple separated for a while, although they eventually reconciled.

Indeed, according to Dr. Schover, most partnerships do survive cancer. However, if there were sexual or relationship issues before diagnosis, the cancer may magnify these problems or give the couple a convenient reason for their emotional and sexual difficulties. And in Dr. Schover's view, the sexual problems that can arise—which affect up to 50 percent of all women being treated for breast cancer—may persist for a long time if they are not addressed, either through counseling or through renewed communication between the partners.

As a young woman with breast cancer, then, you're faced with a twofold task: to come to terms with your new body and to learn how to feel comfortable physically and sexually with others.

Changes in Body Image

If you're like most young U.S. women, by the time you're in your late teens, you've spent a certain amount of time coming to terms with your breasts, from their first dramatic appearance at puberty through your discovery of your female body in your teens to your creation of an adult sexual and social life. You've already had to relearn your body through two major changes: from childhood to puberty, and from puberty into adulthood. It's a huge challenge to relearn it again so soon—to come to terms with a lumpectomy, a scar, or the loss of one or both breasts. The challenge is all the greater if you felt that your breasts were the one part of your anatomy that you were not ambivalent about.

"I was always very well endowed," says Joy. "My breasts were always a part of enjoying summertime in bathing suits, being able to go out with people and have a nice time and wear nice things. I had really tried very hard to lose weight right before I was diagnosed with breast cancer, and

I'd been successful. In the 3 years prior to my diagnosis, I was growing to appreciate my body. I had just started to understand breasts and how great they can be."

Then came cancer, and a mastectomy. "Losing my breast so early in life was a total letdown," Joy says. "You think you're being cheated."

Cindy felt even more strongly that her breasts were central to her self-image, especially after she won a beauty contest, Miss Seoul Korea, that involved her making promotional visits to Planet Hollywood restaurants and being featured in commercials and banners for the suntan lotion Hawaiian Tropic.

"I felt wonderful about my body," Cindy recalls. "And I was always totally obsessed with my breasts. I had really, really nice breasts. A full C size. Men adored them. Even girls were like, 'Wow, you have great breasts.' To be Asian and have such big breasts was unusual. I felt great about it."

For Cindy, breasts were central not just to her body image but to her entire sense of who she was. "I definitely had an attitude about it. I got my first training bra in fourth grade. By eighth grade, I was close to a D cup. It's almost like I was damned for concentrating all my energy on my breasts."

Cindy's pride in her breasts was countered by feelings of frustration about her weight. "I was kind of stocky and round in high school," she says. "In college, I lost all my weight. I became anorexic." Eventually, Cindy overcame the anorexia, won her beauty title, and got engaged to Joseph, whom she describes as "a hunk."

"I have pictures of me 3 months before I was diagnosed—and let me tell you, I was a little hottie," she says. Then Cindy was diagnosed, had a lumpectomy, and began undergoing chemo and in vitro fertilization, so that she and her fiancé could freeze embryos for their future child-bearing. As a result of the two treatments, Cindy started to gain weight. The combination of losing part of her breast and losing her glamorous shape seemed like a double blow to Cindy—an almost unbearable attack on her sense of self.

For many young women, the initial rage, despair, and sense of betrayal can sometimes give way to a new appreciation of their physical selves. It's a transition that Joy says happened slowly as she went from feeling cheated when she first learned of her diagnosis to later feeling grateful to her body for enabling her to survive.

"After the mastectomy was complete and I was home recuperating, I remember being really grateful to be alive," she says. "I remember thinking that life was very precious, and I had enormous gratitude for the

Leslie Mouton, Going Public

I didn't cry when I was diagnosed. I didn't cry when I had surgery. I cried when I knew my hair was going to fall out. I thought, "I'm going to look sick now. I'm a news anchor. I have to go on the air. I can't look sick."

I dealt with the hair loss pretty well once it happened. But losing all my hair was something I just didn't expect. And the false eyelashes, I never got used to. It took me an extra half hour to get ready for the news. I'd think I'd have it just right, then I'd get the glue out, and the eyelash would be crooked and I'd have to start all over again. I was so afraid I'd be reading the news and one would pop off—or, worse, halfway off. My co-anchor came up with a code in case one of my eyelashes started drooping. He said, "Leslie, if I ever say 'coming unglued' or 'lashing out,' you'll know to check your eyelashes!" Luckily, he never had to say those words.

I spent a ton of money on my wig. My thought was, "I'll shave my head, put my wig right on, and no one will ever know. I won't skip a beat."

Then, 2 weeks to the day after my chemo started, I was in the shower getting ready for work. It was 3 A.M., and clumps of hair were coming out. And I sat there and cried. I had tried to prepare myself for it, but I couldn't. Nothing could have prepared me for that moment when the clumps were falling out in the tub. My husband was still sleeping, and I woke him up and said, "Today is the day." He got up, put his arms around me and gave me a kiss, and said, "I'll see you tonight with clippers."

That night, my husband, my daughter, my friends and I had a big hair-shaving party. And when it was all over and I looked in the mirror, I screamed at first. And then I looked again, and again, and I realized it was still me. I was so afraid of losing my hair and that a part of my identity would fall out with it. But inside I was the same person. Maybe even a better person. I didn't have to do all the primping and preening—I got to look on the inside. And I learned to love what was on the inside.

You have to love yourself first. That's number one. If you can't come to terms with how you look, how is anyone else going to?

people around me. And the simplest things—a beautiful blue sky, dipping my feet in the water (because I couldn't go swimming yet)—just very simple things that I could enjoy—they all meant so much. You would think, 'They just cut off a body part; I must be in extraordinary pain.' But I wasn't in pain. I was thankful that I could get out of bed and help myself, and I felt that I was a pretty strong gal. I knew I could continue to live my life without a breast." Although Joy continued to feel anger that her innocent and carefree self had been "stolen," she also felt wonder and gratitude for the body that continued to live on. Indeed, finding ways to love your body, feeling that you are in partnership with it rather than at war with it, can be very helpful to both your physical and your emotional recovery from breast cancer.

Tracy Pleva Hill, diagnosed while breast-feeding at age 32, felt that she was far more concerned for her husband and her 18-month-old son than for her own physicality. She also felt relatively unconcerned with how other people viewed her. "I was just like, 'I have to deal—now you deal,'" she says. "There are a lot of people I feel very comfortable around, and we make jokes about my breasts and my implant. And there are some guys that I'm friends with, and with them, I'm like, 'They're lookin' okay, aren't they?' And then I'll ask, 'So is one looking a little bit lower than the other?' I even offered to show my reconstruction job to some of the women at work. To me, the fact that I've had a mastectomy is just not important. I don't think it reduces my femininity at all. I just don't."

Aquatia Owens, also diagnosed at age 32, says that she felt traumatized by the physical changes brought on by her cancer and chemo. But she also reports developing a hard-won sense of serenity about her physical self.

"To mention breasts in a sexual way—I don't look at them that way," she says frankly. "I just want them to look good under my shirt. But if one of my breasts has to go, it has to go. You're losing your hair, throwing up, losing weight—your whole self-esteem is affected. You look terrible, you feel terrible. And you look out your window, and you see your friends, your colleagues, having a great life. And that's sad, that part is almost devastating. You have to be very strong-willed to say, 'That's gonna be me. I'm gonna be out there again.'"

Finding her equilibrium wasn't easy for Aquatia. "I kept myself busy," she says, "but the whole time, my self-esteem was shot. On the surface, I was strong, but internally, you just want to say, 'When am I going to be back to my normal self?' And it takes a long time. Because you are judged by what you look like, and how you feel, and how sexual you look. And you have to change that perception of yourself. That's the hard part. Going through something like this, you have to go inward, because physically, you have nothing to look at—you're a mess, physically. So you have to take care of your soul."

Hair, Baldness, and Wigs

For most young women with breast cancer, losing their hair is a big issue. Yet women deal with it in widely different ways, and they report that their attitudes tend to change a great deal as they go through the process.

"I've got a great hair loss story," says Tracy. "My hair starts falling out, and falling out, and falling out. And I'm pulling it out because it's fun. And it finally gets to the point where it just looks terrible, and my husband comes home from work, and I said, 'You just gotta buzz my head.' He said, 'I don't think I can do that.' 'Yeah, yeah, you can. Get your buzzer out, 'cause you're buzzin' my head.' And I've got my head in the sink, and I said, 'When I look up in the mirror, how badly am I gonna cry?' He goes, 'I don't think you will.' And I look up. Okay, I look pretty good. And my son was down for a nap, and I put a baseball cap on, and I walk in the room and I'm holding him. He's a year and a half. And I take the baseball cap off, and he gives me this weird look. I let go of him and say, 'Jason, is it okay that Mommy looks like this?' He says, 'Yes.' And he leans over and kisses the top of my head."

Tracy points out that she's always had short hair, so her "cancer haircut" looks good to her, "like a cool, hip, New York haircut." Now, though, she's letting her hair grow, because "I think my husband wants me to put all this behind us. He's used to me with longer hair. So I'll let it grow."

Still, says Tracy, it's an odd experience making the transition back to a precancer sense of her body and her hair. "My husband and I went on vacation to Mexico, and I had to get waxed," she says. "It was devastating—bikini, eyebrows, legs. I couldn't believe I'd been hairless for 6 months, and now I was ripping hair out of my body."

Like Tracy, Kelly Douglas took a playful approach to the changes in her body image. She actually enjoyed the prospect of being bald as another quirky look that suited her artistic image and her creative job at a toy company, and, like Tracy, she had her husband shave her head.

"You want to look, but you don't want to," says Kelly, who was 24 when she was diagnosed. "And I'm like, 'Is my head going to be really lumpy? Misshapen? Am I going to have to deal with this forever? Well, OK, not forever, but what's going to seem like forever.'

"And then part of me was like, 'It's done.' And I think mostly I was just so relieved to have the hair gone, since it was falling out. It just feels more comfortable and clean. Definitely kinda weird though."

Mark, who'd been married to Kelly for 2 years when she was diagnosed, says, "I think it was a situation where we'd had so much change since Kelly's diagnosis with cancer that it was one more step in that change that we knew was coming. In a way we were looking forward to it, because it's one more step toward recovery."

For Mark and Kelly, having Mark shave Kelly's head took on several added layers of meaning. "It was symbolic of her body changing again, and symbolic of me participating in that with her," says Mark. "And to let her know that I was here to support her—whatever it takes. And really, that's been my mantra—'whatever it takes'—through this whole process."

Tony Mattox found it a bit more harrowing to cope with his wife's hair loss, perhaps because Leslie herself was so devastated by the prospect. "We knew it was coming, but we really had no way to prepare for it," he says. "She just woke me up out of a deep, deep sleep. It was such a shocking way to wake up. And it was shocking to see it finally happening."

Tony did his best to be supportive to Leslie, who was tearful and distraught. But after she left for work, he says, "I sat on the edge of the bed for 45 minutes to an hour, just thinking and thinking. I was just sitting on the bed wondering, 'Now what? What is she going to be thinking the rest of the day? Should I have even let her go to work? Is there anything I can do to make this easier on her?'"

Mark and Tony were particularly supportive partners, but not all women report such good experiences. "Joseph never made me feel very good about myself," Cindy says. "He'd look at everything like, 'Okay, one more shot. This is almost over with.' He just wanted it to be done. I felt like a burden." This sense of being a burden was intensified because Cindy felt both that she wasn't very attractive and that Joseph didn't think she was.

"When I was bald and fat," she recalls, "he said he still thought I looked great—but I knew better. You know how men check out other women? Well, I'm fine with that up to a point. But when I had cancer, this woman stepped into the subway, all decked out in designer clothes and colorful sandals. And then there was me. I was wearing a scarf on my head because I was bald. I was sweating and pale, and I was going to radiation to burn myself. And he kept looking at *her*. After that I didn't want to go outside with him."

Aquatia Owens felt that she could trust her partner throughout the process of diagnosis, treatment, and hair loss. It was her own reactions that changed, she says, not his.

"We met as friends—we were friends first," she says of the man who was with her when she was diagnosed at age 32 and to whom she got engaged when she was a 4-year survivor at age 36. "That was a very

Tips for Coping with the Changes in Your Body

- *Stay in touch with yourself.* Give yourself some quiet time each day to connect to your own body—and your own feelings. Write in your journal, draw pictures that express how you feel and how you see yourself, or just sit and meditate. Whether you feel like you love or hate your body, enjoy or despise your new look, it's important that you let yourself experience whatever emotions come up. The more fully you feel each emotion, the more flexible and open you can be to a wide range of experiences.

- *Honor your own feelings.* Now that breast cancer has come into the national consciousness to such a great extent, there can paradoxically be pressure on each young woman to be a "heroine," a "super-survivor" who meets every challenge with a smile and never feels discouraged, angry, or resentful. Yet blocking out your feelings is a sure-fire recipe for depression—that helpless, hopeless condition in which you simply feel numb and miserable. There's no right way to go through any part of this experience, including the losses and changes associated with your body and your appearance.

- *Find a support system.* Did you know that the best predictor of whether or not people will undergo posttraumatic stress syndrome after combat or a disaster is whether or not they have a support network? Turning to friends, partners, family members, support groups, coworkers, and anyone else who will support you during this difficult time can make a huge difference.

- *Keep talking with your partner.* Although your partner isn't going through the same kind of trauma you are, he or she is still facing an overwhelming challenge. It's important for both of you to be able to share your feelings with each other. As we saw in Chapter 6, it's also important for your partner to have a support system of his or her own, to vent feelings that may not be appropriate to share with you. Urge your partner to be as open with you as possible, while finding friends and loved ones who can also listen.

- *Remember that your feelings—and your decisions—can change.* Maybe you, like Leslie, will begin by wanting to wear a wig and conceal your baldness from the world. Or maybe, like Kelly, you'll find it fun and interesting to experiment with being bald. Either way, you may discover that your feelings change. Try to stay open to your journey's twists and turns, and remember the mantra that applies to pretty much every aspect of your experience: This too shall pass.

good foundation. That helped us get through this. I never doubted him—even when I had no hair. I remember walking around the house in hats and scarves, and he said, 'I know you have no hair.'"

For Aquatia herself, though, losing her hair was more traumatic. "You learn a lot about yourself when you lose your hair," she says. "You realize your hair tells a lot about you."

"I had never bought a wig before. I still wanted to look cool going through all this. And I couldn't find a wig, and I was devastated. I remember doing this alone. I was on a street corner in Manhattan, looking through the yellow pages, trying to find a place that makes wigs. And when you walk in, you have to explain to the person why you need a wig, and I wasn't really comfortable at that point talking about what was going on."

"However," Aquatia says, "either luck or fate stepped in, because I found a woman and she was great. She loved my bald head. She made three wigs for me, and I looked beautiful in those wigs. I loved my wigs! I still have my wigs."

For Aquatia, the specially made wigs became a symbol of finding her own beauty, even during a difficult time. For Robyn Mitchell, diagnosed when she was a 30-year-old single mother living in Casper, Wyoming, the wig was a symbol of her gloomy prospects.

"There's only one picture of me with the wig," she says. "I didn't feel like myself. I didn't want pictures. I felt like used goods." Now Robyn is beginning the second year of a relationship, and she says, "There is hope out there. Don't think you're no good. There are men out there who will understand." But even though she is active with the American Cancer Society and the Young Survival Coalition, she still doesn't like to look at objects that remind her of her cancer—or her hair loss. "Once, my son and I were in the garage," she says, "and we found this fleece hat that I wore all the time during treatment. He said, 'Oh, I remember this hat. You wore this a lot.' I said, 'Yeah, but I'm not going to wear it any more.'"

For some young women who are going through breast cancer, hair loss and changes in body image can be devastating. But some women who feel enormous pain can eventually find a new relationship to their bodies and their hair. "I tell other women, we have a perspective and a self-love that others don't have," says Robyn. "And I know I have better hair than I had before!"

Dating and Meeting New People

For many young women with breast cancer, it seems way too daunting even to make a new friend, let alone to date or to begin an intimate sexual relationship. When Roberta met Lee, for example, she was 27 and had been diagnosed with cancer 6 months earlier. She'd already had a mastectomy and reconstructive surgery, and she had recently begun chemo. She had made a point of keeping up her social routine, but she wasn't interested in meeting anyone new.

The night Roberta first met her future husband, her chemotherapy treatment had been especially difficult. "I should have been at home in bed, rather than out in a bar," she recalls. But she'd agreed to meet her friend Russ, and Russ had brought along his friend Lee. Both Lee and the others who were there that night remember an instant attraction between the couple. But Roberta has no memory of the meeting.

"Lee and I must have talked—I don't really remember," she says. "All I wanted was to get home and go to the bathroom where I could get sick in the most dignified manner."

When Lee called the next day to ask Roberta out, Roberta was "completely baffled. Didn't he know that I had cancer? I couldn't date. I was damaged goods." Although Roberta told her friends that she was returning Lee's call only to avoid being rude to "Russ's friend," she actually found it a bit thrilling that someone could be attracted to her despite the cancer. "I didn't think I would ever go out with him, but I was excited about the prospect of flirting."

Roberta assumed that Lee knew all about her breast cancer, but, in fact, Russ had never mentioned it to him. "She had that special glow about her," Lee said later. "I just didn't know it was the chemo glow! But there was nothing, absolutely nothing, to indicate that there was anything wrong with her physically or mentally—with respect to the disease, with respect to worries. She put on a very normal face."

For her part, Roberta thought that her cancer was the most obvious thing about her. "You don't really think of yourself as a person," she comments. "You sort of think of yourself as a disease. And you forget that outside people still view you differently. You tend to read your concerns into what everyone thinks. You assume they feel sorry for you. You assume they're just trying to be nice. And it just astounded me, it was just such a bad point in my life that I just couldn't imagine that anyone would want to ask me out, or date me, or even really get to know me. It's like— it's more trouble than it's worth, why bother?"

Because Roberta seemed so vital and energetic, so unwilling to make any concessions to either the cancer or the chemo, Lee vastly underestimated the effect that the disease was having on Roberta's sense of herself. "She would bring a pillow to work, so if she was worn out by chemo, she could go to sleep under her desk," Lee recalls. "She would go out party-

Joy and Vasu Simha Met 5 Years after Joy's Diagnosis

Joy: *I'd always had body-image issues, and I had gone to a support group where I had met another woman who had learned to love her body by standing in front of the mirror and telling herself she was beautiful. So one day I decided I would test her exercise. Every day I would stand in front of the mirror and tell myself I was beautiful. At first, I didn't believe it. But slowly and gradually, I began to believe it.*

Then I took up sculpture. I took a lump of clay one day, and I created this image of my body. And I was like, "Oh, my God. That's really amazing." I don't have a right breast, and the model I made doesn't have a left breast. It's a mirror image.

I loved that piece, but I kept it hidden, because it was really personal for me. Then when I met Vasu, and I thought that he could be the man of my dreams, I decided that the sculpture was probably the best way to introduce him to what my body looked like. So I showed him the sculpture, and he said, "Looks good to me." So I knew it was fairly safe showing him my body for the first time.

Vasu: *I think early on, when we were just friends, she mentioned that because of cancer, she'd had a mastectomy. I didn't really know what a mastectomy was, how much of your breast it took off. I didn't know, but I didn't care. It didn't really bother me.*

Joy: *I could tell right away it didn't bother him. I could tell he would be fine seeing my body, and it let me feel safe. I knew that I would be safe. That he wouldn't run away and scream.*

ing, she would go out with friends." So when Roberta told Lee that she didn't want to be dating anyone, it came as a complete surprise: "It was a very different face than she showed in public."

Roberta was attracted to Lee, but from her point of view, dating was out of the question. To Roberta, cancer was a sign "written on her forehead" that marked her as unfit to date. But to Lee, the more time they spent together, the more Roberta's cancer was just one small part of a woman whom he had grown to love and found beautiful.

Today, Roberta notices a similar disjunction in other young cancer survivors. "You look at the women who have a little buildup or a little scar, and they'll be like, 'Everyone can see!'" she says. "If they wear a dress, they worry that the scar sticks out. And you look, and you're saying, 'Where?' And then, 'Oh, OK, yeah, it's there.' But if you're going through it, it sometimes seems like the whole world can tell."

Sex and Sexuality

When you consider how exhausting, frightening, and debilitating it is to have cancer, surgery, chemo, and radiation, it's not surprising that the experience leaves many young women feeling less sexual. Add to the mix an often dramatic shift in body image, the hormonal changes brought on by various treatments, and the effect of the experience on a sexual partner, and you can see why women find that their sexuality is affected by their breast cancer, at least for a while.

Dr. Schover points out that there are two aspects to sexuality: physical and emotional.

On the emotional level, she says, women may feel insecure about themselves and their bodies, and this can dampen their sexual desire and/or make them uncomfortable sexually with either old or new partners. To explore this issue, she and her colleagues surveyed breast cancer survivors who had had breast reconstruction (plastic surgery to replace a breast after a mastectomy), comparing them with women who had undergone breast conservation (lumpectomies that allowed women to retain most of their original breast).

"I was surprised at how similar the women in the two groups were," comments Dr. Schover. "The surgical technique used had very little bearing on sexual satisfaction after breast cancer."

What was important, Dr. Schover found, was the element of choice. "As long as a woman feels that she had some role in choosing her treatment, women with varying types of reconstruction and conservation adjust well sexually. We found that the only real difference between breast conservation and breast reconstruction was that women with reconstruction were less likely to enjoy breast caressing and were less likely to have that as part of their lovemaking routine." But, says Dr. Schover, "In terms of how often they had sex, and how satisfied they were, the groups were very similar. What we found—and this was replicated in larger studies—was that for young women, the real problem is chemotherapy."

Dr. Schover's observations were borne out by a study of breast cancer survivors in Los Angeles and Washington, D.C., that was published in the *Journal of Clinical Oncology*.[1] Although the mean age of the sample was 55.8 years, the women surveyed ranged from age 31 to age 88. Most of them were living with a partner, including a very small percentage (0.8 percent) who were living with a female partner. About 75 percent of the women in the study were white, 16 percent were African American, and the remainder were listed as "other."

Generally, the report found, the women were functioning well, and their sense of themselves, physically and sexually, was comparable to that of healthy women from the same age groups. However, the report also found a "greater risk of sexual dysfunction" among women under 50 who had undergone premature menopause, and among women who had received chemotherapy. The idea that sexual dysfunction can result from premature menopause and chemotherapy was further supported by a 1996 conference on Breast Cancer in Younger Women sponsored by the National Cancer Institute,[2] which identified breast cancer survivors under age 50 as "a particularly vulnerable group." The monograph discussing the study in Los Angeles and Washington, D.C., acknowledged that many women in the study had problems with their body image but pointed out that these were comparable to the anxieties felt by healthy women of the same age.

There is some good news here for younger women. First, permanent premature menopause is less likely to be a result of chemotherapy and other treatments for women in their twenties and early to middle thirties than it is for women who are already closer to menopause when they begin their treatment. Thus, the symptoms of hot flashes, night sweats, and vaginal dryness—which affect the sexuality of most women, whether they occur as part of a normal menopause or are the result of a medical treatment—are less likely to be permanent in younger women. (For more on fertility and premature menopause during treatment, see Chapter 9.)

Second, if the symptoms themselves are the problem, rather than generalized depression or low sexual interest, relieving the symptoms may help restore a woman's sexual feelings, especially as she recovers emotionally and physically from the traumas of surgery and treatment. This encouraging perspective is supported by the *Journal of Clinical Oncology's* findings of "low to average rates of depression" among breast cancer survivors and "good quality of marital/partner relationships." While the initial effects of cancer, surgery, and chemo or radiation mean that a woman's sexuality can be affected for a while, both her sexual feelings and her relationships have a good chance of eventually returning to normal. Moreover, the report found, "many women reported important positive aspects to their breast cancer experience":

> Throughout the open-ended questions in our survey booklet, many women wrote comments such as: "Many pluses have come about after the treatment and I consider myself a thriver, not a survivor . . . . The small amount of pain I have reminds me I'm fully alive and have two breasts, and am a lucky woman indeed"; "I feel the cancer experience made me take a deep soul-searching into my life and made me face things instead of just letting them continue as

usual. It has given me strength to do what I need to do," and "I am at a better place now and I like myself more now than ever before. Everything good has become acutely better and more appreciated. Everything trivial is not paid attention to. The focus of my life is now on what's good and important." These examples demonstrate the ability of these survivors to turn a serious and life-threatening situation into a positive force in their lives.[3]

However, the report also cited comments from somewhat younger women who had gone through premature menopause, including those of a 40-year-old divorced woman made 2 years after her mastectomy and chemo:

Due to the fact that chemotherapy put me into menopause, I find I have trouble becoming lubricated, have slightly less interest in sex, and experience some pain during and after intercourse. I'm also uncomfortable with my body and my partner seeing my scar and, therefore, find it harder to relax and enjoy sex.

A more detailed report of the same study, published in the *Journal of Clinical Oncology* in 1999, offered a more specific picture of the factors that help determine a woman's sexual health after breast cancer.[4] Not surprisingly, women who experienced vaginal dryness had less sexual interest, as did women with lower body images. Women who had found new sexual partners since their diagnosis or who had fostered better adjustments with their existing partners tended to have more sexual interest, as did women with better mental health in general and those who were premenopausal after treatment.

Interestingly, when the researchers evaluated women's experiences of sexual satisfaction, they found that the major reason for lack of satisfaction was not the woman's own sexuality but rather her partner's sexual problems. Having a good relationship with a partner seemed to be the most significant factor in being sexually satisfied. Having a new partner and experiencing greater mental health in general were also associated with more sexual satisfaction. Factors that didn't seem to matter included having had a mastectomy without reconstruction, having a low body image, or ceasing to menstruate. Women in these categories went on to enjoy just as much sexual satisfaction as their counterparts.

The report also found that women who had been sexually active before they were diagnosed with breast cancer tended overwhelmingly to continue their sexual activity after treatment; only 8.9 percent of women who had been sexually active when they were diagnosed were no longer sexually active at the time of the survey. The researchers concluded that the kinds of sex lives that women had before their breast cancer play a big part in the kinds of sexual activity that women enjoy afterward.

Although the study included few women in their thirties and no women in their twenties, its findings are at least somewhat validated by the stories that younger women tell. Women in strong partnerships, like Kelly, Leslie, Tracy, and Aquatia, had some rocky times, and so did their partners (see Chapter 6). Eventually, though, couples who had been happy before returned to satisfying sexual connections. And women like Joy and Roberta, who had been single when diagnosed, went on to form sexually satisfying relationships with new partners—relationships that both women actually found deeper and more meaningful than any that they'd known before their illness.

Yet it's important not to underestimate the difficulties that may arise along the road to eventual satisfaction. Both Cindy, whose relationship was threatened by cancer, and Leslie, whose marriage remained strong throughout, experienced significant interruptions in their sexuality. "I had no thoughts of sex," Cindy says. "I just wanted him to hug and kiss me." And Leslie's husband, Tony, said that often Leslie didn't want even that much physical contact. Despite her happier relationship with her partner, she might have echoed Cindy's comment: "My nickname is OUCH—because my whole body just hurts."

Loss of Sexual Sensation

Cindy and Leslie both experienced loss of sexual desire. But Francie Coulter, diagnosed with breast cancer just before her 37th birthday, had a different type of sexual problem: loss of sensation. "I could reach orgasm," she explains, "but it didn't feel like anything was happening. My body was numb. I couldn't believe it. I said, 'Oh, God, don't let this be what I'm left with.'"

For Francie, the problem was compounded by the fact that none of her doctors seemed comfortable talking about sexual issues. Nor had anyone warned her about the possibility of sexual problems.

"I know what the doctors are thinking," she says. "They're thinking, 'We're trying to keep you alive. Not having sex isn't exactly life-threatening—that's something you can worry about later.' Knowing that doctors have that attitude makes it even harder to talk about sex with them."

Francie's sense that doctors want to avoid discussing sex is supported by a 1996 article in *Cancer Nursing*. In a survey of 67 women questioned for the article, 82 percent said that they had never been asked about sexual issues by either a doctor or a nurse.[5]

Tips for Coping with Sexual Problems after Treatment

As we saw in Chapter 3, reducing the amount of estrogen in a woman's body is one approach to breast cancer treatment. However, both hormonal treatments and chemotherapy can produce the sexual symptoms that accompany low estrogen levels, including vaginal dryness and atrophy. Marisa Weiss, M.D., founder of Living Beyond Breast Cancer and www.breastcancer.org, offers these suggestions to women for regaining sexual pleasure.

- *Lubricants.* Sometimes you can experience sexual desire and even sexual pleasure, but lack of moisture in the vaginal area and vulva can keep you from enjoying intercourse. If penetration and intercourse become painful, it's easy to lose sexual interest altogether. Lubricating the vaginal area can overcome this problem, making sex generally more pleasurable.

- *Vaginal film.* This product sits inside your vagina, helping you retain your vaginal fluids. Unlike lubricants, which you use only during sex, vaginal film is used a few times a week on a regular basis.

- *Vaginal estrogen.* Doctors are reluctant to give breast cancer survivors estrogen treatments or hormone replacement therapy, for fear that estrogen will promote their breast cancer. But vaginal estrogen, taken as a suppository, seems to remain in the vagina; very little of it migrates into the bloodstream, where it might increase the risk of cancer.

- *Estring.* Another way of promoting vaginal estrogen is through this plastic ring, which sits in the vagina and releases estradiol—a form of estrogen—over a 3-month period. Again, releasing estrogen directly into the vagina seems to minimize the risk of the hormone's finding its way into the bloodstream.

- *Testosterone cream.* Testosterone—the male hormone—is crucial for women's sexual lives as well. Women seem to need a certain amount of testosterone in their systems to be able to achieve orgasm. Testosterone cream is usually applied to the inner arm or inner thigh, although it can be applied directly to the clitoris. Although no long-term studies have been done on how breast cancer survivors respond to testosterone, many women have been willing to risk possible detrimental effects to regain their sexual functioning. There is no commercially available version of testosterone cream, but many "compounding pharmacies" create their own products, which often include a version of this cream.

Fortunately, Francie did feel able to discuss the problem with her boyfriend, whom she'd been dating for a year. "We were wildly in love," she says. "When you've been together for only a year, you want everything to be perfect. And when you enter into cancer treatment, it can be very discouraging. I thought maybe we should take a hiatus and I should go through it by myself. But that wasn't realistic. And he was great. He was wonderful."

Still, Francie remembers, "I feel like I failed my partner. He didn't have any resources or anyone to talk to. I bought a book about breast cancer for him, but I never gave it to him. Because we were dating and not married, I wasn't sure what I could expect from him."

Francie found it especially frustrating that her problem was neither desire nor the ability to achieve orgasm, but simply the fact that her physical sensations were replaced by numbness. Eventually, her chemotherapy ended. "The feeling started to come back within 60 days," she recalls.

"Now I'm at the point where I even find humor in the situation. The most important thing," Francie says, "is for women to know what to expect. I think women should be prepared."

Finding Your Way

For young women with breast cancer, there are no easy answers to the changing questions of sexuality and body image. It's important to focus on the solutions that work for you. Having breast cancer will almost certainly bring profound and lasting changes to your sense of self and your body image, particularly if you have a mastectomy. But the stories of young survivors suggest that these changes can be positive as well as negative and that their ultimate outcome can have a lot to do with your confidence in your choices. What this means is that if your relationship to your body and your sexuality is not working for you, don't settle for less than full satisfaction. Reach out to your partner and your friends; find a support group; get counseling; or find your own unique ways to reconnect to your body and your sexuality: yoga, dance, meditation, massage, long walks in a beautiful environment. Give yourself time—but don't wait too long. Studies show that most sexual issues either were resolved within a year of treatment or else were never resolved. It can be challenging to reclaim your physical self after the trauma of breast cancer, but the stories of young women survivors suggest that the effort to rediscover your body and your sexuality is well worth it.

CHAPTER 8

"Do I Want Another Breast?"

The Pros and Cons of Reconstruction

Roberta Levy-Schwartz couldn't have been happier with her reconstructive surgery. "I do believe I have one of the most gorgeous plastic surgery jobs ever done," she says. Yet despite her pride and pleasure in the work of her plastic surgeon, Roberta, diagnosed with breast cancer at age 27, felt a great deal of anxiety the first time that she was intimate with Lee, the first man she dated after the surgery. "You're pretty sure that no matter how good it is, it's not good enough," she says. "It's not what it was before."

When Karen Sattaur first had her mastectomy, not only didn't she want reconstructive surgery, she wasn't even interested in a prosthesis. "It wasn't important to me," says Karen, who was diagnosed when she was 34 years old. Karen relates her initial lack of interest in a prosthesis to her preoccupation with her husband and two children. "I put my bathing suit on, and it was obvious that I was missing a breast," she recalls. "I would go to the pool and meet women—I was bald, too—and I'd talk to other women about how important it was for us to take care of ourselves. Of course, we didn't spend nearly enough time on that— maybe 5 minutes a month. We all spent our lives on our children and our husbands, and we put things for ourselves on the back burner." Eventually, though, Karen's feelings about forgoing the prosthesis changed. "It was very strange," she says. "Now I feel so weird without one."

Joy Simha had no ambivalence at all about not getting reconstructive surgery after her mastectomy, which she had when she was 26, single, and an avid kayaker. From Joy's point of view, she had already spent far too many hours away from the whitewater rapids that she loved. "I realized reconstruction didn't really fit in with my kayaking lifestyle," she explains. "It might jeopardize my ability to use certain muscles. I was just sick and tired of doctors, and sick and tired of treatments. For all the different reconstruction options, I learned what I would have to do to recover, and for me, I realized that if I'm going to take unpaid time off from my freelance work, I'm going to Europe, I'm going to kayak another river, I'm going to do something really fun. I'm not going to sit in a hospital! So for me, reconstruction has never been enough of a priority to make me want to go back to the hospital."

Prostheses and Reconstruction Methods: Assessing Your Options

Once you've worked out what type of surgery and treatment you're going to have, you're faced with another set of options: prostheses, breast implants, one of the many different types of flap reconstruction that are now available, or no cosmetic response to your surgery. Different choices are appropriate for different women—and, as Karen's story shows, the same woman may make different choices over time.

As with so many decisions about your breast cancer, there are two keys: knowledge and self-knowledge. You need to know all the different options that the science of plastic surgery now makes available. And you need to know yourself—what concerns you have about your appearance, your comfort, the time you spend in the hospital, and your recovery time.

Going without Prosthesis or Reconstruction

Some women choose not to disguise their mastectomies in any way. This is a rare choice, but it seems to work well for the women who make it, at least for a while. Those without prostheses, however, may find themselves feeling uncomfortable. Karen Sattaur, for example, says that 3 or 4 months after her mastectomy, she finally gave in and was fitted for a prosthesis. "It's just something I have to wear now," she says, although she adds, "I'd like to not feel like I have to wear it."

Karen compares her relationship to the prosthesis with how she felt about buying a wig to cover her baldness. "I was mortified that I was bald," she recalls. "I felt ashamed. I had so many negative feelings. I knew it wasn't my fault, but that didn't make me feel better."

Then one day she went to her chemo appointment wearing a wig and makeup "and trying to feel as good as I could. And a girl came and squatted down in front of me and said, 'Karen, that just doesn't look like you.' I thought, 'Screw you. It took me an hour this morning to get ready.' And then I really looked at myself, and I thought, 'She's exactly right.' I took the wig off, threw it in the closet, and never wore it again. If you can't look at me with a bald head, don't look at me."

For several months, it was important to Karen to affirm her sense of being complete "just as she was" by not wearing a wig and not getting a prosthesis. Eventually, of course, her hair grew back, and after a while she did get a prosthesis. Now she's considering reconstruction as well. For Karen, as for many women, responding to breast cancer was a long and complicated process, and different decisions were right at different times.

Prostheses

In most parts of the United States, you'll be offered a prosthesis while you're still in the hospital, either through the American Cancer Society's Reach to Recovery program or from a company that sells prostheses. You may keep this first prosthesis for a while—in theory, they last from 1 to 2 years—or you may want to explore other looks after you've been home for a few days. For example, some women whose remaining breast is relatively small find that if they wear loose-fitting clothing, they don't need a prosthesis. Others like to button up sweaters over another shirt. You may want to experiment with the clothes you have to find out how they fit you now. And, after trying out your old wardrobe with your new body, you may decide that you need a bigger, smaller, or differently shaped prosthesis than the first one you chose.

Prostheses, also known as breast forms, can be bought from medical supply houses, in lingerie stores, or through a mail-order catalogue; you can also have them custom-made. Your hospital or cancer center may also have a specialty store that sells prostheses. In theory, your insurance should pay for prostheses, but it's a good idea to check with your company to find out its policies. If you're on Medicare, you should be able to get a prosthesis every year or two, as long as your doctor writes you a prescription.

These days, prostheses are made with nipples. If the nipple on your prosthesis is not as prominent as the one on your real breast, you can buy a separate nipple to attach to it.

Some women get special swimming prostheses, but if you have a high-quality silicone breast form, it's probably already waterproof. "I coached

Joy Simha

When I decided not to have reconstruction, I did things a bit sloppily. I stuffed my shirt with cotton, and it was fine—well, no, actually it was horrible. I was in the hospital and they didn't have a prosthesis big enough for me. You know, they send you home with this foam falsie, but they didn't have anything big enough for me. The woman kind of gave me a bag of cotton and another falsie, and it was really awful.

My first follow-up appointment, I went to the breast surgeon and the scar was feeling fine. And she gave me a prescription for a prosthesis, and I went to the boutique, and there was a woman working in the boutique who spent a lot of time with me, having me try on all different sizes so I could see what I would look like. You know, no woman's breasts are symmetrical: You are always bigger on one side and lighter on the other. And so what's important when buying a prosthesis is what shape is comfortable for you and what size you need—and why should your false one be bigger than your real one? Why should you carry extra weight?

Wearing a prosthesis is not so bad. It's a little difficult when you go shopping for clothes. You know, a lot of clothes are really low-cut. And what you don't realize is that with the prosthesis, your cleavage starts higher than you think. But I never really wore a lot of low-cut clothing that showed a lot of cleavage before breast cancer . . . so there's no reason to start now!

a high school diving team," says Karen Sattaur. "The day I got my prosthesis, I dove into the pool, and by the time I came up, my prosthesis was down by my belly button. The kids fell over laughing. I said, 'Hey, kids, here's the deal: If you notice this happening, you need to let me know.'"

Prostheses are made in different sizes, both to accommodate different women's breasts and to match different types of operations. If you've had a wide excision, you can get a small filler—a shell that can be placed inside your bra. If you've had a simple mastectomy, you can find a slightly less full prosthesis; for a radical mastectomy, you can get a fuller form.

"The first one I got weighed about 50 pounds," says Karen Sattaur. "I thought, 'You have to be kidding me.' It was just the funniest thing. My kids would put it on their head and walk around. I walk in the door, take it off, and put it on the dryer. So kids in the neighborhood will ask, 'What's that?' My son Damon will say, 'My mom's breast.'"

Tips for Choosing a Prosthesis

- *Consider comfort as well as appearance.* Some women will find that a prosthesis that matches their remaining breast is too heavy for them. Check out the lightweight prostheses, which are also made of silicone but which weigh less than the standard prostheses. If you're an especially active woman, you might prefer a self-supporting prosthesis, which sticks directly to your skin and may feel more secure than a regular prosthesis, which simply rests inside your bra cup.

- *Choose the method of purchase that's most comfortable for you.* Some women prefer shopping by mail order to preserve their sense of privacy, but mail-order shopping makes it harder to try on a wide range of products. You might enjoy shopping at a boutique or fancy lingerie store, or you might find the fashionable atmosphere a painful reminder of your loss, especially soon after your surgery. You also have the option of shopping at a medical supply store; this may help you to focus on the prosthesis as a medical necessity, but some women find it depressing to associate their prostheses with wheelchairs and artificial limbs. Experiment with the approach that works best for you— and think about taking a friend, lover, or partner with you for moral support.

- *Be prepared for your feelings to change.* Many women who choose prostheses report moving on to reconstructive surgery after a few months or years. Other women make different choices with regard to their prostheses, coming to prefer comfort over appearance or seeking a sexier, more playful look than they were ready for at first. You'll need to replace your prosthesis every year or so anyway, so you can use each new occasion as an opportunity for experimenting with your options. And knowing that you'll have other chances to choose may make it easier to settle on an initial decision—after all, you can always change your mind!

Making Decisions about Reconstruction

Thanks to advances in plastic surgery, it's possible for women to have their breasts reconstructed after a full or partial mastectomy. Most women wait several weeks or months after their mastectomies to get reconstructive surgery, but the latest trend is to perform both the mastectomy and the reconstruction during the same operation. That way, the woman never has to be without breasts.

As women like Roberta can testify, it's possible to have reconstructions that look extremely natural and can barely be distinguished from real breasts. Yet despite their appearance, reconstructed breasts don't function the way real breasts do. You won't experience sensation in the reconstructed breast, and it may take time for you to accept it as an integral part of your body.

Women have various reactions to reconstruction. Many women feel that restoring their missing breast(s) enables them to go on with their lives. They report that they feel more "balanced" knowing that they have two breasts of relatively similar size. Many women find it reassuring to feel the familiar sensation of a breast beneath each arm. Certainly having reconstructed breasts makes it easier to buy bathing suits and other kinds of revealing clothes. And having two breasts means that you can throw on a T-shirt or a bathrobe, braless, without worrying about looking uneven.

On the other hand, some women feel that reconstructing a breast is a kind of denial. The reconstructed breast can never take the place of the real breast, and for some women its presence may be a reminder of their loss. Some women feel that they need time to mourn their lost breast(s) and that getting reconstructive surgery, especially during the same operation as the mastectomy, interferes with the mourning process. "I think I should have delayed reconstruction to come to terms with my mastectomy and then had reconstruction and come to terms with that," says Susan Kolevsohn, who was 22 when she was diagnosed with breast cancer.

Susan says that she had immediate breast reconstruction because she hadn't been told that she could have reconstructive surgery later. Now she has to deal not only with the loss of her real breasts, but also with the integration of two new breasts into her body image. "It's been very confusing," she says, "because they're not mine. And they never will be. I have to come to terms with that. I have to come to terms with the fact that I've had a mastectomy and now these things are there."

As Susan considers her experience with reconstruction, one theme keeps recurring: her lack of preparation for the process. "My doctor wanted me to wake up feeling whole," she says. "But that wasn't how it turned out. When I woke up, I was petrified. I couldn't feel my chest. No one told me it would be like that. I was hysterical. I thought I'd died. I said something to my gynecologist, and she said, 'What did you expect?'"

Susan also found that her reconstructed breasts didn't look the way she'd expected them to. "I was shocked when I saw the reconstruction," she says, "even though the plastic surgeon said, 'We'll fix it.' At that time, I was just blocking everything out emotionally. I was trying to be brave, concentrating on the practical stuff. I didn't have much of an emotional reaction—just, 'What are we going to do to fix this?'"

Now, 4 years after her operations, Susan feels that she is finally having the emotional responses she'd avoided at the time. "Sometimes I just feel really sad that it all happened," she says. "My mom's worried that I'm going to be depressed. There's mourning for the part of the body that I've lost. I didn't realize I'd have to mourn."

For Susan, being a young woman with breast cancer intensifies her sense of isolation and sorrow. "I'm not sad all the time like I was before," she says, "but every once in a while I'll think, 'No one else my age is like this.' And the loneliness comes back."

Another drawback of reconstruction is that it usually involves spending more time in the hospital. Even when the reconstruction is done during the same operation as the mastectomy, a woman may need to return to the hospital to have work done on her original breast, to help it match the reconstructed one. ("I've been talking to my reconstruction surgeon about ways to even me out a bit," says Tracy Pleva Hill, who is otherwise delighted with her reconstructive surgery.) And since having both operations at once is a relatively new development in plastic surgery, most women still don't have that option, especially if they live outside of a major metropolitan area.

"I consider reconstruction every single day," says Karen Sattaur. "But I want to wiggle my nose and have a breast appear. I don't want another surgery. I don't want to be in pain any more."

Nevertheless, Karen is strongly leaning toward the reconstruction. "It's important to my kids," she explains. "As weird as that may sound, my son wants to know when I'm going to get my breast back. I'm 36. If I were 80, I'd probably have the other one off."

But Karen doesn't just want reconstruction for her children's sake. She also expects plastic surgery to restore the figure she had before childbirth. "I was a cute little B before I had children," she says. "Now I'm a saggy C at best! I'm excited about getting my little B's back."

Unlike Susan Kolevsohn, Karen likes the idea of immediate reconstruction and says that the only reason she didn't have the dual surgery was that her cancer was so far along by the time she had her mastectomy. "If I'd had reconstruction right away, I could have had dimpling from the radiation and the chemo," she explains. "I didn't have 6 weeks to heal after surgery—I needed chemo immediately. So the doctors recommended no reconstruction, and I went along with it."

As Karen talks about her experience, she keeps returning to her wish to be done with medical treatments of all kinds. "I want to have it over," she says bluntly. "I'm tired of being hurt. Poked." Karen is also tired of the prosthesis, which, she points out, she's lived with for 2 years.

The Plastic Surgeon's View

Many plastic surgeons feel strongly that reconstruction can make an enormous difference in a woman's self-image and sense of well-being, and they recommend it highly. "I think for most women reconstruction is very important," says Carlin Vickery, M.D., who is in private practice in New York City. "Even for women who don't think it's important, who say, 'I don't want reconstruction; this isn't important to me.' Many women will come back to me later and say, 'I had no idea how important this would become to me.'"

Dr. Vickery points out that having a mastectomy without reconstruction serves as a constant reminder of cancer. "Every time you bathe, every time you turn around in the mirror, every time you go to get dressed, you have to think about the fact that you have breast cancer. You have no ease with which to dress. If you have one side with a breast and the other side flat, it's very difficult to find clothes that fit. Every blouse has to be carefully thought about, every bathing suit has to be carefully thought about. And that's just what the external world sees. When you dry yourself off in the mirror and you see a scar across your chest, it reminds you that you have cancer."

Edward Luce, M.D., agrees. Dr. Luce is the chief of plastic surgery at the University Hospital of Cleveland and president of the American Society of Plastic Surgeons. In his view, reconstruction is an extremely important part of helping young women recover from the psychological effects of breast cancer, especially, he says, "if reconstruction can be accomplished at the same time and in the same setting as the mastectomy."

Dr. Luce feels that young women may want breast reconstruction even more than older women, because they're still experimenting with their body image, seeking new partners if they're single, and holding themselves to higher standards for how they look. But ironically, because of their busy lives, young women may not have the extra few days they need for the highest quality reconstructive surgery. "I had a 33-year-old patient," he recalls. "She was part of a two-income family. And they had two girls, one 6, one 3. When we talked about reconstruction, she elected to have the most simple procedure because she could not take time away from her job and her family to get the more complex, albeit better, reconstruction."

Tips for Working with Your Plastic Surgeon

- *Be clear about what you want.* Many plastic surgeons are focused on helping women achieve a particular body image—and may assume that you want to look like a young, big-breasted woman with firm, upright breasts. If you want your surgeon to help you attain this image, that's terrific. But if you prefer being flat-chested, having smaller breasts, or going with a more natural look as you age, you may need to speak up. Be sure your plastic surgeon is sensitive to your needs, especially if you want something unconventional.

- *Be aware of your plastic surgeon's perspective—literally.* Your surgeon works on you when you're lying down, and so he or she sees you from above. Breasts that look right from this angle don't necessarily look the way you want them to when you're standing or sitting. So make sure that you and your surgeon have the same idea of the goals you're both striving for—before you go into the operating room.

- *Have realistic expectations.* Most of us have strong feelings about our breasts and the role they play in our body image. So getting a new breast or breasts can seem like a chance to construct breasts of the shape and size we've always wanted. Be aware, though, that the rest of your size, shape, and age will remain unchanged. While it may be exciting to fantasize about looking different, achieving a new body image, or recapturing a look from an earlier time in your life, you may want to think carefully about how much of that fantasy you want to (or can) turn into reality. Work with your surgeon to make cosmetic choices that go with the rest of your body, choices that you'll be happy to live with for a long time.

- *Be aware of your own emotions.* As Susan Kolevsohn, like many women, found, there is a certain amount of mourning that goes with losing a breast. Plastic surgeons, like most physicians, are naturally focused on the positive—what they can do for you, how they can help. That's their job—and they deserve gratitude for it—but no matter how beautiful your new breasts look, they won't be the same as your old breasts. Make sure you get the support you need to help you come to terms with this reality, and to help you make realistic decisions about your surgery.

Given the satisfaction that Dr. Luce sees among women who have had reconstruction, he finds it upsetting that only 15 percent of all women with mastectomies make that decision. "I think it's appalling," he says frankly. In Dr. Luce's view, young women who might benefit from breast reconstruction are being steered away from reconstructive surgery. And when they do get the surgery, he believes, they're urged to have simpler, less costly procedures. In part, he says, this may be because many physicians still aren't comfortable with the latest, most complicated reconstructive techniques. And, he says, "Not to take a cynical view, but it may also be because many insurance companies offer the same reimbursement for both simple and complex types of reconstruction." Under those circumstances, Dr. Luce believes, there might be a "natural temptation" for a doctor to recommend a less costly procedure.

"As a result," Dr. Luce says, "women without good insurance coverage tend to have an even lower reconstruction rate. But coverage for reconstruction is federally mandated. Insurance companies have to cover it." Insurance coverage for surgery on the unaffected breast is also federally mandated if it's needed to help the two breasts match. So Dr. Luce urges young women to look into all the reconstruction options that may be available before they make a decision, and to insist upon the choice that is best for them.

Like Dr. Vickery and Dr. Luce, J. Grant Thomson, M.D., also believes that reconstruction can be of crucial importance to a young woman's sense of comfort with herself. According to Dr. Thomson, an associate professor at the Yale School of Medicine and director of microsurgery in the plastic surgery section, "Studies indicate that breast reconstruction is important for the social well-being of women in general. But in my impression, it's even more important for younger women."

Dr. Luce relates how much reconstruction means to the young women he treats. "When women come in for their pre-op consultation, it's gloom and doom," he says. "Then I start talking about reconstruction and different methods, and you can see that as the consultation unfolds, there's a glimmer of hope sitting there."

Dr. Vickery reports a similar experience. "When my patients realize what reconstruction can mean to them, it's a wonderful feeling," she says. "You walk into the room and see their faces light up. That's really my measure of success—when I see patients smile. Many of my patients send me wedding invitations or birth announcements, and then I know I helped them get back to their lives."

However, at least one study contradicts the notion that reconstructive surgery plays a major role in breast cancer survivors' sense of well-being. A group of researchers led by Julia H. Rowland surveyed 1957 breast cancer survivors from two major metropolitan areas 1 to 5 years after their diagnosis.[1] "Earlier research has suggested that conservation or restitution of the breast might mitigate the negative effects of breast cancer on women's sexual well-being," write Rowland and her colleagues. However, they argue, this earlier research failed to compare women who underwent lumpectomies, women who had mastectomies, and women who had mastectomies plus reconstruction.

When Rowland and her colleagues compared these three groups of women, they discovered that the most important factor in a woman's response to breast cancer surgery was the type of surgery that she had. Women who had lumpectomies tended to feel better about their bodies and to see themselves as more attractive than women who had mastectomies, with or without reconstructive surgery. Yet after 1 year, even the type of surgery tended to matter less to a woman's quality of life than her age or her exposure to adjuvant therapy.

Although Rowland's study included some younger women, most of the women she surveyed were in their forties, fifties, and sixties, so it may be, as the plastic surgeons suggest, that reconstruction is more important to younger women. As with virtually all areas of breast cancer research, much more work remains to be done where young women are concerned. The lesson that you can draw from the Rowland study, however, is to listen to yourself and your own instincts. A plastic surgeon may refer to evidence that reconstructive surgery will make you feel better, and he or she may well be right. But take your time, think through what you want and need, and, if at all possible, find some other young (or middle-aged) survivors to talk to. Then make the decision that is right for you.

The Two Types of Reconstruction

There are two basic approaches to reconstruction: using implants and using materials from your own body (also known as flap reconstruction). Reconstruction with implants is a more established and better-known technique, and most plastic surgeons are comfortable with it. Flap reconstruction is a newer technique that is less well known among plastic surgeons, but it is considered to produce more natural-looking breasts. Implants take less hospital time and less recovery time; flap reconstruction is a longer, more involved process. Different types of potential side effects are associated with each technique. In both cases, there will be scars that will fade with time.

Pros and Cons of Reconstructive Surgery

Pros

- Your breasts will look more the way they did before.
- You may be able to go braless without worrying that your mastectomy will show.
- You have more clothing options.
- You may feel more comfortable showing a more "normal" looking body to an old or new sexual partner.
- Your bodily sensations—such as the feeling of having breasts under your arms—more closely resemble the way you felt before your mastectomy. (Although the sensation in your arm itself is likely to be the same as before surgery, you are unlikely to have any sensation in your new breast.)

Cons

- You have to undergo more surgery, with all the time, money, and physical discomfort that that involves.
- If only one breast is being reconstructed, you may want further surgery done on the natural breast, so that the two match.
- Having reconstructed breasts makes some women miss their original breasts more, not less.
- It may be disconcerting to have breasts that have very little physical or sexual sensation.
- You run the risk of getting breasts that don't look right to you, or breasts that look normal through bras and clothing, but not when you are naked.

Reconstruction with Implants

An implant is an artificial substance—either silicone or saline—enclosed in a silicone envelope. The procedure for both types of implants is the same: An implant is placed behind the pectoralis muscle on your chest, and the skin is sewn shut over it. Because the implant is behind the muscle, it can't give you a very large breast—only a bulge as it pushes the muscle out. Therefore, this technique tends to work better for either small-breasted women or women who have had double mastectomies and are happy with reconstructive surgery that gives them smaller breasts.

Getting implants put in during the same operation as your mastectomy won't add any extra time to your hospital stay (as opposed to other methods of reconstruction, to be discussed later in this chapter). If you have implants put in during a separate operation, that's done as outpatient surgery, and you can go home the same day. No matter which method you choose, you will have to return for a second operation to reconstruct the nipple and areola; this is performed with local anesthetic and does not require a hospital stay.

Breast Implants with Expanders

Although you might theoretically choose to have breast implants inserted after a mastectomy, in fact, your plastic surgeon will be far more likely to recommend a modification of this technique known as breast implants with expanders. According to Dr. Luce, "Using implants alone after mastectomy is very, very uncommon. The complication rate of this surgery is higher because the tissue is not ready to have the implant placed in there yet. I never, ever recommend it. With implants, I always recommend having the tissue expanders put in first." Indeed, says Dr. Luce, "I haven't put an implant in without an expander since the expanders were developed 20 years ago."

When you are getting implants plus expanders, an empty sack is inserted behind your pectoralis muscle, and, as in the ordinary implant procedure, the skin on top is sewn shut. The sack, however, contains a tube and a valve, enabling your doctor to inject saline into it over the next 3 to 6 months. As the saline expands your breast, the skin on top stretches. When you've got a breast of a size that pleases you, the sack is taken out and replaced with a permanent saline or silicone sack of the same size.

The advantages to this procedure are that you can find out what size you are comfortable with and you have a chance to stretch the skin and muscle gradually, enabling you to obtain a larger breast. The disadvantages are that the procedure takes time and can be uncomfortable. Your actual hospital stay, however, is no different from that with the regular implant procedure.

Kathy Burgau planned to have children after she recovered from breast cancer, and thought that she'd have reconstructive surgery after childbirth was over. But Kathy loved playing softball and doing other sports, so she "just wanted to be rid of that thing in my bra. It was always in my way." As a result, she had an expander put in, an option that posed less risk to her athletic activities than the more complicated flap procedures. "Before scheduling my surgery, I made sure it wouldn't interfere with a softball or volleyball game. And less than a month after the expander went in, I was back in action."

The Silicone Controversy

The use of silicone inside some breast implants, and for the envelope enclosing all types of implants, has become controversial. Silicone is a synthetic plastic made of silicon, oxygen, hydrogen, and carbon. In the early 1990s, women began to complain of health problems that they attributed to silicone-filled implants. In 1992, the FDA banned silicone-filled implants for most women on the grounds that the manufacturers of these devices had not provided enough information to demonstrate the implants' safety.

No conclusive studies had proven that implants were *not* safe. The public's perception, however, was that they were not, and numerous lawsuits were filed against various manufacturers. Without ever admitting that silicone implants were dangerous, three manufacturers agreed to a global settlement in 1994, setting up a $4.2 billion fund for women with implants who had developed serious autoimmunological diseases such as lupus and rheumatoid arthritis.

As a result of the controversy, silicone implants are restricted to certain groups of women, one of which is women who choose reconstruction after a mastectomy. Saline-filled implants are available without restriction.

Although there is no definitive word on the safety of silicone-filled implants, Dr. Susan Love, among others, is critical of the FDA's ban. "Despite the testimony of hundreds of women who attributed their health problems to the implants, recent studies have not been able to demonstrate a connection," she wrote in the 2000 edition of *Dr. Susan Love's Breast Book*. Implants may interfere with mammography in healthy women, and there is some concern that implants make it harder to detect a recurrence of cancer on the chest wall; however, such recurrence is rare.

So if you decide to get breast implants, you face a choice: silicone or saline. Remember that both types of implants use a silicone envelope, so in both cases, you're putting an artificial substance into your body and leaving it there for several years. (Other types of envelopes are currently being researched, but they too are made from artificial substances about which we have no long-term data.) If silicone implants leak, you're exposed to potentially dangerous silicone. If saline implants leak, you're exposed only to salt water.

However, when saline implants leak, they collapse completely, which means a second surgery. Silicone implants, on the other hand, become "encapsulated"—small, hard, and rocklike—when they collapse, through a process known as "capsular contracture." And some women find that even in their ideal state, silicone implants feel *too* hard and firm—particularly if they do not match a softer, sagging remaining breast.

Lanita Hausman, Diagnosed at Age 32

It took about a year to finish the whole reconstruction process. I remember sitting on the plastic surgeon's table and she was tattooing the nipples on—it was the last thing she had to do—and I had this great idea to get a real tattoo. And I said, "If a person decided to get a tattoo, would it hurt anything?"

She said, "You won't hurt anything I've done."

I said, "I've been thinking about getting a tattoo." My cancer was on the right side, and I wanted a pink ribbon tattooed above the breast. She thought that was a fabulous idea. She said, "You can make an appointment with the tattoo artist and come in here first, and I'll shoot you up and numb the area."

I was this little preppie living in New York City at the time. I had my walking shorts on, and my camel coat and my little leather briefcase and my little cardigan sweater, and my perfectly coifed bobbed hair. I went down to the East Village and rang the doorbell at this place—and at the top of the stairs this woman opens it and her hair's a quarter of an inch long, every imaginable place on her face is pierced, you can see tattoos on the exposed parts of her chest and arms. And she looks at me and says, "Can I help you?"

I said, "Yes, I'm here to get a tattoo." She was really neat because I told her why I was there, and she free-handed it and worked with me to get it the way I wanted. This summer I went back to the Village to have it touched up. It hurt a lot more because the nerve endings are starting to regenerate. She started, and I was like, "Whoo-hoo, this is tough."

I'm proud of it. It was the punctuation at the end of the sentence. I wanted to make an exclamation: I'm done, and this is my way of honoring that. I'm very proud of that.

YSC public relations codirector Jeannine Salamone, herself a young breast cancer survivor, comments, "Silicone implants are more lifelike and feel more natural to touch. Roberta [Levy-Schwartz] and I have talked about this. Her silicone implants are much more 'real' than my saline implants."

Dr. Luce, on the other hand, refuses to use silicone implants. "I use saline. Period," he says, stressing that his choice stems not from health concerns but because "I know that silicone implants have problems with hardness and capsular contracture. I don't feel much enthusiasm for them."

Drawbacks to Breast Implants

Breasts with implants tend to remain firm and hard. If you have two implants, you may find the total effect somewhat unnatural. If you're trying to match a remaining breast, you may find that while your remaining breast droops, sags, and changes shape with age, your silicone breast remains the same. This change may not be noticeable under your clothes, but it may be quite apparent when you're naked. For many women, this leads to having more surgery on the remaining breast, to help both breasts match. Some women who were comfortable not wearing a bra before find that they need to wear one so that their old breast can match their new, higher breast.

Any surgery brings the risk of postoperative infection. Breast implants make such infections more difficult to treat, and in some cases, an infection may necessitate having the implant removed.

Finally, implants don't last forever, and sometimes, once they're in, there are unforeseen problems that make replacement necessary. If you turn out to be a poor candidate for implants, you'll end up needing flap reconstruction anyway. And even if your implants do work well, some doctors estimate that they last only 12 to 15 years—which means that if you're in your twenties or thirties, you may need your implants replaced at least once or twice over the course of your life.

What the Plastic Surgeons Say

Many plastic surgeons recommend silicone implants for elderly women who aren't worried about the possible long-term effects of the silicone, who don't mind the fact that the implants last only 12 to 15 years, and who may be less concerned about how their bodies look in the nude. The procedure is also popular with younger women who have children at home and who are unwilling to sacrifice the 5 days plus extended recovery time needed for flap reconstruction. It is easy to locate plastic surgeons who are familiar with the implant procedure, but finding surgeons who are familiar with the alternatives, especially if you live outside a large metropolitan area, can be difficult. Also, your insurance company may favor the implant procedure, which is cheaper and requires a shorter hospital stay than flap reconstruction. However, plastic surgeons who are adept with flap reconstruction vastly prefer it to reconstruction with implants, because it produces more natural-looking breasts.

Both Dr. Luce and Dr. Thomson urge caution to women who are considering implants. They are concerned about capsular contracture, the possibility of contraction or collapse of silicone implants, especially for younger women, who will be living with the implants for a longer time.

**Pros and Cons of Breast Implants
(Compared to Other Reconstruction Methods)**

Pros

- They require a shorter hospital stay.
- The procedure is shorter, requiring less time on the operating table.
- The procedure is less expensive.
- It may be easier to find surgeons who are skilled in and comfortable with this method.
- Implants are less likely to affect shoulder muscles and other muscles than flap reconstruction—making it easier to continue with athletic activity.

Cons

- If there is postoperative infection, it is more difficult to treat.
- There is less chance of matching a remaining breast, and so more surgery may be required.
- There are possible long-term effects of having silicone inside your body.
- There may be problems with leaks and breast collapse.
- Implants may need to be replaced.
- Breasts with implants tend to look and feel less natural.

"The longer you have an implant, the more possibility there is for capsular contracture," says Dr. Thomson. Dr. Luce adds that while saline implants may also deflate, they can be replaced in a relatively simple outpatient procedure.

Clearly, if you are considering the implant method of reconstruction, you should discuss the procedure in detail with your plastic surgeon and get his or her estimate of how long your implants can be expected to last. You might also find out from your surgeon what is involved if replacement is necessary.

Flap Reconstruction

The newest form of breast reconstruction surgery, and the one that produces the most natural-looking breasts, is flap reconstruction, which uses material from the woman's own body to reconstruct a missing breast or breasts. In this procedure, the doctor creates a flap—skin, fat, and muscle—using tissue taken from another part of the body, such as the back or abdomen. Technically, tissue can also be taken from the buttocks, but according to Dr. Luce, "It's a method that has never had widespread acceptance because of the asymmetry and deformity of the buttocks that results."

There are a number of different types of flap surgery. In *pedicle flap reconstruction*, the tissue stays attached to the original site by its pedicle—the feeding artery and vein—so that the original blood supply can continue to feed the living tissue. The flap is tunneled beneath the skin to the chest while still attached to the pedicle, which may also include a nerve, providing some limited sensation in the newly constructed breast. The flap tissue either creates a small breast mound or is used as the pocket for an implant.

Free flap reconstruction involves the surgical removal of tissue from the abdomen, thighs, or buttocks. This tissue is then transplanted to the woman's chest. Through microsurgery, the blood vessels in the transplanted tissue are reconnected to the blood vessels in the breast region. This procedure is the most complicated of all the flap reconstruction techniques, as it requires the plastic surgeon to be experienced in microvascular surgery.

Both types of flap reconstruction are vastly more complicated than the simpler implant technique, and both types leave scars in two places: the location from which the tissue was removed and the newly reconstructed breast. The surgery also takes several hours longer than the implant.

The great advantage of flap reconstruction is that it produces a far more natural-looking breast that is made of flesh, not silicone. The breast created through flap reconstruction, while it will not have the internal sensation of a real breast, will feel "real" to the touch and will sag and droop the way a real breast does, making it more likely to match a natural breast. If flesh and tissue have been taken from the abdomen, in a so-called TRAM (transverse rectus abdominis muscle) flap, the procedure is like a tummy tuck, in which fat is taken from your midsection. In both an actual tummy tuck and a TRAM flap, you'll emerge from surgery with a flatter stomach area.

Both Dr. Luce and Dr. Thomson vastly prefer flap reconstruction to implants. "The use of a patient's own tissue is a preferable method of reconstruction—it's more natural-feeling and natural-looking," says Dr. Luce. "I would suspect that over the long haul, the patient's own tissue is more durable. That just makes intuitive sense."

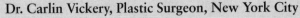

Dr. Carlin Vickery, Plastic Surgeon, New York City

If you're young, at some point you'll have to come to terms with the fact that no matter how good the breast reconstruction is—and I think we've made enormous strides over the past 20 years, our results are very natural—it is never going to be your original breast. The sensation will not be the same. And even though we have learned to do mastectomies through very small incisions, there will be some scarring, and portions of your breast will be reconstructed. So it may take you a period of time and a period of grieving before you integrate that into your body and introduce that into any intimate relationship you have.

There's no question that right now our feelings about our bodies, be they male or female, are hypercritical. So if you add to that the fact that you've now had a mastectomy and you have a reconstructed breast that is not perfect, no matter how good I make it, that can be a big mountain for you to climb, especially in urban centers, where there is a tremendous premium placed on physical appearance.

But if you do have reconstruction, in my experience, it gives you a terrific sense of well-being. We first make the breast mound, then later put on the nipple, and then get color on the nipple. And as this process continues, it's amazing to see how my patients are transformed. All of a sudden, they're coming in with a big broad smile. And after we do the nipple and the areola, they'll say, "I didn't think that was important, but I can't believe how great it looks." Having breast reconstruction means that you can get up in the morning and look in the mirror as you get dressed, and not have the first thing that screams out to you be "breast cancer." My patients tell me they feel "whole" again—that's the word that gets repeatedly used.

"My personal bias is that flaps are far superior esthetically," says Dr. Thomson. "I try to steer almost every patient toward flap reconstruction unless there's a contraindication."

Drawbacks of, and Contraindications to, Flap Reconstruction

Flap reconstruction is definitely a longer and more complicated procedure than implants, and this may be an obstacle for some surgeons and some women. Many surgeons are simply more comfortable with a shorter, simpler operation. Many have not mastered the microvascular surgical techniques required for this challenging procedure. For some women, there are medical reasons not to remain under anesthesia for the 6 to 8 hours that a flap reconstruction involves. And some women have had surgery in the place where the flap would normally come from, making it impossible to harvest tissue from that area. Finally, some women are simply too thin to allow for an easy harvesting of tissue from other parts of the body.

Cynthia Rubin, the YSC president, did eventually have a TRAM flap reconstruction, using fat from her stomach—but because she was so thin, she had to gain weight first. Susan Kolevsohn was also too thin for a TRAM flap, so she had the same operation with material taken from her thigh. Susan had the added concern of needing to have both breasts reconstructed because of her bilateral mastectomy.

"I had a thigh tissue flap, and I now realize that I was too thin at the time to have the reconstruction I did," Susan says. "There wasn't enough tissue to make a full breast, so my breasts ended up low on my chest, and flat. It was really weird. There were dents everywhere. On my thighs, too." The problem wasn't fixed even after a second surgery, and Susan also suffered from infection. She finally went to another surgeon, who used silicone implants to fix the dents in Susan's breasts and did as much as she could to fix Susan's thighs. "But she couldn't fix it completely," says Susan ruefully. "My thighs look different now. I have to wear loose-fitting pants. Now I'm left with a big dent on my thigh, so my legs look heavy. A lot of my body issues were complicated by that."

Dr. Thomson says that problems like the ones Susan had are relatively rare and that even for thin, athletic women, it's generally possible to find some tissue to harvest. "We can usually squeeze it out," he says. "We can usually make the belly really tight and use that tissue. I once had a patient who was a beauty pageant winner who had breast reconstruction—and we did a TRAM flap on her, taking tissue from her belly. She looked at the tummy tuck as an added benefit of going through this."

Pedicle Flap versus Free Flap Reconstruction

Pedicle flap reconstruction is easier than free flap reconstruction, and more surgeons are trained to do this procedure. However, for a pedicle flap, the plastic surgeon can use only tissue from an area that can easily reach the breast—the abdomen or the back, rather than the buttocks or thighs, which are also available with the free flap technique. Also, when the tissue is tunneled through the body in the pedicle flap procedure, a lot more of the body surface will be disturbed, possibly leading to more long-term complications. These complications are uncomfortable but rarely dangerous. You do run the risk, however, of losing some strength in your abdominal or back muscles. Some patients find that their ab-

Pros and Cons of Flap Reconstruction (Compared to Implants)

Pros

- Flap reconstruction tends to look and feel more natural.
- If you have one remaining breast, your reconstructed breast is more likely to resemble it, because it's made of your own tissue.
- Flap reconstruction will age similarly to the other breast.
- There is no danger of an implant's collapsing or contracting.
- Your own tissue may be more durable than any implant.
- No artificial materials are being put into your body.

Cons

- The surgery takes longer than the implant procedure.
- You will need a longer hospital stay and a longer recovery time than with implants.
- Fewer surgeons are comfortable and experienced with these procedures.
- For women without insurance, the procedure is more expensive than that for implants.
- There is scarring elsewhere on the body, in addition to the breast.
- Pedicle flap reconstruction may impair the strength of back or abdominal muscles and/or make the abdomen more sensitive.
- You will not be able to do any heavy lifting for at least 6 weeks—a consideration if you have young children at home or a job that requires lifting.

dominal area is extremely sensitive after this operation, so that they are unable to wear waistbands, or extremely weak, so that they have to wear panty girdles. Taking tissue from the back runs the risk of weakening your back and shoulder strength, which might interfere with your ability to engage in mountain climbing or competitive swimming. You may also need to have more physical therapy after pedicle flap procedures.

Plastic surgeons generally agree that the more active and athletic patients are, the lower their risk of losing muscle strength when this procedure is done. "I've had world-class tennis players come for TRAM flaps, and we've taken muscles from the lower abdomen," says Dr. Vickery. "And because we have refined those operations further and further, at

Roberta Levy-Schwartz

For me, perception was reality. And because you can see your breast and look down on it, you could say, "What if?" I just needed to know it was not there. So, I had a prophylactic mastectomy on the other side. Now I have two implants.

Before my breast cancer, everything about my body was the way God gave it to me. I think that once that changes, you're just scared. And I think Lee made that very easy for me. He just said, "What's the problem? I don't really understand. You're beautiful." I was beautiful no matter what. I'm still amazed that no matter what I do, he thinks I'm beautiful. It's just amazing. I think that's the best advice I could give any man dealing with breast cancer—just like you never tell a woman she's fat, she's always perfect. At the time, all I needed to hear was that it was perfect, and I was gorgeous, and I needed to hear it repeatedly, over and over, and in 68 different ways. I just needed to be reassured. It wasn't a big deal for him. Which is amazing.

The trepidation is that you're going to open your shirt or your world—and to a certain extent, your breasts become your world for about a year while you manage to get them healthy again—and that someone's going to cringe and say, "Look at that, oh, my God," and reel away from you, sort of like they did with the Elephant Man. And Lee just didn't. He just kind of went, "Okay, you're gorgeous. This is all you've been scared about? Let's move on, let's get married." I think it took me a while to get over that shock.

this juncture, we can do it with almost no muscle taken out. Patients can anticipate that they can go back and do exactly what they were doing beforehand." Indeed, says Dr. Vickery, if she didn't believe that patients could fully recover from flap reconstruction, she would not advocate the procedure.

Radiation and Reconstruction

Although it has been uncommon for young women who have received radiation therapy to then get reconstructive surgery, it is possible—and it's becoming far more common. Dr. Thomson recommends that women who want implants wait at least a month after radiation before they have reconstructive surgery. However, he personally recommends flap surgery rather than implants for women who have had radiation, since, as we have seen, implant surgery usually involves tissue expanders. "The problem with putting a tissue expander under irradiated skin," explains Dr.

Questions to Ask Your Plastic Surgeon about Reconstruction

- Am I a candidate for breast reconstruction?
- When can I have reconstruction done?
- What types of reconstruction are possible for me?
- What should I expect to pay for each option? What does my insurance cover?
- What type of reconstruction do you think is best for me? Why?
- How much experience do you have with this procedure?
- What results are realistic for me? Can I see a picture?
- Will there be scars? Where? How large?
- Will flap surgery cause any permanent changes where tissue was removed?
- How closely will the reconstructed breast match my remaining breast?
- How will my reconstructed breast feel to the touch?
- Will I have any sensation in my reconstructed breast?
- What possible complications should I know about?
- How much discomfort or pain will I feel?
- How long will I be in the hospital?
- How long is the recovery time?
- How will my activities be restricted after surgery, and for how long?
- How much help will I need at home to take care of my drain and wound?
- What do I do if I get swelling in my arm (lymphedema)?
- Do you have other patients who have had the same surgery that I can talk to?
- Will reconstruction interfere with chemotherapy?
- Will reconstruction interfere with radiation therapy?
- If I get implants, how long will they last?
- What kinds of changes to the breast can I expect over time?

Questions provided by the American Cancer Society and the National Cancer Institute.[2] See the Resource section for more information.

Thomson, "is that the radiation causes scarring of the skin and muscle of the chest wall, which makes the skin tight and hard to move."

An alternative method of reconstruction for women who have had radiation therapy, or for whom a TRAM flap cannot be used, is called the back tissue or latissimus dorsi flap; it uses muscle and skin from the upper back. Either the latissimus dorsi muscle alone or the muscle and its overlying skin can be transferred from the back to the front of the body to make a breast. Because the latissimus dorsi flap is smaller and thinner than the TRAM flap, this procedure almost always requires an implant to give the new breast the volume and shape it needs. When the back tissue is transferred, a pocket is created where an implant can be inserted during the same procedure. While this procedure may cause some cosmetic unevenness to the back, back strength and function are typically not affected. Jeannine Salamone had reconstruction with saline implants after her radiation therapy, although her surgeon warned her that the irradiated side of her breast would be much firmer than the unirradiated side and that the two sides wouldn't exactly match. However, says Jeannine, "I'm happy with the results."

Coping with Reconstruction

If you're like most patients who undergo reconstructive surgery, you'll come out of surgery feeling exhausted and in pain. After all, doctors have been working on your breast and another part of your body—abdomen, back, buttocks, or thighs—for several hours. You'll be given continuous pain medication through an IV that you can control with the push of a button. You'll spend the first 1 or 2 days in bed, using a catheter to urinate. On the third or fourth day, you'll be able to walk around a little, and by the fifth or sixth day, you'll be ready to leave the hospital. Your chest will feel numb, but the area from which tissue was taken will be quite painful. Most women have a second operation for touch-ups and to make a nipple, but this second round of surgery is far simpler, less exhausting, and less painful.

Doctors differ on whether you'll need physical therapy after a flap reconstruction and if so, how much, but most doctors prescribe physical therapy for typically 4 to 6 weeks, depending on the woman's previous physical condition and her goals for after the operation.

As we've seen, your responses to reconstruction may differ depending on whether you've had immediate reconstruction (getting your new breast rebuilt while the old one is being removed) or whether you've chosen to separate the two procedures. Certainly there is no time limit on reconstruction, although proponents of immediate reconstruction, like Dr. Thomson, point out that having the two operations at the same time

Cynthia Rubin, YSC President, Diagnosed at Age 36

Originally I didn't have enough fat to have a TRAM flap, so I was told I'd have to have an implant. So at the time of my mastectomy, I had a tissue expander put in. I knew I couldn't have the real implant until after radiation.

The tissue expander sat really high, and I felt like it was right under my chin. It looked like a baseball sitting in the middle of my chest. I had already gained about 5 or 6 pounds because of the steroids I was taking and because of the premature menopause caused by my treatment. So I asked the plastic surgeon how much more weight I needed to gain to get a TRAM flap. She said, "I try never to recommend gaining weight, but probably about 6 or 7 more pounds." Even then, there wasn't much tissue that they could take for the reconstructed breast, so I ended up having a small reduction on the other side to make my two breasts match. And I'm so happy with my results.

A year and a half went by from mastectomy to reconstruction. It's a very difficult thing to go back a year and a half later and have major surgery. And since I got a free flap, it was 7 hours worth of surgery. I kept thinking, "This is vanity." There were all these really cute plastic surgery residents at the hospital, and they would come and look at my breasts every day. They were younger than me, and I would tease them. I asked them, "Do you think this is a crazy thing to do?" They didn't know what to say. I said, "You're going to be plastic surgeons soon; you have to figure out an answer to that question."

I remember feeling that I was being a bad feminist, thinking that I was vain. Breasts shouldn't be important to me—the liberated, modern woman that I am. It's like a face lift, it's purely cosmetic. And you find yourself asking, "What is femininity?" We shouldn't be defining whether we are feminine by our breasts. I've never been a girlie girl—I've never been into hair and makeup, and here I am having 7 hours worth of surgery to have a breast. And I'm thinking, "I am so shallow." But psychologically I felt like something was taken from me. And I wanted it back.

means that surgeons do not have to deal with scar tissue in the breast area, which makes reconstruction easier and sometimes more attractive.

In Dr. Vickery's opinion, one of the most important factors in coping with reconstruction is—as with many aspects of breast cancer—your support system. "The people who have good support are going to have an easier time," she comments. In fact, Dr. Vickery recommends support

Tips for Making Decisions about Reconstructive Surgery

- *Find out everything you can.* Check out the Resources section. Read *Dr. Susan Love's Breast Book.* Talk to your plastic surgeon—and to one or two others, if you're concerned about getting a broader picture. If at all possible, talk with women who have had the various procedures, and find out what worked—and didn't work—for them. It can feel overwhelming to research reconstructive surgery when you have so many other medical decisions to make and procedures to cope with. But knowledge is power, and when you know your options, you're far more likely to make a decision that you'll be happy with now and in the future.

- *See for yourself.* Ask your surgeon to show you pictures of different types of reconstruction. And, if you can, ask women who have had the procedures to show you the results. "In the YSC, we often show our various types of reconstruction to newly diagnosed women trying to make decisions," says YSC president Cynthia Rubin. "Asking survivors for a 'show and tell' is really helpful."

- *Mobilize your support system.* Many women expect that the time they will most need support is during the initial diagnosis and treatment. But the reconstruction process also requires a support network, both to support you in your decision and to help you recover from any surgery you decide to have. If you feel your friends and family are looking for concrete, useful ways to offer their support, you might ask them to help you research your surgical options, and then discuss your choices with them. A support group, particularly one of young women, will also help you both make good decisions and cope with the results of your choices.

groups even to patients who come in with great support networks. "Even if women have a family, it's good to hook up with someone who has been down the road," she says. "It is hard for family members and other close friends to hear about it all the time, but you may have a need to go over it. And you don't want to wear out the people who are closest to you."

Making Your Decision

As we've seen throughout this chapter, deciding what kind of reconstructive surgery you want—or even whether you want it at all—is a complicated decision. In his book *The Breast Cancer Wars: Hope, Fears, and the Pursuit of a Cure in Twentieth-Century America,* Barron H. Lerner, M.D., explores the decades of feminist debate over reconstruction options. One of the most passionate voices in this debate was that of author and activist Audre Lorde, who chronicled her encounter with breast cancer in *The Cancer Journals* in 1980. Lorde, who was diagnosed with breast cancer in 1978 at age 44, resented the implication that her goals should be to conceal the absence that was once her breast, to make herself attractive to men, and to participate in the socially imposed silence around breast cancer. In Lorde's words, she opposed "the path of prosthesis, or silence and invisibility, the woman who wishes to be 'the same as before.'"[3]

A similar attitude was expressed by Deena Metzger, a writer and spiritual healer who was diagnosed with breast cancer in 1977. A famous photograph of Metzger, nude from the waist up, arms outstretched, face turned joyously up to the sun, graphically reveals the difference between Metzger's full breast and the flattened area marked by a mastectomy scar. The photo was reproduced in many feminist publications, including *Our Bodies, Ourselves* and *Her Soul Beneath the Bone*, a book of poetry on breast cancer.[4] Metzger's gesture was echoed in a 1993 photograph that appeared in the *New York Times Magazine*, in which supermodel Matuschka (diagnosed at age 37) revealed her mastectomy scar.[5]

Perhaps the value of listening to these other voices is simply to remember that you have lots of choices—and that some of your choices are not necessarily permanent. Diagnosed with breast cancer at age 26, Joy Simha chose not to have reconstruction because "for me reconstruction has never been enough of a priority to make me want to go to the hospital." Today she's a nursing mother who is less concerned than ever with replacing her missing breast. Yet she is most comfortable thinking of her decision as part of a process—a process that very easily might have gone differently and may yet be transformed:

"If I had decided to have the mastectomy right away and done all the reconstruction research, I probably would have had the reconstruction. I might have had two matching perky breasts. I might have been a supermodel today! But at the time, it wasn't the issue I needed to deal with, so I didn't deal with it. Because, you know, every decision you make, you make at your own comfort level, and for me, that was my comfort level. I don't know what it's going to lead to. In 5 or 10 years, I might still decide to have reconstruction. We'll see what happens."

So, as you make your decisions, trust yourself and go at your own pace. Remember: There's no time limit on reconstructive surgery. You can have it any time, at any point. And even if you get implants, you can always have them removed and undergo the more elaborate reconstructive procedures. It's your body. Make your choices according to the values and the timetable that are right for you.

CHAPTER 9

"This Is My Miracle Baby"

Dealing with Fertility, Pregnancy, and Breast-Feeding

Kathy Burgau had been married for 3 years when she was diagnosed with breast cancer at age 26. "We were supposed to have a baby and in the spring build a house," Kathy explains. "I finally met with the oncologist in December. He asked, 'Do you want children?' My husband is the youngest of fourteen, and I'm the youngest of five. Both our mothers are from families of ten. So, yes, we wanted children!" Because women getting chemotherapy run the risk of infertility, Kathy went through an elaborate and expensive fertility procedure to enable her to freeze several embryos before she started treatment—a procedure that had to be carefully monitored to make sure it wouldn't promote her breast cancer. "I had the last fertility procedure on a Monday," Kathy recalls. "Friday I was supposed to start chemo. I had to go through a bone scan again to make sure my cancer hadn't spread because of the estrogen they had given me." Five years later, Kathy's cancer has not recurred, and she and her husband have finally built their house. "The baby is next!" Kathy says. "We're still looking at the spring."

When Joy Simha was diagnosed with breast cancer, having children was the least of her concerns. "I think having children was mentioned very briefly," Joy says. "But having kids was not a priority because I was single. I was 26 years old. I had always said that if I met the man of my dreams and fell in love with him and could not live without finding out what our children would be like, then I would have children. But if I

209

never met him, and I just was living my own life, and was happy to be alive and healthy, and children weren't in the cards, then that would be OK, too."

~~~

In addition to her breast cancer, Roberta Levy-Schwartz had a rare medical condition that might have made pregnancy very risky for her. "It's really funny when you call a gynecologist to schedule a prenatal visit, and they say, 'Are you high risk?'" says Roberta. "And what they mean is, 'Are you a high-risk pregnancy? Have you had miscarriages? I'm not a high-risk pregnancy, but I am a high-risk person!" Yet despite her cancer and a host of other possible complications, Roberta was able to become pregnant and give birth to Rena, her daughter. "I still wake up thinking, 'This is not possible,'" she says. "I still have to see the rattle next to my bed to realize that I did have a child. A lot of people come up to me and say that Rena is a miracle and that it's incredible that this is possible. I don't know if Rena is a miracle, but I know that it's incredibly special that I'm sitting here today. Hundreds of women with breast cancer tell me that they are Rena's aunt. I feel like I have hundreds and hundreds of godparents for this child. It seems that Rena, in her 3 months, has touched them more than anyone in their lives. That Rena has inspired them to go on to the next place that they can be. I guess that is a miracle."

Coping with the Challenges: Breast Cancer Survivors and Motherhood

Young women with breast cancer differ from older women in lots of ways, including their relationship to fertility, pregnancy, and child-rearing. If you want to become pregnant, you may wonder how tamoxifen and chemotherapy will affect your fertility. You may also be worried about the possibility that the pregnancy will make your cancer worse, that you'll pass on the "breast cancer gene" to your daughter, or that you might not live to see your child grow up. And if you choose not to have children—or have discovered that you can't—you may find yourself struggling with the consequences of that reality.

These already complex issues become even harder to deal with when you discover how hard it is to get information about them. Because such a small percentage of breast cancer survivors are young women, very few studies have addressed these issues, and the studies that do exist tend to be unreliable. The collective wisdom of women survivors can also be hard to come by: Existing support groups tend to focus on older women, who are at the end, not the beginning, of their childbearing years.

Sometimes doctors simply don't have the answers. Dr. Jeanne Petrek of Memorial Sloan-Kettering Cancer Center in New York City is currently engaged in an extensive study of the effects of pregnancy on breast cancer survivors. In fact, she's one of the nation's experts on the subject. Yet even she is at a loss when her patients ask her for guidance.

"When a woman asks me if I am certain that it's safe to get pregnant after breast cancer treatment, I tell her I don't know," Dr. Petrek says frankly. "And that's what I have to say to be honest. If a woman asks me if she can use hair dye, I can tell her, 'It's been studied. They didn't find any risk of recurrence. Period.' So some trivial issues have been put to rest. But the important issues have not."

Sometimes young women simply don't know what questions to ask. "I ended up taking a type of chemotherapy that was more dangerous for my ovaries," says Joy. "I didn't even know to ask if there was a chemotherapy that could be less detrimental to my fertility. The main focus of the doctors was putting me through the least invasive treatment. But perhaps it would have been a better concern to pay attention to my fertility."

In Joy's case, everything turned out fine: When she was 33, she gave birth to a healthy baby boy, whom she was even able to breast-feed with her one remaining breast. But Joy is painfully aware that her doctors were not concerned about her fertility—largely, she thinks, because they were used to dealing with older women.

Coping with your relationship to fertility, pregnancy, and childbearing can be difficult anytime in life. Dealing with these issues when you have breast cancer can sometimes seem overwhelming. The first step, though, is finding out what the medical community does and doesn't know.

Preserving Your Fertility

Kutluk Oktay, M.D., is one of the nation's leading experts on fertility and breast cancer. A reproductive endocrinologist at Cornell University's Weill Medical College, he has helped many young breast cancer survivors conceive.

"Fertility is immensely important," says Dr. Oktay. "I've had many patients tell me that they were more upset to hear that they would not be able to have children than to hear that they might die from cancer."

Dr. Oktay began his research when he noticed a serious gap in existing medical knowledge. The field of oncology focused on cancer patients, and fertility medicine dealt with fertility issues in healthy adults. But virtually no work had been done on the fertility issues specific to young women with cancer.

Dr. Oktay has worked on two new procedures that may enable young breast cancer survivors to preserve their childbearing capacity. To understand why these procedures are necessary and how they work, let's start with a closer look at the threats to fertility posed by standard breast cancer treatments.

Fertility and Chemotherapy

Every woman is born with a fixed number of eggs, which are stored in the ovaries. Once she enters puberty, a hormonal signal is set off each month, directing the ovaries to release a single egg. If the egg is fertilized, she gets pregnant; if it is not, she menstruates. When her ovaries run out of eggs—usually in the late forties or early fifties—a woman goes into menopause.

But chemotherapy, which is designed to target rapidly growing cancer cells in the body, can also trigger a kind of "self-destruct" mechanism in a woman's eggs. If too many eggs are destroyed, a woman's body may "understand" that she has gone into menopause. Her ovaries stop functioning, and menopausal symptoms—hot flashes, fatigue, mood swings—may result. The woman also loses her childbearing capacity.

The younger a woman is, the more eggs she still has stored in her ovaries, so this kind of premature menopause is far less likely in younger women. The dangers to fertility are more significant for women over 35, and still more significant for women over 45, who are only a few years

---

Aquatia Owens

No one tells you that you can't have a child. But it's scary. I went to a breast cancer conference last month and attended the session on fertility. There were women there who were pregnant. But I've been taking tamoxifen for 5 years, and they don't have any results on people who've been doing that. I finished tamoxifen a couple of months ago, so now I'm asking myself, "Do I want to risk my life to have a child?" My husband, Jim, was adopted, and we are open to adopting, but I think I'd like to try to have my own child. But I'm scared. Before I try to get pregnant, I need to find someone who knows more about tamoxifen and what kind of danger I may be putting myself in. The whole point of the tamoxifen was to block the estrogen in my body, and I know getting pregnant is going to make my estrogen levels go high. Is that something I should do? I don't know.

away from menopause anyway. However, some younger women, particularly those with preexisting fertility issues, may also undergo permanent or temporary menopause or develop other kinds of fertility problems as a result of the chemotherapy.

Not all types of chemotherapy affect fertility in the same way. And, as Joy found, doctors who are used to treating older women may not even think of preserving fertility as a primary goal. Not nearly enough research has been done on the long-term effects of chemotherapy on fertility, and new chemo regimens are being developed all the time. So if preserving fertility is a concern for you, discuss this issue with your doctor.

Fertility and Tamoxifen

Another common treatment for breast cancer is tamoxifen, which has a kind of paradoxical hormonal effect that isn't yet fully understood. To understand what we do know about tamoxifen, we have to start with a closer look at estrogen.

Estrogen is the female hormone that signals our bodies to fulfill their female functions. This female hormone gives us our secondary sex characteristics—breasts and pubic hair—and it has a profound effect on our bodies generally, including our genitals, skin, hair, blood vessels, bones, and pelvic muscles. Estrogen also plays a big part in the female monthly cycle. When we're ovulating, estrogen causes our uterine and vaginal linings to thicken, preparing them to receive a fertilized egg so that a pregnancy can proceed. And when a pregnancy does occur, estrogen signals our bodies to stop ovulating, which is why estrogen and estrogenlike substances have been used in oral contraception.

Tamoxifen is one of those estrogenlike substances; indeed, it was originally used as a birth-control drug in England. When tamoxifen was first thought of as a treatment for breast cancer, researchers believed that it worked by blocking the effects of the body's natural estrogen. They thought that the body's own estrogen promoted breast cancer, whereas tamoxifen—an "imitation estrogen"—did not. Tamoxifen, they believed, took over the body's estrogen-receptor sites—the chemical places where estrogen needed to "land" in order to be effective. With tamoxifen taking up most of the receptor sites, the body's own estrogen had nowhere to go, so it simply passed out of the bloodstream into the urine and was expelled from the body.

Now researchers understand that it's not that simple. The body doesn't have just one type of estrogen-receptor site; it has two, known as "estrogen receptor alpha" and "estrogen receptor beta." So there are three ways in which estrogen can affect us: It can act on our alpha

213

Randi Rosenberg, Diagnosed at Age 32

When my chemotherapy was over, my oncologist and I really struggled with whether I should get tamoxifen. We really didn't know what the long-term effects were. We didn't know what the efficacy was in younger women. So we really struggled with whether this was going to be the appropriate treatment for me. I was also concerned about fertility issues—keeping in mind that when I was diagnosed, I was 32. When I finished treatment, I was 33. By the time I would finish the 5-year course of tamoxifen, I would be 38 years old.

I was not happy about the fact that the choice of whether to have children might not be mine to make. The fact that this drug and this disease would dictate to me whether or not children were in my future was a very frustrating and very scary proposition to me when I was making that decision.

But tamoxifen has such a good efficacy rate that my oncologist really felt it was in my best interest to try it, and we could make the decision 2 years out, 3 years out. If we wanted to start a family, we could think about suspending treatment.

Meanwhile, I derived a great deal of hope from the fact that both Joy and Roberta were going through pregnancies at the same time. That was such a monumental thing. It represented happiness. It represented life. It proved that there is most definitely life after breast cancer. It really offered so much hope to the rest of us that it can be done.

receptors, on our beta receptors, or on both. These sites are located throughout the body in different combinations. That's why estrogen affects so many parts of the body in such widely different ways, causing cells to grow in some organs while inhibiting cell growth in others.

Tamoxifen also has widely differing effects on various body parts. In some organs, tamoxifen blocks the effects of estrogen. In other organs, it heightens that effect. Although scientists don't fully understand all the ways in which tamoxifen operates, it seems to block estrogen from causing breast-cell growth, thus inhibiting breast cancer. But it also blocks the estrogen receptors in the brain, fooling the brain into thinking that the body doesn't have enough estrogen and causing the brain to send out signals to make more. Thus tamoxifen stimulates excessive estrogen production, which in turn stimulates—and in some cases overstimulates—ovulation.

As a result, if you take tamoxifen for a long enough time, you become dependent on it. As with most oral contraceptives, you may have trouble regaining your own natural cycle after you stop taking the medication. Usually this loss of fertility is only temporary, and normal ovulation resumes soon after tamoxifen treatments stop. But in some cases, 3 to 5 years of tamoxifen treatment can seriously compromise the body's ability to ovulate, especially if the woman has also lost numerous eggs during chemotherapy. Doctors refer to chemotherapy as an "insult" to the ovaries. Tamoxifen can magnify that insult.

Fertility Procedures

We might think that a woman whose fertility is compromised by chemo and tamoxifen could simply undergo one of the many fertility procedures that are now available. The most common procedure, and the model for most of the rest, is the procedure known as in vitro fertilization, or IVF. In IVF, the woman is usually given hormones to regulate her cycle and increase the number of eggs she releases. (Remember, in a normal cycle, the woman releases only a single egg each month.) The harvested eggs are combined with sperm in a petri dish (a small glass dish) to form embryos—the beginnings of life. Of course, not all eggs will be successfully fertilized. But doctors hope that out of the many eggs they have harvested, they can create several embryos.

Two or three of these embryos are then reinserted into the woman's womb, where, it is hoped, at least one of them will attach. (If more than one attaches, the woman will become pregnant with twins or triplets.) If the pregnancy doesn't take, another set of embryos can be reinserted the following month, and this can continue until either the doctor runs out of embryos or the woman gets pregnant. Embryos can also be frozen and reinserted at a later point—currently, up to 7 years after they are created.

In theory, then, a woman who was about to undergo chemotherapy could undergo IVF and then freeze the embryos, planning to reinsert them several years later, after the chemotherapy and tamoxifen treatments had ended. That way, even if the chemo destroyed many eggs and the tamoxifen impeded ovulation, a woman might still be able become pregnant. However, IVF is an uncertain procedure with widely varying success rates, though most specialists believe that between one-third and one-half of all women under 35 who attempt IVF can expect an ongoing pregnancy that results in a live birth. And both IVF and most other current fertility procedures (whose success rates are even lower) involve giving the woman heavy doses of estrogen.

Kathy Burgau, Diagnosed at Age 26

When I got diagnosed, my oncologist worked with a fertility specialist all weekend to figure out what they could do without raising my estrogen levels. The fertility doctor said he could do the in vitro. I could start the drugs immediately because I had just started my period. It was going to cost $10,000. They taught me how to give myself the hormone shots. We left the hospital and we had to pick up medicine. One bottle was $290.

On the way home, Perry, my husband, wouldn't talk to me. I started crying. He said, "Why are you crying?" I said, "We can't afford it." He said, "Quit crying." I said, "Well, they told me I have cancer. Now I can't have children." He said, "I don't care what we have to do. We'll live in this apartment the rest of our lives. I'll sell the pick-up, I'll sell the sleds—I want us to have a family." So I gave myself the shot.

I was injecting myself with a medicine called Lupron. What the Lupron does is, it takes control of your hormones, so you cycle when it wants you to. I got my period right after Christmas. Then I had to start Metrodin. I had to give myself three shots of Metrodin a day, $50 a shot. For 10 days. So, $150 a day. Insurance would not cover it. Everyone wrote letters—my doctors, me, my work—saying that my disease was taking my fertility away, but the insurance wouldn't pay.

I got an estradiol check every day. They'd check my blood. Every 200 points is an egg. They wanted to see how high I'd get. That was 1997, the worst snowfall Minnesota has had. The doctor was up in Fargo, about an hour's drive away from where we were. So we got stuck in Fargo many times, trying to get up there through the snowstorms. On Friday, they'd check my estradiol—it was 2000, so I had, like, 10 eggs. That weekend we stayed at my brother's because we were worried about the snowstorm. It was almost like I had morning sickness, my ovaries were so big. Sunday night, Perry gave me a shot of another med—it makes your eggs break loose so they're floating, like letting loose to go into the uterus. The shot was in my butt. Because he didn't hit a vein, he had to do it again. The little shit!

They did my estradiol the next day, and it was up to 5400, so I had 27 eggs. That's the highest they've ever had. They called me "Fertile Myrtle"! They do a vaginal ultrasound and then they go in with a needle, and the needle goes through your body and into the ovary, and back out of the ovary. They squirt fluid in and that loosens the eggs, and then they suck the eggs out through the needle.

> *They got 27 eggs. Of those, 24 were good. When they put Perry's sperm with it, 18 took.*
>
> *I had been on the pill for 10 years. And here to have 18 embryos take, they were like, "Oh, my God." Out of all the procedures, that was the most painful!*
>
> *But now, 5 years later, I'm about to quit tamoxifen, and we've got our house. So this spring, I'm going to try to get pregnant.*

Estrogen helps doctors control the woman's ovulation cycle so that they can plan when to harvest her eggs. It also stimulates excessive ovulation. In fertility procedures, working with the normal one egg at a time is considered far too slow. Harvesting eggs from a woman's body is painful, time-consuming, and expensive, so doctors don't want to do it more often than they have to. And for the woman who is about to undergo chemotherapy, it's particularly important to harvest multiple eggs, since this may be her last chance to ovulate. Yet the estrogen given to a breast cancer survivor to stimulate hyperovulation might also promote the young woman's breast cancer.

Studies of cancer incidence following infertility treatment are contradictory for general populations and virtually nonexistent for breast cancer patients. One study involving nearly 30,000 women found higher incidence than expected for breast and uterine cancer within 12 months of exposure to fertility drugs with IVF. Overall incidence of cancer, however, was normal.[1] Another study of approximately 5500 women in England found no link between ovarian stimulation and increased breast cancer risk.[2]

IVF and other fertility procedures can be exhausting, uncomfortable, and sometimes painful as the excess hormones play havoc with the body, mind, and emotions. In addition, for breast cancer survivors, unlike healthy women who have IVF, there is the tension of knowing that this procedure is a one-shot deal. Eggs are usually harvested sometime between the woman's operation and her commencement of radiation or chemotherapy, with the woman painfully aware that this may be her last chance to conceive.

Some women, like Kathy Burgau, feel so strongly about preserving their ability to have children that they're willing to go through the whole process. Kathy's IVF procedure, conducted in 1997, involved a complicated set of hormone treatments designed to minimize her exposure to estrogen. Still, Kathy and her doctors understood that the fertility procedure had a massive effect on Kathy's hormones and posed at least some risk to her life.

New Fertility Procedures

As we've seen, IVF poses lots of problems for breast cancer survivors. Moreover, IVF relies upon the creation of embryos—fertilized eggs. Although embryos and sperm have been successfully frozen, unfertilized eggs are far more difficult to freeze. Therefore, women without partners have to either find a sperm donor or risk being unable to preserve their genetic material.

However, two recently developed procedures offer new options for breast cancer survivors. One is to remove ovarian tissue and freeze it, thus keeping it safe from the effects of the chemo, and then reinsert it into the body when the cycle of chemotherapy is over. This procedure involves minor surgery. The patient is put under general anesthesia, and a laparoscope—a long, thin device—is inserted through the patient's navel. The laparoscope enables the doctor to see the woman's ovaries without making a large incision; instead, tissue can be harvested through small incisions made along the bikini line. The whole procedure takes about an hour, and the woman can usually go home a few hours later.

A second, simpler procedure developed by Dr. Oktay is proving successful. He removes the woman's ovary, cuts it into little pieces, and then returns it to the body immediately by inserting the pieces under the skin of the forearm. The eggs continue to grow, and eventually they can be harvested from the arm for IVF.

"The forearm is a protected site," explains Dr. Oktay. "If women are getting radiation, they can raise their arms away from it. And if the cancer comes back, the eggs are protected, because they are far away from vital organs. Also, having the ovaries in the arm makes them very easy to monitor."

Although this approach is currently available to only those few women who have access to the small number of specialists trained in the technique, Dr. Oktay hopes that the treatment will eventually become more widespread. Like most advanced fertility techniques, Dr. Oktay's method has a relatively small chance of resulting in a pregnancy, but it does seem to point the way toward another future possibility for young women with breast cancer.

Coping with Fertility and Childbearing

Making decisions about having children can be stressful at the best of times. For young women with breast cancer, the decision-making process can be particularly difficult. Likewise, facing a loss of fertility is often difficult, even if a woman is comfortable with the prospects of adopting, fostering a child, or living a child-free life.

Cynthia Rubin says that it's important to separate feelings about children from feelings about fertility. "I'm not someone who always had a master plan," she says. "I didn't say, 'I have to get married by such and such an age. I have to have two kids, two cars'—I never lived that way." Cynthia lost her fertility as a result of her breast cancer treatment, as she'd been told she might, and today she feels sure that not having children was the right decision for her. Yet she also feels a kind of sadness about losing her fertility.

"I wasn't dying to have kids," Cynthia says bluntly. "But I think one of the things cancer does is make you feel like a total failure. From a biological point of view, why are we here? To reproduce and live as long as we can. It's survival of the species—not the philosophical view of 'why are we here,' but the biological outlook. So as a woman, you feel like you're a failure. You feel worried about a loss of femininity."

Still, Cynthia says, "Kids are always an option, because there are other ways to have children. And there are lots of women who are infertile for a variety of reasons. People have different feelings about what infertility means, but I still consider parenthood an option. I never felt the specific need to pass on my own genes."

Getting Pregnant after Breast Cancer: What Are the Risks?

Even if you know you can get pregnant, you face another tough question: Should you get pregnant? Breast cancer survivors face three big versions of this question:

1. Will getting pregnant increase my risk of breast cancer?

2. Am I passing on the breast cancer gene to my daughter?

3. How do I feel about having a child whom I might not be around to raise?

Will Getting Pregnant Increase My Risk of Breast Cancer?

Unfortunately, the best medical answer to this question is, "We don't know."

There are some things we do know. Pregnancy involves a thousandfold increase in the amount of estrogen in your body, and, as we've seen, estrogen appears to promote the growth of breast cancer cells. Breast surgeon and national breast cancer expert Dr. Susan Love explains,

> From an epidemiological standpoint, there is a higher risk of breast cancer during and right after pregnancy. So it is not uncommon for women to get cancer while they are pregnant or shortly thereafter,

219

when their hormone levels are much higher. Whether those hormones are causing the breast cancer or pushing it along, we don't really know, though it probably is related to hormones. The irony is that after pregnancy, the tissue matures and the woman is less susceptible to hormones.

Dr. Love adds that the high level of estrogen and progesterone may not necessarily cause breast cancer, but "it certainly causes the cancer to grow faster."

Dr. Jeanne Petrek, a breast surgeon at Memorial Sloan-Kettering in New York City, explains that pregnancy will not cause cancer cells to spread throughout your body: By the time you have been treated, the cancer either has or has not metastasized (spread). Sometimes, though, it has spread in the form of tiny cells known as micrometastases, not in the form of full-blown metastases that settle in your lungs or bones. These micrometastases may have already spread to other parts of your body and be lying dormant. Perhaps chemotherapy has rendered them unable to grow, but they still remain alive. If they remain small and weak enough, the body's own immune defenses may be able to hold them in check. "But the hormonal or other unique aspects of pregnancy might possibly encourage these cells to grow and divide," says Dr. Petrek. And since there's no known test that can detect the presence of micrometastases, there's no way for a woman to know whether, by becoming pregnant, she is potentially giving these inactive cancer cells a huge hormonal boost, waking a danger that would otherwise have remained dormant.

Several studies do exist that seem to indicate that there is no increased risk for pregnant breast cancer survivors. But it turns out that those studies aren't very reliable. So Dr. Petrek has begun a major long-term study to find out just how safe it is for a young woman with breast cancer to become pregnant. Her first step was to review existing studies on breast cancer and pregnancy. In 1997, she coauthored an article published in the journal *Cancer* that argued that the previously published studies offered no basis for concluding that pregnancy was safe for breast cancer survivors.[3] Then as now, she stressed that pregnancy is not necessarily unsafe—it's only that no reliable research has vouched for its safety.

For one thing, Dr. Petrek points out, many of the existing studies are retrospective. Rather than starting from scratch to follow the progress of a randomly chosen group of women, a retrospective study interviews doctors about the cases they recall. Of course, doctors use their medical

Roberta Levy-Schwartz, Pregnant 5 Years after Treatment

Lee made me promise, point blank, that this wasn't going to be one of those ER episodes where I was going to die on the table and they would save the baby. This was a decision that "I am number one; please, God, let the baby be healthy and normal," but no matter what, I was going to survive and be with Lee.

records to assist their memories. Nevertheless, they may have "recollection bias"; that is, they remember those patients who survived—and whom they have seen more recently—more readily than they remember those patients whom they have not seen for many years or who have died.

Dr. Petrek also explains that many of the previous pregnancy studies dealt with extremely small samples of women, and that they have other flaws as well. She hopes that some of the pressing questions on women and pregnancy will be resolved when her own long-term study, which looks at 5-year survival rates for mothers after delivery, is completed.

There is a study that was released in 2002 that is far larger and more reliable than any previously published research has been. Scientists at the Fred Hutchinson Cancer Research Center, publishing in *Cancer Epidemiology, Biomarkers, and Prevention,* looked at 1174 women in western Washington state who had been diagnosed with invasive ductal breast cancer (the most common form).[4] All the women were under the age of 45, making this the largest group of young women with breast cancer ever studied. However, this was a study of women who had given birth *before* their diagnosis, not after.

Still, the results are sobering for young breast cancer survivors who are thinking of getting pregnant. The study found that women diagnosed with breast cancer within 2 years after giving birth had twice the risk of dying from the disease as women with a less recent or no history of childbirth. The women in the study were all diagnosed between 1983 and 1992 and were then followed for an average of nearly 9 years. At the end of follow-up, 48 percent of the women who had given birth within 2 years of their diagnosis had died, compared to only 23 percent of the women who had never given birth and 24 percent of the women who had given birth at least 5 years before being diagnosed. It also seemed that tumors were far more aggressive in the women who had recently been pregnant than in the other women.

It isn't clear what these results mean for women who get pregnant after, rather than before, their diagnosis. However, the study certainly seems to suggest that the massive infusion of estrogen that pregnancy represents does indeed make breast cancer tumors more aggressive.

One other factor that women with breast cancer might take into account is the age at which they get pregnant. Dr. Love says that, "From a breast cancer standpoint, the younger you are at your first pregnancy, the lower your risks. The theory is that the breast tissue isn't fully developed until you've had a full-term pregnancy. And when that tissue is more fully developed, it's less susceptible to carcinogens." Likewise, figures from the National Cancer Institute reveal that among women who are pregnant or who have just given birth, breast cancer occurs most often between the ages of 32 and 38,[5] suggesting that earlier pregnancies may make breast cancer less likely.

But this protective effect of early full-term pregnancy is complicated for young women carrying BRCA1 or BRCA 2 mutations. In fact, one study published in *The Lancet* finds that pregnancy is a risk factor for hereditary breast cancer. Researchers studied women who had all developed breast cancer by the age of 40 and determined that "carriers of the BRCA1 and BRCA2 mutations who have children are significantly more likely to develop breast cancer by the age of 40 than women who are nulliparous." The study also concluded that each pregnancy is associated with an increased cancer risk in genetic mutation carriers.[6]

Am I Passing On the Breast Cancer Gene to My Daughter?

Once again, doctors just don't know as much as they'd like to about the role of genetic factors in breast cancer. They do know that there are "breast cancer genes" that may make it more likely that some women will get breast cancer. But, as we saw in Chapter 1, more than 80 percent of women get the disease without having had any family history of it, and there are many women with a family history of breast cancer who have no signs of the disease.

Dr. Petrek recommends that women get tested for the gene if they are concerned about passing it on, particularly if they were diagnosed as teenagers or in their very early twenties. "Only 10 percent of all women with breast cancer have BRCA1 or BRCA2, the 'breast cancer genes,'" she explains. "But if you're diagnosed when you're young, you're considered far more likely to have them. We think maybe about half of the really young breast cancer patients may be carrying BRCA1 or BRCA2. So a lot of young women ask for a blood test, which is a fairly simple test, but expensive. For some women, though, it's worth it, because it sets their minds at rest that they are not passing on a breast cancer gene to their children."

Lanita Hausman, Decided to Adopt

Before I was diagnosed, we talked about having kids in some future sense. I'd say, "Well, I'll have one at 28." But then 28 came and I was afraid. Even before I was diagnosed, I knew I had a family history of breast cancer. I didn't want to pass it on. So then we said, "OK, I'll have one at 30. Then at 35." I'd never been around kids anyway. Tom was more open to the idea. I didn't want to have my gene pool out there, because it seemed so likely that, given my family history, I had the breast cancer gene. And I was worried that if I had a baby, and I had even one latent cell of breast cancer inside me, the estrogen increase of pregnancy would cause that cell to grow. Eventually, we made plans for adoption.

How Do I Feel about Having a Child Whom I Might Not Be Around to Raise?

This is perhaps the most difficult question of all, since there is no medical study—nor any prospect of one—that might help answer it. For some women, having a child without some assurance of their own survival just feels wrong. These women may choose not to have children at all, or to wait until they've had 5 cancer-free years, when their chances of survival have vastly increased.

Cindy Kim, age 28, says that being diagnosed with breast cancer has completely changed her ideas about having children. "Before cancer, I just wanted to have babies," she says. "It was my number one goal. It's what I wanted more than anything in the world. I thought, 'If I can't have babies, I won't have chemo.'"

But as the disease progressed, Cindy's feelings began to change. "Now I'm scared to death of babies," she says vehemently. "I don't want them. Subconsciously, I think I'm trying to talk myself out of it. I'm just so scared that I'm going to have a recurrence while I'm pregnant, and that I'm going to die and leave my children behind. I haven't dealt with that. I go to a shrink, but they just want to talk about death. Well, I don't want to talk about death any more! I want to talk about the daily things that happen that I'm suppressing."

"I really think I have posttraumatic stress disorder. I have night sweats, chills. I have these dreams where all these dead people are touching my arm. They're saying to me, 'Let's go.' I had this dream the other night where my whole loft apartment was filled with 2 feet of water, and I wanted to see what was under the water. I could see that it was clear—

that there was nothing there—but I dipped my head under anyway and looked. And when I did, it was a mile deep, and there were sharks everywhere, and they were all coming after me. Can you imagine me having kids with this going on? We have three embryos ready to go, but I just can't even go there right now."

For other women, though, having a baby is a leap of faith, an assertion that they *will* live to raise their child, no matter what it takes. Or having a child may represent another kind of faith: a belief that life is worth living on any terms, and that now is all we have. "We know that life is very precious and that you take every day and do what you can with it," Joy says simply. "And hopefully my child will be healthy and happy and he'll have everything he needs."

Joy also feels that having had breast cancer has helped to make her a better mother. "I've really learned that you don't sweat the small stuff," she says. "And if it isn't a deadly disease, you know what? It's all small stuff. Whether he eats his peas or doesn't eat his peas is really not going to be an issue in this house! Breast cancer puts it all into perspective."

Having Breast Cancer during Pregnancy

According to the National Cancer Institute, once in every 3000 pregnancies, a woman is diagnosed with breast cancer either during her pregnancy or within the year. That means that about 15 percent of all breast cancer survivors under 40 were diagnosed during or soon after their pregnancies. And researchers believe the incidence of breast cancer during pregnancy may be increasing as more women delay becoming pregnant.[7]

One such woman was Charnette Messé, who was diagnosed with breast cancer at age 31, the day before she found out she was pregnant. She and her husband, Tom, already had a 3-year-old, Gabrielle, and since their daughter's birth Charnette had been trying to get pregnant again.

Despite her diagnosis, the news that she was pregnant came as a joyous relief. "I had prayed to God that if I had to die, could He please give me a baby so that Gabrielle would not be alone," she says. "I felt like this was God working a miracle for me. I wasn't afraid of the cancer any more when my doctor told me I was pregnant."

For women like Charnette, though, breast cancer treatment can be difficult. First, the tumor is likely to be larger, according to Dr. George Sledge, professor of medicine and oncology at the Indiana University Cancer Center. When the tumor is bigger, it requires more urgent treatment—and more radical surgery.

Charnette Messé, Receiving Chemo While Pregnant

It's been very scary because people have sent me stories of women who have been diagnosed while pregnant. And both of the mothers I read about died after giving birth. I look at them as very inspirational, though, because they went ahead and gave birth anyway. But, of course, I think about that—how long am I going to have with my new baby?

My philosophy is that life, though unpredictable, is beautiful. That's so important to me. Even though my life is the way it is right now, my life is still beautiful. I've lived a beautiful 31 years. When we are faced with our greatest turmoils and greatest fears, we still have to look at the beautiful side of life. And what's so beautiful about life—is life. The life inside me right now. And my daughter Gabby. Life is the most beautiful thing, and if we would just understand that, it really would be a beautiful world. That's what I live by. That's what I stand by.

But even if your tumor is smaller, you probably won't be able to have a lumpectomy, since that procedure is usually followed by radiation therapy. Radiation while you're pregnant, however, would damage the fetus.

Sometimes women request a lumpectomy and offer to wait for their radiation therapy until after they've given birth. But their cancer is probably too aggressive to allow them to wait, according to Dr. Petrek, because pregnancy itself can make your cancer more aggressive.

Dr. Petrek, author of the chapter on breast cancer and pregnancy in *Diseases of the Breast,* a major medical textbook[8] explains that pregnancy creates a large network of ducts, lymph vessels, and blood vessels in the breast—a network that can help the cancer to spread even faster than usual.

According to Dr. Sledge, ideally, surgery would be followed by chemotherapy. However, most doctors are reluctant to prescribe chemotherapy during the first trimester of a pregnancy because of the increased possibility of fetal abnormalities. Second and third trimester chemotherapy is currently considered safe by most physicians,[9] although few long-term studies have been done on children born after chemotherapy. The most thorough study to date followed 84 children whose mothers received chemotherapy during pregnancy (including 38 who were treated in the first trimester). After 19 years of analysis, researchers found no congenital, neurological, or psychological abnormalities in those children. Although the mothers had cancers other than breast cancer—leukemia, Hodgkin's disease, and malignant lymphoma—researchers say this is evidence that "chemotherapy at full doses can be safely administered" during pregnancy.[10]

According to Dr. Eric Winer, director of breast oncology at Dana-Farber's Gillette Centers for Women's Cancer in Boston, "We have some moderately reassuring information about beginning chemo in the second trimester. We know of many women exposed to chemotherapy who deliver what appear to be healthy babies. Whether these children are at increased risk for health problems 30 and 40 years down the road, we can't say yet."

Because treating breast cancer during pregnancy is so difficult, many doctors were once eager to terminate those pregnancies. That response is no longer the norm—but once again, the data are simply lacking. Dr. Petrek reports that some small retrospective studies suggest that there is no benefit from therapeutic abortions (abortions done for health reasons) in these cases, but, she says, these studies are small and imprecise and, in her opinion, offer an insufficient basis for forming a medical opinion.

Charnette is planning to receive chemotherapy while pregnant, a treatment that for her evokes both fear and hope. "In a way, I'm looking forward to starting the chemo," she says, "because I hope it's going to help me medically. I think my baby is a miracle baby as it is, and I don't think God is going to let anything happen to my baby. Everything that I've been told is that when you're in the second and third trimesters, the baby will do well."

"These are intensely personal decisions," says Dr. Sledge. "One woman who hears about the medical data may say, 'I don't want to stay pregnant.' Another woman may make a different choice. Our job as doctors and health-care professionals is to help guide women through this very difficult decision, and to explain all the knowns and unknowns that we are dealing with."

Abortion and Breast Cancer

Few questions in medicine may be more controversial than whether abortion increases a woman's risk of developing breast cancer. At least 80 research studies worldwide have collected data about breast cancer and reproductive factors such as childbirth, menstrual cycles, birth control pills, and abortion. Approximately 30 studies have examined the risk of developing breast cancer in women who have had abortions. As we discussed in Chapter 4, having a full-term pregnancy early in a woman's childbearing years is protective against breast cancer, and a woman's age at menarche and menopause also influences her risk for breast cancer, with earlier onset of regular menstrual cycles and later age at menopause associated with higher risk.

The question is: Is there a link between pregnancy termination and breast cancer? The answer is: The scientific evidence is inconclusive and inconsistent. The best approach to this highly emotional and highly politicized topic is to consider the science behind the existing studies and to understand why the question is being asked in the first place.

The theory linking abortion and breast cancer is based on the idea that abortion disrupts the hormones associated with pregnancy. Pregnant women experience a surge of sex hormones (estrogen, progesterone, and prolactin), which stimulate immature breast cells to mature into fully differentiated cells in the breast glands in preparation for lactation. Some studies conclude that if this cell proliferation process is artificially interrupted, hormone levels drop dramatically, and the possible protective effect of differentiation is lost, making the cells more susceptible to carcinogens and, therefore, to cancer.[11]

One of the most widely recognized studies showing a link between breast cancer and abortion was conducted by Janet Daling, Ph.D., at Seattle's Fred Hutchinson Cancer Research Center and appeared in the *Journal of the National Cancer Institute*. For the study, 1806 women (845 with breast cancer and 961 without) in Washington state were interviewed about their reproductive histories, including abortions. Researchers discovered that among women who were 45 and younger, the risk of breast cancer among those who had had abortions was 50 percent higher than among other women. The study found no link between breast cancer and spontaneous abortion or miscarriage, but it did conclude that there was a greater risk for women who had their first induced abortion before age 18.[12]

In 1995, a year after this study was published, Louisiana became the first U.S. state to require abortion clinics to inform potential patients that induced abortions may increase breast cancer risk. And in 2001, a Pennsylvania teenager sued the New Jersey doctor who performed an abortion on her, alleging that had she been made aware of the "breast cancer link," she never would have had the abortion. Both examples highlight the social and legal implications of this type of research.

Even proponents of Daling's work, however, point out that case-control studies are not best suited for determining whether abortion increases breast cancer risk because they are too small to eliminate chance or other unidentified risk factors as the reason for their findings. That's why more weight is given to cohort studies, in which a group of women, some of whom have had abortions, are followed to see who develops breast cancer.

One such study, published in the *New England Journal of Medicine,* looked at all Danish women born between April 1, 1935, and March 31, 1978, some 1.5 million women. Instead of relying on the women's answers to reproductive questions, the scientists turned to Denmark's national abortion and breast cancer registries. They found no increased risk of breast cancer associated with abortion.[13] A similar analysis of Swedish women who had had legal abortions before the age of 30 found no association between first-trimester abortion and breast cancer in young women.[14] (Earlier reports of the Swedish statistics had suggested that there might be a link; however, later analysis showed that the early reports were faulty, largely because women who had breast cancer were more likely to report the abortions that they had had, while women without breast cancer tended to underreport their abortions.[15]) Finally, a study that compared 3200 U.S. women with breast cancer to a cancer-free control group of 4844 found that "the risk of breast cancer is not materially affected by abortion."[16]

Ultimately, research findings have been inconclusive. In an effort to sort through the inconsistencies, the American Cancer Society and the National Cancer Institute have reviewed the studies and reached the same conclusion: There is no proven relationship between abortion and breast cancer risk.[17] That said, the NCI is funding at least six other studies examining complete pregnancy history, including induced and spontaneous abortion, in relation to the risk of breast cancer. NCI researchers admit that it is possible that an increased or decreased risk could exist in small subgroups of women. "For example," says an NCI report, "the large Danish study found a slightly lower breast cancer risk in women with abortions occurring before 7 weeks' gestation, and a slightly higher risk in women who had abortions at 7 or more weeks."[18]

Whether these findings quell or increase the uncertainty you may have over this issue, it may be helpful for you to understand how difficult it would be to put this issue to rest once and for all. A definitive answer to the question "Does abortion increase breast cancer risk or doesn't it?" would require a large randomized controlled trial—considered the "gold standard" of scientific research. But such research will never be possible, because in a randomized controlled trial, researchers, not patients, would decide who would get an abortion, in order to minimize any other differences between the two groups of women that could affect breast cancer risk.

Breast-Feeding after Breast Cancer

There is some evidence that breast-feeding may reduce the risk of breast cancer. A study in the *New England Journal of Medicine* found that both pre- and postmenopausal women who breast-fed for about a year and a half reduced their risk of breast cancer by 30 percent.[19] However, no data are available on women who breast-fed after breast cancer treatment.

If you have at least one remaining breast, you probably will have the option of breast-feeding, which is certainly healthy for your baby and may be emotionally satisfying for you. If you've had a single mastectomy, pregnancy won't cause any changes in the chest area where your breast used to be, but your remaining breast will go through all the usual changes of pregnancy, growing larger as you prepare to lactate. A breast that has undergone lumpectomy and radiation is also likely to go through the usual changes. However, since irradiation damages some of the milk-producing parts of the breast, the irradiated breast is likely to grow somewhat more slowly than the other breast and will have little or no milk production.

Women can breast-feed with either one or two functioning breasts. However, breast-feeding will make your breast grow larger, so if you're using one and not the other, you can expect them to become markedly different in size. Your breast-feeding breast may stay somewhat larger even after breast-feeding is over. If this is a concern, you can have it reduced by plastic surgery.

"It gives me sheer pleasure to see Anand using the breast the way a breast was supposed to be used," says Joy. "At one time, I had a lot of anger toward my breasts, and I wanted to have both of them removed. Now, 7 years later, after I've had my son and he's breast-feeding, I'm really, really glad I still have one breast and I can do that for him. That I can give him mother's milk. It's a miracle."

CHAPTER 10

"I Want to Dance at My Son's Wedding"

When You've Got Children at Home

When Karen Sattaur was diagnosed with breast cancer at age 34, she had a 4-year-old son and a daughter who was about to turn 2. Living in West Palm Beach, Florida, the only women she knew with breast cancer were older women, and she was desperate to connect to other young mothers who had shared her experience. When she found a Web site dedicated entirely to the issues of young women with breast cancer, she was overjoyed. "Anyone else out there going through this with little ones?" she wrote in her first posting. "Some days I just want to lock them in the closet so I can sleep! Or just do nothing. . . . Sometimes I have no juice to play, read, clean, . . . and I feel guilty. They do not understand that I feel yucky and simply don't want to. I hate putting them in front of the television, but thank God it's there!"

Two years later, Karen said, "The older the kids get, the harder it is. Because they have a better understanding of what this can mean. They understand loss better. When I was first diagnosed, I cried for 3 weeks. I was feeding them chocolate cake for breakfast. Then I said, 'Karen, get a hold of yourself. Get up and fight. Make a conscious decision that you are going to live, and do everything in your power to do that.' It's horrifying to think that I have these two beautiful children and I could leave them. But let's face it, we're all going to die someday, and none of us ever knows when. So I look at my illness as that I've been given advance notice. I have to make sure I do everything I can for my children in case I have to go."

Tracy Pleva Hill faced a double challenge: First she was diagnosed with breast cancer; then, after a mastectomy and a course of chemo, she saw the cancer come back. Throughout it all, she had to care for her son, Jason, who was only 12 months old when Tracy was diagnosed. "I told every doctor I saw that I wanted nothing more than to dance at my son's wedding," she says. "It became—and continues to be—my ultimate ambition. I focus on this every day when I'm on the brink of tears thinking about my fate and as I help other young women deal with their diagnoses."

❦

When Ellen Feig was diagnosed, she was 36 years old, with a 5-year-old son, Benjamin, and a 2-year-old daughter, Sammi. "The most important issue at that moment was how to explain to the kids what was wrong with Mommy," she says. Her son had already lived through Ellen's bout with lupus 2 years previously, but, says Ellen, "This seemed different—my life genuinely seemed to be up for grabs. I knew that I had to tell the kids something—after all, the house had become a maelstrom of crying relatives, constant phone calls, and sadness. Intuitively, they knew things were not right. Yet how to say it?"

Caring for Your Children While Caring for Yourself

Raising children is a handful for any woman. For a woman who's undergoing breast cancer treatment the challenges can seem overwhelming. Women with breast cancer struggle to find the energy to deal with their active toddlers and inquisitive older children. They look for ways to tell their children about what's wrong and to help their children handle the possibility that Mommy might not be there any longer. They look for ways to be there for their children—and to let their children be there for them, as much as is possible or appropriate.

Mothers with breast cancer also find that their children are a powerful reason to keep going. Wanting to see their children grow up—or even finish kindergarten—can multiply a woman's will to live while making her painfully aware of the preciousness of every moment.

Talking with Your Children

Mothers with breast cancer agree that it's important to bring children into the process as early and as honestly as possible. It may be tempting to think that you can protect your children from having to cope with your illness. But, according to H. Elizabeth King, Ph.D., a child psychologist who is herself a breast cancer survivor and the mother of two children, even very young children are old enough to understand that something scary is going on in the household, whether the grown-ups talk about it or not. "They pick up the emotions of their parents and the other adults," Dr. King says. "You can't get a diagnosis and not react with fear, anxiety, and stress—and your kids will pick up on it." Therefore, Dr. King advises, parents should talk directly to their children, so that the children can express their fears directly.

"For children of any age," she says, "I'd have a short conversation with them to give them the basic facts. 'Here's what's going on—the doctor says something is wrong with Mommy, and she may have to go into the hospital, and she might take medicine and look funny for a little while, and we wanted you to know.' If they're younger than 5, your kids will remember it for maybe 24 hours. Older kids will retain the information longer. Either way, you've set the stage, and now you can bring it up in the context of daily life."

In Dr. King's experience, a child's first question is almost always, "Are you going to die?" She advises parents to respond to the question as directly as possible.

"What I told my children—and what I would recommend to other parents—was, 'No, I'm not going to die. I'm seeing a doctor, and they're going to treat this. My dying is not something you need to worry about. If anything changes, I'll tell you.' Because when a child asks, 'Are you going to die?' they mean next week or next month. So what they're looking for is reassurance. I believe that even with the worst prognosis—like the one I had—most women are looking at surviving for at least a few years. And for a child that's a lifetime. To give them the burden of death if it's 1 or 2 or 5 years away is a horrible burden. And unnecessary, I think."

Moreover, says Dr. King, by the time they're 7, most children have heard the word *cancer* and have at least some idea of what it means. "They've heard of someone who has it," she says. "Or they've seen it on TV. Or a teacher has had it, or a classmate's parent. When I was diagnosed, my friends and I discussed this, and we realized that all of our children had had some experience with the word *cancer*, whether with a friend or a teacher or a grandparent. Cancer is very prevalent in America. So in all likelihood, your children have already heard the word *cancer*, and they know it's a bad thing." This makes it especially important, in Dr. King's view, to address the topic with your children as directly as possible, to give them room to ask questions about death if they choose to, and to share with them as much information as they can handle.

"The more honest and reassuring a parent can be, the more helpful it is to a child," she says. "My being a doctor helped in some ways, but dealing with this issue in my own household was also a massive learning experience for me. I talked at length with my friends—some of whom are also mental health professionals—about how to talk to my children, what to tell them, and when to tell them. But none of our plans worked out! My son came home and saw me wearing a bandage from the biopsy

Dr. H. Elizabeth King, Child Psychologist, Breast Cancer Survivor

My son was 7 years old when I had to tell him I had breast cancer, and that's when he started drawing Kemo Shark. It was strictly his idea. We had talked about my chemo and all its side effects. He was always asking me, "Why can't you come to dinner?" and I'd have to explain that it was because the chemo made me feel sick to my stomach. And he'd tell me, "If the doctor gave you that medicine, he must've made a mistake." I'd try to explain to him that the medicine was good for me, but sometimes it also made me feel bad.

He came up with the idea of the shark eating the cancer cells. He would take his picture of Kemo Shark on trips with him, and he'd draw Kemo Shark going places with him. It became a real ally, a real friend. I told him, "This is great! When I get well, we'll make a comic book." I had a very poor prognosis. And it was very traumatic for my children. So I think he chose a shark—the scariest thing he could come up with—to treat the scariest thing he could ever imagine. Sharks are huge and scary and mean—they're the perfect thing to fight cancer.

I was really struck by the lack of materials that were out there for children, to help them understand and cope. So, when my treatment was done, I told my son, "We're going to make Kemo Shark into a comic book to help other people." And that's exactly what we did.

and asked me what it was for and if I had had surgery. Although I had planned a more careful introduction for him, he just jumped right into it. In retrospect, I think the fact that a friend down the street had just been diagnosed made him more alert and sensitized to the problem."

Dr. King reminds parents that different children will deal with your breast cancer in different ways. While her 7-year-old son was eager to talk, her 12-year-old daughter, "usually a Chatty Cathy," refused to talk to her mother or anyone else about her mother's illness. "The children reacted totally differently from what I would have predicted," says Dr. King. "And you should know that if your children also react in an unpredictable way, you shouldn't be unnerved by it—that's just part of being a child."

Dr. King says that different children also have different concerns. "My son was hung up on how I got cancer. He decided it was contagious. Because the woman down the street had been diagnosed 2 weeks earlier, it made sense to him that she got it first, then I caught it. When I said, 'No, it's not contagious,' he would ask, 'Well, how do we get it, then?' I'd have to say, 'I don't know.' And he would come back with, 'Well, if you don't know, how do you know it's not contagious?'"

Dr. King believes that breast cancer was especially disturbing for her daughter, who was just beginning to face her own growth into womanhood, because it raised questions about her own relationship to her body, as well as bringing up issues about how other people saw her. One of Dr. King's daughter's friends also had a mother with breast cancer, and the friend's main concern was not being known as "the girl whose mother has breast cancer."

"I think it's very difficult to figure out exactly the right thing to do," Dr. King says frankly. "Even if you do what the experts say, your illness may affect your children in unexpected ways."

Getting Professional Help

Although Dr. King is herself a child psychologist, she is not quick to recommend that parents seek professional help for their children. "If it's possible, have the child get help from the adults who are already around the child," she advises. "See if you can draw upon friends' parents, teachers, ministers, rabbis, and people like that." However, she says, if your child has symptoms such as insomnia, difficulty concentrating, bouts of crying, or periods of becoming extremely withdrawn for more than 3 weeks, you need to consult a psychologist or counselor.

Maintaining Continuity

Another way in which parents can help their children through this time is to try to support their children's activities as much as possible. Encourage your children to continue visiting their friends and, if possible, to have their friends visit them. "That can be tricky," Dr. King says, "but some families hire sitters to come and help with the kids, so that their children can have friends over." If your son or daughter is on the soccer team or is taking swimming lessons, finding ways to get them where they need to go and motivating them to stay involved will provide them with a sense of normalcy and give them more opportunities for peer support.

What Your Children Understand

Of course, children of different ages can cope with different levels of information. As you think of ways to tell your children about what's happening to you, it can be helpful to know what children of various ages are able to understand.

Beth Brokaw, Diagnosed at Age 37

My children were ages 2 and 7 when I was diagnosed with metastatic cancer. I talk with them as openly as I can. They know I have cancer, and they know about the treatment. The doctors have just put me on a new chemo, and I will lose my hair any moment now. And my daughter's birthday is this week—she's having a slumber party—and she said to me, "I hope you keep your hair for the party."

When I lost my hair the first time I was diagnosed as metastatic, I wanted to normalize the experience for them. I told them my hair was going to fall out, and I said to them, "Okay, you're usually not allowed to pull Mommy's hair, but this time you are." And they thought it was so much fun. They kept it for a doll. We made it an experience that we shared together, so they wouldn't be frightened by Mom being a bald-headed woman. It's been a little more of a challenge to know what to tell them about death.

I don't know how long I'll live. A week or a month is a long time in a child's development process. I don't know how much to prepare them for my death before it cracks their universe. When it comes up, we talk about it. But I haven't fully pushed it in their face. I've never said, "Mommy's gonna die." My debate is how much should I prepare my kids for my death when I don't know myself how long I have to live. I've tried to help them have a normal life, while being as open as I can about what's going on. The toughest thing is knowing how to deal with death.

My daughter is a quiet introvert—she doesn't ask a lot of questions. And I have to be thoughtful and careful about when and how I bring things up. We were walking home from church once, and I was talking with a Sunday school friend about what causes cancer. And I said, "No one really knows, but it might be the environment, it might be the cancer gene." And she looked at me and said, "Mommy, I sure hope I don't have the cancer gene. But I sure am glad I have the good grades gene." It was a lovely way for her to express what she was feeling—that you get good and bad genes from your parents.

My son, on the other hand, is a very verbal little guy. He's much more of an extrovert. He came home the other day and said, "Daddy, is Mommy gonna die soon?" So we talked to him. We said, "She's not dying now. But she may die sooner than Daddy and other people because of this disease. But we don't know when that might happen."

Children Age 2 or Younger

Very young children are likely to pick up on the fact that the grown-ups around them are scared. At this age, children have no real concept of death, says Dr. King, but they may somehow realize that death is what their parents are suddenly afraid of. Although children of this age don't understand the permanence of death, according to Dr. King, "They are terrified of the word."

Children who are too young to conceive of death may need even more comfort and reassurance than older children during crises, and you may need to repeat your explanations many times, in many different ways. Very young children also may not understand the permanence of the problems you're facing. Explaining that "Mommy is too tired to play right now" may make sense on a one-time basis, but a very young child may not be able to retain this information.

It can be painful having to tell a child over and over "not now" or "Mommy already said no!" If possible, have a substitute to offer. If Mommy can't give a big hug, can she give a small one? If you can't play a running game, can you read a book or cuddle gently? If you can't do something, is there another loving adult who can? (If you've been pregnant with one child while raising another young one, you'll already be familiar with this technique!)

Children Ages 3 to 5

Children of this age understand the concept of "something bad," but not of death itself. "They know Mommy is sick and she has to have an operation," says Dr. King. "But there's no true understanding of what it means to be diagnosed with cancer or that it is life-threatening."

At this age, children do have a sense of their own bodies, though, so they can grasp the idea of being hurt, being sick, or even losing a limb. They just can't understand the permanence of death. Perhaps because they can grasp how troubling death is without really understanding it, they're prone to guilt and anxiety about whether they've caused the "bad thing" to happen, whether that bad thing is their mother's illness, her fear of death, or death itself. Children of this age are still figuring out the difference between their wishes and reality, so they are especially prone to "magical thinking"—believing that they've caused something simply by wishing for it. After all, when they were infants, didn't they wish for food, dry diapers, and hugs—and somehow, those things all magically appeared?

Now they're old enough to realize that sometimes they're mad at Mommy and wish she would go away. It can be frightening and guilt-

Leslie Mouton

It was dinnertime at our house, and it started like most nights. My 2–year-old, Nicole, was sitting in her highchair pulled up to the kitchen table. She always sits in between me and her father. She is the designated food blesser at our house. Once she learned the dinnertime prayer, she would have it no other way—she says it every night!

This night, it started like every other night: "Dear Lord, bless this food and allow it to nourish our bodies; we love you, Jesus," but where the "Amen" usually goes, she added in a little extra thought of her own: "and bless Mommy's boobie, Amen!"

I just about dropped my fork, and my chin did drop about 2 inches! My husband, Tony, looked at me, and I looked at him, and then we both looked at Nicole. "What a beautiful thing to say, Nicole," I told her. She responded, "It'll be okay, Mommy, Jesus will make your boobie all better!"

It wasn't until that moment, the night before I was scheduled for surgery to have a cancerous lump taken out of my left breast, that I realized how much my little 2-year-old baby understood. I guess I thought she was too young to realize what was going on. Boy, was I wrong!

When I found out I had breast cancer, I tried to ease the fears of my husband, relatives, and friends, but I never even thought about how it would affect my 2-year-old daughter. Little ones are brighter than we think, and acutely aware of what's going on around them.

How could she not know something was going on? Our phone was ringing off the hook, flowers were arriving every 10 minutes, and I kept telling people not to worry about me, I would beat this and be okay!

Nicole never asked questions, and I didn't even think about telling her I had breast cancer. But I should have. She did show me subtle signs that she too knew that something was wrong. She was clingy, more so than [she usually was]. And my baby girl, who had slept through the night since she was 3 months old (I know, I know, I'm very lucky!) suddenly would wake up in a terror two or three times a night. We finally had to make her a little bed by our bed. We told her that if she couldn't sleep, she could crawl into that bed next to ours. Every morning we would wake up to find her snuggled in blankets by our bed—sound asleep.

Obviously she sensed that something was wrong with Mommy— and I should have been up front with her from the start.

I'll never make that mistake again. The night she blessed my boobie at the dinner table, I decided it was time for us to have a heart-to-heart about Mommy's cancer. I was very up front about it. I told her Mommy's boobie is sick, but doctors are going to help make it all better. I explained to her that when I came home from the hospital, I would be in bandages, and very sore on my left side. She asked me if we could still give big hugs. I told her we would have to give little hugs for a while, and she would have to lie on my right side when we cuddled at night to read books before bedtime. She crawled onto my lap and asked if she could touch my hurt boobie. I said sure, but after today, she would have to take special care when she's around it. She gently placed her hand on my breast, "We can have big hugs tonight, right, Mommy?"

"Right," I said, and she threw her tiny arms around my neck, squeezing as hard as she could.

The week that followed surgery was tough on Nicole. Every night she asked me if I was all better, and if we could give big hugs again. When the bandages finally came off, and I was feeling better, I went straight to her arms. "I'm ready for big hugs, Cole Bug," I said. She gasped, her eyes widened, and she ran over to me, threw her arms around me, and not only gave me giant hugs, but a big sloppy kiss on my cheek! "Now you're all better, Mommy?" she asked.

Then I had to prepare her for what was next. I had to explain that while I was no longer sore from surgery, I still had to take medicine to make sure I was well. That medicine, I told her, would make Mommy very sick for a few days, but she shouldn't worry when I'm in bed. I explained it's all part of making me well, so I can be here for her for a long, long time to come!

She thought about it for a minute, and said, "That's okay, Mommy, I'll take care of you."

I knew the chemo would make my hair fall out, so I also had to decide how I would help Nicole cope with that. I didn't want her to be freaked out about her mom going bald, but I also didn't want to hide it from her.

Tony and I decided we would make it a big event. A party, something she would find fun, not frightening. So the day my hair started falling out, we had a hair-shaving party! Our family and friends came over, and we made it a big event. I told Nicole that the medicine I was taking for my boobie makes my hair fall out, and I let her grab a handful out of my head. She thought that was pretty neat! We tied braids in my hair and laced each one with pink ribbon—memory locks for all to keep.

Then one by one, the braids were cut. Nicole, with the help of her daddy, cut off the first one. She clapped and smiled! After the braids came the clippers. Again, with her daddy's help, she was the first one to buzz my hair off. She counted "one, two, three, four!!!" and buzzed away!

When it was over, she looked at me and said, "That was fun, Mommy. Can we do it again tomorrow?"

"No," I told her, "this is a one-shot deal!"

From that night on, Nicole never questioned me about my hair. She accepted me bald, and loved me just the same. When she drew pictures of our family, she would say, "Look, Mommy, I gave you hair!" I would say, "Thank you, sweetheart, it's beautiful. And you know, Mommy's hair will grow back real soon!"

I've learned that children know more than what we teach them, and they take their cues from our behavior. How we react to life's most challenging times sets the example for how they will act. If we are up front with our children, and let them know that we are okay with what's happening, they remain secure and stable.

By the way, about 1 week after surgery, Nicole was back in her bed and sleeping through the night. "Bless Mommy's boobie" became a normal part of her dinnertime prayer for months. But today, 1 year after diagnosis, with hair back on my head, the dinnertime prayer has returned to normal, and so have our lives!

provoking for them to find out that Mommy is indeed going away to the hospital or for treatments that leave her tired and sad—or to sense that the adults around them worry that Mommy may be going somewhere and not coming back.

So when you're dealing with children aged 3 to 5, you've got two challenges: helping the child understand what's happening to you and to your family and making sure that the child knows that he or she didn't cause any of it. It can be hard for adults to remember how personally young children take everything. Watching for feelings of guilt or fear in your preschoolers can enable you to help them cope with a situation that is difficult for all of you.

Children Ages 6 to 8

Children this age share many of the difficulties faced by younger children in grasping the nature of the crisis that has hit their family. They sense that if they lose their mother, their whole world—indeed, their whole

Juanita Lyle, Diagnosed at Age 32

I really wanted my kids to understand what was going on with me. But it was hard because my husband had such a hard time dealing with it—he couldn't even say the word cancer. *When I was diagnosed, my husband told our son, "Don't tell anyone your mother has breast cancer." That was an incredible burden for my son to carry with him, an incredible secret for him to try to keep. I always thought it was important to talk about the cancer and be open about it. It's hard enough figuring out what to do as a parent to explain cancer, but it's even harder when Mom and Dad don't agree on an approach. And that's the way it was in my house.*

To help my kids understand what was going on, I let them be there sometimes when I was taking chemo. I had my doctor talk to them and explain things as best he could. At the same time, I wanted to make sure their lives were as normal as possible. I didn't want them to think I was going to die. I wanted them to continue with all their activities. I made sure I was still going to their soccer games and letting them have friends over, even though sometimes I felt lousy. My son always jokes with me that on many mornings when he knew I was feeling just awful, I'd still catch him before he went out the door, to make sure his hair was brushed and he had all his stuff for school.

I wanted to prepare my kids for the possibility of my death without making them feel like I was going to die—which was a hard fence to straddle. We talked a lot about God. And mostly we didn't talk about death, we talked about life.

After my hair fell out from chemo, I was sitting on the edge of my bed crying and my son came along and saw me crying and he said, "Mom, why are you crying?" I said, "For the first time in your mother's life, she's being very vain." I said, "I don't know how I'll deal with not having hair." And he made the most profound statement. He said, "You know, Mom, don't worry about that because we still have you." Then he found a health article in a magazine one day, and he came to me and said, "Mom, I found this article about hair." It was an advertisement for men who have bald heads. He said, "You should call this number, Mom; this might give you your hair back." I was so tickled. It was the sweetest, most comical experience I've ever had.

identity—will be shaken. Like their younger brothers and sisters, they may feel guilty or fearful for having "caused" the family's problem through their own "bad" feelings.

However, children at this age are better able to ask questions, to explain what they're thinking, and sometimes even to share their feelings. The challenge in dealing with children of this age is to cope with their strong feelings while you are still coming to terms with your own emotions.

Because children aren't as strong as adults, they can't always handle emotion as soon. At this age, it may take children a day, a week, or even several weeks to process what you're telling them or to take in the crisis that they sense around them. They may need to reassure themselves that their whole world *won't* fall apart before they feel safe experiencing their sadness, loss, or fear. Before expressing themselves directly, they may cry for a long time about seemingly small matters, be fearful of things that never used to frighten them, or show a lot of emotion about seemingly unrelated people or events.

Furthermore, to kids this age, parents still seem all-powerful. (Feeling that our parents are *still* all-powerful is something that even grown-ups struggle with!) It's hard for a child of this age to believe that a grown-up does anything against his or her will. On some level, your child may understand that you have to spend more time at the hospital or resting in bed, that you just can't do all the things you did before. But it may be hard for him or her to really believe that this is beyond your control—and the idea that anything is beyond your control may also be quite frightening.

The challenge in dealing with children of this age is to let them have their whole range of feelings—anger, sadness, frustration, fear—without giving them the idea that you're going to fall apart or sink under the weight of their emotions. Of course, you want to focus on the positive, and you want to help your children to do so, too. But the more space you can give them for the full range of their feelings, the more easily their good feelings will flow.

Karen Sattaur, Diagnosed at Age 34

I have a 6-year-old, Damon, and an almost-4-year-old, Marie. When I was diagnosed, my son was 4 and my daughter 1½. My son and I are very similar and very close. He knew what was going on. We chose to tell him just about everything you could tell a 4-year-old. We got books. Kidskonnected.com sends a package out to the children of newly diagnosed mothers. They sent each of the kids a teddy bear and a book called Kemo Shark. *It's a wonderful little book. It talks about what chemo does. It was so helpful. We read it quite a bit.*

The day my hair fell out, my kids stood next to me as my mom shaved my head. We all cried. They saw that this made me sad. They had to see that this hurt, but they also saw that it wasn't going to be the end of things. Adversity hits us, but how do we deal with it?

Damon said, "Mommy, I love you anyway."

My son goes to the school where I teach. He's in kindergarten. When my hair started falling out again, I said, "Damon, I have to tell the kids at school what's happening to me." I said, "I want you to know that the kids in your class will say things like, 'My grandma had cancer and she died.' They're not saying it to be mean, they're saying this because they also loved someone who had cancer."

"Mommy, I'd be so sad if you died."

We just sat in the garage and held each other and cried.

It's hard because I know that as my kids are getting older, they have a fuller understanding of the significance of what is happening. My kids have never lost someone they love. Their grandparents are still alive, and so are their aunts and uncles. They've never been to a funeral, and it wrecks me to think mine might be the first one they go to.

The books use the word dying. *It's not appropriate for my kids. They can ask about it. But I'm not going to tell them ahead of time. People have asked, "Have you taken Damon to therapy?" Hell, no. I think bringing in a therapist before a child is ready can do more harm than good.*

Mommy's going to be kicking with both feet out of the grave, I promise you that. I'd like to talk to the young moms out there. I'm always getting questions, "What do you say, what do you do? I just want my life to be normal." My answer is, "Your life will never be the normal you knew." As much as that makes me angry, it's the truth. But your cancer doesn't have to be doom and gloom, it just has to be. And the way the mom handles it is the most important thing. Sometimes I'm short, not pleasant; I may not like myself. My kids are like, "Dang, Mom!" But I keep going.

The day after I came home from my mastectomy, my son said, "Will you pitch to me?" Peanut butter and jelly had to be made, and diapers had to be changed—and I wasn't going to be the thing that brought my family to its knees. I thank God for them.

Children Ages 9 to 12

As Dr. King found with her daughter, breast cancer is hard for older children because it seems to affect their whole identity. Children this age are very much aware of the differences between themselves and other children, so that having a sick parent may seem to change the child's entire sense of self.

Moreover, girls in this age range are beginning to understand that someday they will be women, with breasts and other aspects of a female identity. An increasing number of 11- and 12-year-olds are entering puberty these days, and associating their growing breasts with their mother's dangerous and debilitating illness can be a blow to their own sense of themselves as budding women.

Robyn Mitchell, Diagnosed at Age 30

My son Nicholas was 3 when I was diagnosed. I potty-trained him through my chemo.

It was pretty challenging being a single mom. During chemo, my day care called and said, "Your son has a 103 fever." I was very susceptible to any illness because my white count was so low. But I said, "I've got to go get him." I knew I had to take care of myself. But I had to be a mom, too. I said, "If I get sick, then he and I will just both have to be sick together."

When I lost my hair, that freaked him out a little bit. He'd say, "Mom, go put your hair on." There were times I'd just be lying on the couch and he'd say, "Mom, feel better." After chemo was done and I was feeling like a whole person again, I was like, "Thank goodness Nicholas has his mom back." I felt like I was missing out, too.

I was very fortunate to have the support I did. I was living with my mother. She was a great help. She told Nicholas, "Mommy's sick right now." He just adapted to what was going on.

If I was feeling bad, my sister would come and take him. She came over with three bottles of antibacterial soap and wanted to make sure that everyone in the house used it. She told everyone, "If you're sick, you don't come in this house."

My friend was a godsend, picking Nick up and dropping him off at day care. Walking into day care is like walking into a germ dungeon, especially when my white count was down so low. So she offered to do it.

Living with my mom, I didn't have to worry about grocery shopping. My family recognized that I was feeling sluggish, and they'd say, "Let me take Nick to the library or the park." But then you get that mommy guilt—"I should be out there." But you have to take care of yourself. You have to rest. My advice is, listen to your body and take care of yourself. Being a mother, you think you're the one who has to take care of everybody—but if people want to take care of you, let them!

Both girls and boys of this age are just beginning to understand that they too can die. So knowing that a parent is sick reinforces these pre-teens' fears about their own mortality. To children of this age, cancer may seem to be an invariably fatal illness, whatever your actual prognosis.

These issues are especially challenging because 9- to 12-year-olds are preparing for the power and independence that will come with being teenagers. This is a time when children are finding out how much they *don't* need their parents—yet their mother's illness and the prospect of her death reminds them how much they still *do* need mommy and daddy.

Children of this age may sometimes need to "feel like babies" when their parents are sick—even if their parents also need to lean on them a little bit, expecting them to help around the house or with younger siblings. It's reasonable to expect children of this age to pitch in, and to be gracious and polite to friends and relatives who have come to help out. But it's important to let them know that they're allowed to be sad or angry, and that feeling helpless and despairing is not somehow "letting Mom down."

Coping with the Daily Demands

Whatever the age of your children, you may be looking for ways to help them cope with your illness while somehow rallying your own energy to continue mothering:

1. *Draw on your support networks.* Now is the time to call on friends, siblings, parents, coworkers, and neighbors. Find out who can do what, and make a special effort to find out who can spend time with your children. Despite your best efforts, you're just not going to have your normal levels of energy for a while, and providing an "extended family" for your children may enable them to continue with their favorite activities, even as you cope with your own recovery. Your children's school may be an ideal place to turn for support, and getting teachers and counselors involved can help children deal with their emotions when they are away from home. It's also reassuring to children to recall that their circle of loved ones is very large. Mom may be the *most* important person in their lives—but it's nice to know there are *lots* of important people.

2. *Communicate with your partner.* As we saw in Chapter 6, this period is stressful for both of you, and stressful times often lead to communication shutting down or going awry. Especially where your children are concerned, it's crucial that you and your partner keep communicating, so that you can share the burdens—and the joys—as much as possible.

244

Tracy Pleva Hill, Diagnosed at Age 32

I want my son to know that I had a hand in making him a good person and a happy person, and that I've set him on the road to having a happy marriage and a happy family life. And I want to know that I've given him values and a sense of wonder, and that I've opened his mind to different things and helped to put a good person on the earth. Whose only legacy will be that he's another good person who opened the store door for someone. That's the kind of person I want to raise.

But when the cancer came back, I got really scared because I didn't see myself dancing at his wedding. I was just praying that I could walk him to kindergarten. And I needed to get back that image of me dancing at his wedding. That's where I want to be. I want to walk him to kindergarten—but I really want to be at his wedding.

My mother promised me, when I was just beginning to come to terms with my disease, that I would indeed dance at my son's wedding. "You and I are going to do the silliest dance at Jason's wedding," she told me. "Even if we both have to use walkers to do it."

I'm holding her to it. I plan to do the chicken dance.

I can just see it. I'm in a platinum ball gown—and I still have a pretty good body. And my son is blond and tall and built like his father—not massive, but solid—and my son's eyes are sparkling. And I just see me standing very close to him. I see Jeff, my husband, standing on the side, smiling. And then I just see me collapsing in Jason's arms. He's got to hold me up, because I can't believe I actually made it. This is the goal. And I really hope I don't ruin that girl's wedding day by trying to take it over. God bless the girl who gets that boy! Because after all I built him up to be in my mind, she's going to have a handful to deal with. I just picture myself being so happy and so proud of him. Just seeing my boy all grown up. That's what I want to see—my boy all grown up.

3. **Communicate with your children.** In any busy family, it can be a challenge to find "quiet time" where your children have the space to share thoughts and feelings that are troubling them, to ask questions about things that puzzle them, and to express the love and appreciation that they feel. In a family that is coping with a mother's breast cancer, finding this "quiet time" may seem almost impossible—and yet it is supremely necessary. You may need to figure out when your best times of day are and plan to set some of those aside as "just hanging out" time with your children.

4. *Figure out what's important, and discard the rest.* This isn't the time to worry about repainting the bedroom or keeping the living room spotless. Of course, some household chores just have to be done, even at the worst of times, and other tasks are crucial to your sense of well-being and order. But anything you can let go of, do. Save your energy for the people and activities that mean the very most to you—anything else just isn't worth it.

5. *Keep checking in with yourself.* As we saw in Chapter 5, journals, meditation, and other kinds of physical or spiritual practice are great ways to stay in touch with yourself, your emotions, and your sources of strength. Making this quiet time for yourself can help you focus on what's truly important to you in your relationships with your kids. Karen Sattaur decided to start a journal for her children, noting important family events, "So that if I'm not here, my kids will have a record of our time together." She also writes her children letters for future occasions, in case she's not there to enjoy them. Other mothers have found that this quiet time has awakened their intuition, so that they can better sense what their children might need—or what they need from their children.

6. *Give yourself a break.* If there is ever a good time to try to be superwoman, this isn't it. As Karen Sattaur found, there will be times when you won't be at your best, when you'll be short-tempered, grouchy, or insensitive. Forgive yourself, move on, and keep doing your best. The kinder you can be to yourself, the better life will be for your whole family—especially your kids.

Looking toward the Future

For many mothers, the hardest part of coping with breast cancer is looking toward a future in which they may not live to see their kids grow up. This pain can be a blessing as well as a curse, though. Many breast cancer moms say that the wish to be there for their kids is the strongest thing that keeps them going.

Journaling for Your Children

Karen Sattaur started a journal for her kids:

"I write to them when events happen—when my daughter rides her bike, when my son lost his first tooth. It's not about cancer. I also write letters for things I may not be here for. My daughter's first period. Her getting breasts—how will she feel? For my son, I just want him to be kind. I just want Damon to be his own person, and to look out for the underdog, and to have a kind and loving heart. I imagine him wondering, 'How do you treat a girl? How do you get your first girlfriend?'"

Here's an excerpt from one of the letters that Karen wrote to her children:

August 27, 2001

Dear Damon and Marie,

I was sitting in the dentist's office the other day reading an article about a young girl who lost her mother at age 14 of breast cancer, and I haven't been able to stop thinking about it. As I sit here, I am 35 and you two are 5 and 3, respectively. I do not know if I have 8 years left of my life. My cancer is back; it has spread to the lymph nodes in my neck, and I am soon to start another round of treatment.

The article I was reading was about this lady's mother who just disappeared one day, probably to go into a hospital and never return. The mother never left her a note of good-bye, or anything for her children to hold on to in the years to follow. I don't want to write this letter and the many more I am sure to write before I die. Now, understand that I have more of a will to live than any other person I know, but I am not sure what fate has in store for me.

I want you to know that you both are my shining stars, and I love you so desperately. As I sit here typing this, I am crying so hard I can barely see the monitor, hurting about leaving you so early. When I was diagnosed with breast cancer last year, you two were the things that made me fight, and you are still my motivation. I will fight this disease to the bitter end, and hopefully within that fight, they will develop a cure that will save my life.

To my sweet medium-sized angel Damon: You just started kindergarten 2 weeks ago, and what a fantastic job you are doing. I feel so proud when I see you walk past my classroom and you are so well behaved and confident. I know you are a role model for the other kids in your classroom with how smart you are and how kind. I also get such wonderful reports from other teachers about what a pleasure you are to have in class. My handsome, handsome boy with a heart as big as space, your mother couldn't love you any more if she tried. Please try to stay as happy, silly, and confident as you are. I know that me being gone has made you very sad, but if you stop being all the things I adore about you, then the cancer has beaten both of us. . . .

And to my sweet teeny weeny angel Marie: The heart on you is as big as the outdoors. You are so loving, generous, and helpful. . . . You love to laugh and play and help me do whatever it is I am doing at the time. You are always willing to help me fold clothes, or sweep the floor, or help unpack the groceries. . . . You are learning how to catch and kick a ball. You go way down the road and run toward the ball—you don't always kick it, but it doesn't stop you from running back down the street to try again.

Saying I love you seems so inconsequential to what I truly feel toward you two. You are miracles to me, both of you. . . .

Sweet Marie, I am so sorry you are going to have to be concerned with breast cancer in your lifetime. Know that you are in a line of women who were fighters and conquered the disease when they found it early. I found mine early at age 30, but no one would take me seriously because I was nursing and I was so young. You need to find a well-trained doctor compassionate to your needs. Your first tests should be done when you are 20, 10 years before my diagnosis. I hope that by the time this is appropriate for you to read, there is a cure for breast cancer and maybe all you'll have to endure is a shot and that will be it.

I'm going to close this letter for now, but rest assured that there will be more to come. You are the lights of my life, and I love you more than you could ever imagine.

Mommy

CHAPTER 11

"I Wanted to Be Taken Seriously"

Workplace Issues

"For me, it wasn't the cancer I was afraid of," says Leslie Mouton. "I was scared to death that it was going to kill my career." When Leslie was diagnosed with breast cancer at age 35, she was a news anchor at station KSAT in San Antonio, Texas. "The idea of losing my job was daunting," she says. "It was the scariest feeling I'd ever known. Because broadcasting was all I knew. I've wanted to be a news anchor as long as I can remember."

"I was trying to figure out a way to talk about this with the men in my office," says Cynthia Rubin, who had made partner in her New York City law firm 21 days before she was diagnosed with breast cancer at age 36. I wanted to say, 'OK, this isn't about breasts, this is about cancer.' Because my breasts are something I never discuss with the men in my office. And I think for younger women this can be a very difficult situation, especially if you work with men who are older than you."

"There are a lot of reasons that people might perceive you as being weak when you have cancer," says Kelly Douglas, who was working at a toy company in Indianapolis when she was diagnosed with breast cancer at age 24. "Even the week after my chemo, I went to work, but I didn't do full days—I was just too tired. There was even one day when I said, 'I really need to conserve my energy.' I deal with large files, so as my computer is chugging along, I have my head on my desk, because I have 4 more hours, and I really want to make it through the day. But that's weakness. I didn't make a full day of work all week. And how does that make me look, working at this job exactly a year?"

Coping with Workplace Issues

If you're in your twenties or thirties, you are most likely either just getting started in your career or just hitting your stride professionally. Even if, like Cynthia and Leslie, you've already achieved significant career goals, you probably still have the sense that your best working years are ahead of you. If you're in your early twenties, the workplace may still seem like new territory. It's natural for you to still be feeling your way—figuring out how to play office politics, how to get yourself noticed by the people in charge, how to accomplish your personal and professional goals. Or you may still be exploring the world of work, trying out different careers, figuring out whether you're happy with your choices, going back to school or making other work-related commitments.

Being diagnosed with breast cancer brings a whole new dimension to this already challenging arena. You may face a number of problems at work: wanting to be taken seriously; seeking the physical and emotional energy you need in order to do the job; dealing with anxieties about dramatic changes in your physical appearance; and handling the practical necessities of negotiating time off for surgery, treatment, and recovery.

The good news is that many young breast cancer survivors have encountered a flexible, cooperative attitude from their employers and colleagues that they would never have expected. "I was so afraid that having breast cancer would cost me my career, that it would destroy me," says Leslie. "And what happened instead? I was promoted—because, despite everything that I was going through, they knew I was doing a good job." While not every woman can expect the kind of unconditional support that Leslie found at her TV station, her story is a powerful reminder of what can be possible.

Other young women have experienced their breast cancer diagnoses as a kind of wake-up call, moving them out of jobs that they didn't really care about into work that they found more meaningful. When women realize that they are faced with a life-threatening disease, it often moves them to rethink the choices they've made. Confronted with this situation, you may find the courage to pursue an ambition you were reluctant to pursue before. You might decide that the work choices you've made so far were based primarily on money or security or prestige and that having cancer spurs you to make decisions that now seem more authentic, exciting, or worthwhile. You may be moved to stand up for yourself more vigorously at the job you already have, or to seek to do better work there, or to find ways to derive more satisfaction from the work you do. Whatever your response, your first step is to become informed about your rights and your options, and your second, to match them with your own needs.

Leslie Mouton, Anchor, TV News

I'm from Lafayette, Louisiana, good ol' Cajun country. And when I was growing up, I always wanted to be a news anchor, but I had this heavy Cajun accent. I remember I used to sit in front of the mirror when I was young with a newspaper in my hand, practicing getting rid of my accent. So I studied broadcasting in college and interned at a station and was very blessed when I got a job in the small market of Alexandria, Louisiana, which is where I met my husband, Tony. Eventually Tony and I were both working in San Antonio. I felt like everything about life was perfect. We're both doing what we love, we have a beautiful baby girl—finally, life is right where we want it to be. Then I discover the lump in my breast. Now what?

I went through surgery and chemotherapy, and tried to cope with the loss of my hair.

Most of the time I didn't wear a wig when I wasn't at work. But when I was on the air anchoring, I always wore my wig. I even named it—she was Betty. I met so many women who would tell me stories that would horrify me. They couldn't walk in their own house by themselves without a wig—that was so sad to me. For women who are going to be diagnosed tomorrow or the next day, I want them to know that you don't have to fear losing your hair. If I can be here on TV without a strand of hair, you can live your life without the hair. That's why I decided to anchor one newscast bald.

I went to my news director and said, "Jim, there's something I want to do." I was already putting together a three-part series on my story. I said, "The night I do the last part, I'd like to do it bald. I don't want to just introduce the story bald, or pull my wig off and make some dramatic display; I want to do the whole newscast bald to show that it can be okay." He looked at me, put his hands together, and he said, "Okay. If you want to do it, we'll do it."

I will never forget making that walk to the anchor chair that night. I saw Betty in my locker, but I left her there. I kept putting powder on my head to make sure the lights wouldn't cause a big glare. And I was definitely nervous—even though I knew I was making the right decision.

Then the six o'clock news started. The camera started on my coanchor, Steve, so that he could introduce me. It wouldn't have been fair to the audience to just start with me bald. Steve needed to introduce me to give viewers a chance to understand what was happening.

Then the weather anchor got a picture of all of us and made everyone bald in the picture. My coworkers made it fun and light and fine. After the newscast we did an online chat. Hundreds of people all across the world had been watching. It was amazing. It was such the right decision. But it was scary.

It's so tough for young women. There are so many who are single, and they're thinking about dating, finding a man, how they are going to be perceived. I just wanted to say, "We can all get through this. Just because we're young doesn't mean we have to hide or be ashamed. We're fighting something that's not our fault."

Tips for Coping with Workplace Issues

- *Start by figuring out what you want.* As Leslie discovered, it may take time for you to sort out your responses, and these responses may change over time. You may also feel constrained by financial pressures, your partner's needs, your children's needs, and many other outside factors. But if you can start by getting clear about what *you* want—not what you think you *have* to do but what you want to do— you'll be in a much stronger position to make and implement good decisions. *Find out your legal situation.* Is your workplace covered by the Americans with Disabilities Act (ADA) or the Family Medical Leave Act (FMLA)? Does your state have employment protection laws that apply to you? Is there a company policy on breast cancer or other illnesses? (Some companies have personnel policies on AIDS and HIV that may offer you some precedents, either legally or as a matter of policy.) Does your union contract provide any safeguards? (For more about your legal rights on the job, see the next section.)

- *Get your support network in place.* It's always easier to act with the support of others. If you can, figure out whom you can trust and work out a plan with them—or at least assure yourself of their support. Your support network may come from inside or outside of work, or both. Unions, feminist groups, and local cancer organizations may be helpful, along with coworkers, trusted supervisors, family, and friends. *Be clear about your bottom line, your backup plan, and your other options.* It can be nerve-wracking to start negotiating for time off or a lighter workload. Even just telling your boss that you have cancer may feel like a heavy decision. Knowing what you will and won't tolerate, and what other options you have, will help you conduct negotiations with the positive air that is most likely to get you good results.

- *Remember that your attitude makes a huge difference.* Although you can't control other people's responses, you can certainly cue them in the direction you'd like them to go. If you act as though you're not sure whether you have the right to continue at work, your colleagues may start to wonder. If you act with perfect assurance that you're the same wonderful coworker you've always been, even if you need a bit more time off, your colleagues are far more likely to respond in kind. Projecting a genuine belief in yourself will help your colleagues adopt that attitude, too.

- *Expect to be surprised.* The reports of young survivors span the gamut, from the ex-best friend who stopped calling to the once-unfriendly coworker who turned out to be a lifeline. Over the course of your illness, treatment, and recovery, you'll encounter many surprises from yourself and others. These surprises may be both a blessing and a curse, but they're definitely something you can count on.

Your Rights on the Job

If you work at a company with 15 or more employees, you're covered under the Americans with Disabilities Act (ADA). If your company has 50 or more employees within a 75-mile radius, you're also protected by the Family Medical Leave Act (FMLA). In some cases, you will be even better protected under state labor laws. Many aspects of California state employment law, for example, extend to workplaces with only five or more employees. Finally, two federal acts, COBRA and HIPAA, protect your right to continued health insurance coverage.

You can find out more about your rights on the job from the Patient Advocate Foundation (PAF) and the Job Accommodation Network (JAN), both of which are private, nonprofit agencies set up to help people with illnesses or disabilities. (For more information about PAF and JAN, and for other sources of workplace information, see the Resources section at the end of this book.)

Americans with Disabilities Act (ADA)

The civil rights and feminist movements won their battles for several major pieces of federal legislation that protect women and minorities from discrimination on the job. When the Americans with Disabilities Act (ADA) was passed, that on-the-job protection was extended to people with disabilities, which the law defines as "a physical or mental impairment that substantially limits one or more of [a person's] major life activities; a record of such an impairment; or being regarded as having an impairment." The federal agency that oversees the rights of other "protected classes," the Equal Employment Opportunity Commission (EEOC), is also charged with safeguarding the rights of the disabled.

As you can see from the definition, there are a lot of gray areas in the law—gray areas that are continually being clarified via lawsuits and administrative decisions. A famous 1992 lawsuit, for example, determined that people with AIDS could be protected under the act, since their illness substantially limited many of their major life activities and since they were perceived as being impaired. As a woman with breast cancer, you, too, may be considered disabled—but according to Sharon Rennert, senior attorney advisor with the EEOC's ADA division, you might not be. As Rennert explains, it all depends upon how severely your breast cancer interferes with your life:

> The statute does not cover breast cancer. It covers a woman whose breast cancer limits a major life activity. If her breast cancer is caught very early, and there's been no mastectomy, and the cancer has all been removed, and minimal time off is needed, then, potentially, the woman would not be covered under the ADA. Some courts have found that early stage cases may not be covered. If you have a more serious case, it increases the likelihood that it would meet the legal definition of disability.

Your Rights under the ADA

The ADA can help you in two ways. First, it protects you from being fired simply because you have breast cancer. You can be fired "for cause"—for something you actually did or failed to do—but not simply because you have a disease. Second, the ADA requires your employer to make "reasonable accommodations" to your needs, if those accommodations don't cause your company "undue hardship."

Clearly, these are two more gray areas. What kinds of accommodations are "reasonable," and which hardships count as "undue"? While the ADA has to be interpreted on a case-by-case basis, it does provide some details about these concepts. According to "Steps to Resolution," a pamphlet published by PAF,[1] reasonable accommodations might include

- Shifting minor job responsibilities to other employees
- Paid leave time that does not present undue hardship
- Modified or part-time scheduling
- Reassignment to a new position that you are qualified for
- Making the workplace accessible and usable

Undue hardship, on the other hand, "would be changes to the work environment that would include significant difficulty and/or expense. Undue hardship also refers to accommodations that would be disruptive or that would alter the nature of the business."

According to Beth Loy, a consultant with the Job Accommodation Network, fatigue, weakness, and the need for time off for medical treatment are the major reasons that women with breast cancer need accommodation, which might include "flexible scheduling, working from home, or sometimes part-time work. For example, if fatigue is an issue and you have to park far away, you can ask for parking that's closer. Sometimes working at a desk is an issue—you might need forearm support. Or if you have to lift heavy objects, you may need a lifting device."

But what if you work as a mail handler, and lifting 50-pound sacks of mail is a regular part of your job? In that case, redefining your job to eliminate heavy lifting or providing you with an expensive lifting device might be considered undue hardship. On the other hand, if you work in an office and your job sometimes requires you to lift piles of books or files from a low shelf, it might be considered reasonable for your employer to install a higher shelf or to assign someone to come in occasionally and help you move the files.

Likewise, if you work at a small company with rigid shift scheduling, allowing you to leave an hour early on the days you have chemo might be considered an undue hardship. If the work flow at your company is more unstructured, asking for a flexible schedule might be seen as reasonable.

Claiming Your ADA Protection

In order to be protected under the ADA, you must inform your employer that you have breast cancer, and you must request the accommodations you need. You cannot say after the fact that you were fired because you had breast cancer if your company can claim that it was unaware of your condition. Nor can you complain that you were not given the accommodations that you needed if there is no record that you ever asked for any accommodations. You can request that your supervisor keep your condition confidential, if you like. But to claim your rights under the ADA, you must tell your employer what you need and why—preferably in writing.

For many young women, words such as "impairment" and "disability" can be daunting. After all, you're trying to prove your strength and competence, to yourself as well as to your employer. Thinking of yourself as "impaired" or "disabled" may run directly counter to the positive attitude you're trying to cultivate elsewhere in your life.

Tips for Your Letter Requesting Accommodations from Your Employer

- Identify yourself as a person with a disability, and state that you are requesting accommodations under the ADA.

- Discuss the impairments that your breast cancer has created—fatigue, weakness, the need to have frequent medical treatments, the need to recover from surgery, etc.

- Suggest your own ideas for accommodations that might address your condition.

- Request the employer's ideas for accommodations.

- Refer to any medical documentation that you have, including a letter from your doctor affirming that you have breast cancer and describing the ways in which it might affect you.

- Ask your employer to respond within a specific, reasonable amount of time. Ten business days is often a good period.

Based on suggestions made by Beth Loy, consultant, Job Accommodation Network

The terminology may indeed be unfortunate. But consider turning your perspective around, so that you view your actions as powerful and assertive. After all, you're claiming your rights to continue working and recovering from cancer in your own way. What could be less "impaired" than that?

Pursuing Your Rights under the ADA

Your first step under the ADA is to figure out what accommodations you need and then to request them from your employer. If the two of you can work out an arrangement that suits both of you, the matter ends there. If you're not satisfied with your employer's response, you have the option of filing a complaint with the EEOC or with one of the state agencies, which the EEOC refers to as "Fair Employment Practices Agencies" (FEPAs). If you have trouble locating the appropriate agency in your area, ask the Patient Advocate Foundation or the Job Accommodation Network to help you sort through the bureaucracy.

Deciding How Far to Pursue Your Rights

If you do decide to ask for accommodations on the job, you may discover that your employer can find lots of ways to make life hard for you, either deliberately or simply by being insensitive. This can often create a vi-

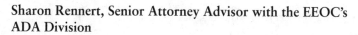

Sharon Rennert, Senior Attorney Advisor with the EEOC's ADA Division

It's important for women to realize that as soon as they know that there's something they need, they should be asking for it. I think that what often happens is that women try to get by without anyone knowing. They won't acknowledge that the treatments are taking a toll.

You might have to ask, "Can I work part-time for a few weeks?" Or maybe you need to ask for the job to be slightly restructured, to say, "Here are the less important parts of my job. I don't have the energy right now to do everything, so how about I focus on the most important parts of my job?" Maybe the less important tasks can be temporarily reassigned.

I think it's important to emphasize that under the ADA, the responsibility is on the woman to request accommodation. It can be hard to ask for what you need. Your relationship with your supervisor can affect whether you feel comfortable asking for accommodations. Or maybe you're in some denial about the side effects you're feeling—you want to believe you can do it all. Whatever your reason for not asking, though, the bottom line is this: If the employer is never told, "I need an accommodation," then you have no legal right to that accommodation. So the moment you realize that you need something, ask for it. It could save you a lot of trouble in the long run.

cious circle in which it becomes difficult to distinguish between legitimate and illegitimate concerns.

For example, if you, like Kelly, put your head down on your desk because you're exhausted from your chemo, your supervisor may chide you for unprofessional behavior. After all, the supervisor might say, the company has accommodated your illness by giving you some time off for the chemo, but your illness doesn't excuse sloppiness or poor office etiquette. You might cringe and agree with your supervisor that your behavior *is* unacceptable; or you might say, out loud or to yourself, "Hey! Being tired after chemo is part of the process of having cancer, and you're legally obligated not to give me trouble about it." Either way, though, you may find yourself reacting to the scolding—overcompensating by trying to do too much; feeling anxious when the supervisor walks through again; worrying unduly about your job performance. Perhaps your extra exertion then makes you even more tired, or you find yourself making mistakes as a result of your anxiety. Now your supervisor points not to your

Tips for Protecting Your Rights on the Job

- *Keep a journal.* Record everything that happens that might relate to your situation. If you've had a meeting with someone, write down whom you met with and what was said. If your supervisor reprimands or praises you, write it down. If your job responsibilities change, or if someone else is asked to do something that would normally be your job, make a note.

- *Save all paperwork related to your job status and responsibilities.* Keep all the memos and other office communications that you get, starting from when you are diagnosed with breast cancer.

- *Write your own letters and memos.* If you've had a meeting with your supervisor, follow up the meeting with a letter or email reviewing your understanding of what just happened. This is both good communication and an effective way to let your employer know that you are keeping track of your situation.

- *Be assertive without being confrontational.* If there was ever a time to be assertive, this is it. Not only will assertiveness help you achieve your desired end, but it will also speak volumes to those around you about the respect you have for yourself.

cancer but to your mistakes, which seems more "objective" and "reasonable"—and legally protected—than criticizing you for cancer-related issues.

Clearly, knowing that you have legal rights is one thing. Deciding how far you're willing to go in pursuit of them is another. After all, having breast cancer is already a lot to deal with. You may feel that you're just not up to fighting for your rights on the job.

Of course, it's your decision. But Rennert urges you to assert yourself and your rights. "If people don't ask for accommodations when they need them, then employers aren't going to realize they may have to give them—and that lets the employer off the hook," she says.

The Family Medical Leave Act (FMLA)

If your employer has 50 or more employees within a 75-mile radius, you may be eligible for protection under the Family Medical Leave Act (FMLA), a law passed in 1993 that entitles you to 12 work weeks of unpaid leave during any 12-month period in response to a serious health condition. (The FMLA also entitles family members to leave to take care

Steps in Exercising Your Rights through the EEOC or a FEPA

- You file a complaint. (Sometimes, just telling your company that you are considering this step can make it more responsive.)

- The EEOC or state agency interviews you to find out what happened.

- You may be advised to enter the EEOC's mediation program with your employer—to bring in a third-party mediator who can help the two of you voluntarily work out your differences. Decisions reached under mediation don't necessarily have the force of law, but mediation may very well solve your problem more quickly and easily than any other option.

- If you or your employer chooses not to enter mediation, or if the mediation process fails, then the agency will investigate. An investigator will interview your employer and probably other employees or witnesses as well. You are likely to be asked to produce medical documents and other relevant evidence. This when having kept a diary really pays off.

- The EEOC or state agency issues a decision as to whether or not it found discrimination. If there was discrimination, a settlement is recommended. However, if you needed an accommodation 6 months ago and your case is only now being settled, you've already suffered from your employer's action. In that case, the EEOC might award you damages.

- If your employer does not voluntarily comply with the EEOC's ruling, the EEOC may choose to bring suit. You may also have the option of bringing a private lawsuit.

of you, as well as granting parents leave to care for newborn or adopted children.) To qualify for the FMLA, you must have worked at least 1250 hours over the previous 12 months. Note that you're eligible for leave on a yearly basis, so if you have, for example, two rounds of chemo treatment over 2 years, you may be able to manage 12 weeks' leave for each.

Sometimes FMLA leave may be taken intermittently. Rather than taking 12 unpaid weeks all at once, you can ask for 1 day off a week or a few hours off each day. In some cases, either you or your employer may choose to use accrued paid leave, such as sick days or vacation time, to cover some or all of the 12 weeks allowed under the FMLA. If you're requesting FMLA leave, make sure you find out what kind of arrange-

Kelly Douglas, Designer at a Toy Company

I've been at this job exactly a year. I had a really good year, but the last couple of months have been plagued. Because of my mastectomy I had to take off 2 weeks, and my biopsy meant that I missed 2 days. That's really hard, especially because industries move so fast and you have timelines—and if you don't meet the deadline, that's a sign of weakness, that you're not up to the job.

When I had the mastectomy, I'd be at work and I couldn't lift things. I'm like, "This is a drag. It's ridiculous. I should be able to move something by myself. I'm usually such a healthy person, and I should be acting more healthy. I shouldn't be sitting around accepting the situation."

I don't like feeling that way. I'm a perfectionist. I want to do a good job—I want to do the best I can. And when I can't, I feel guilty and depressed about it. I think, "Gosh, why couldn't I get this done?" It's really hard, especially when you first start a job.

ments your employer is making. You don't want to discover later on that you've used up your sick leave or vacation time if you didn't intend to do so.

While you're on FMLA leave, you must be given the same group health insurance coverage you had before, "on the same terms as if the employee had never left work," according to the Patient Advocate Foundation (PAF). In some cases, your employer may be entitled to ask you to pay your own premiums, however, so again, check with your company on this matter. However, your coverage while on FMLA leave cannot be considered COBRA coverage.

If your health benefits expire while you're on FMLA leave, your company has to notify you of your COBRA benefits and give you a letter that you can use to protect your coverage under HIPAA. (For more on COBRA and HIPAA, see the next sections of this chapter.)

When you come back from an FMLA leave, you have to be given either your original job or an equivalent position with equivalent pay, benefits, and working conditions. Your company cannot deprive you of any benefits as a result of your leave. However, if you were a highly paid "key" employee, your company may have the right to refuse to give you back your original job, on the grounds that the company cannot afford to do without someone in your position and that it is not possible to replace you for 12 weeks only. A key employee must be among the highest paid 10 percent of employees within 75 miles of your work site. If your company does consider you "key," it has to notify you of this and tell you that it is planning not to restore your job. You also have to be given a reasonable chance to return from your leave before forfeiting your position.

To take advantage of FMLA leave, you have to give your employer 30 days' advance notice if "the need is foreseeable and such notice is practicable," according to PAF. You may also need to provide medical certification before your leave and periodic reports during your leave. In some cases, your employer might ask you to see one or two other physicians for second and third opinions, with costs covered by the employer.

If you use your FMLA leave intermittently—say, around your chemo, or in response to your varying energy levels during treatment—you are supposed to schedule your time off "so as not to unduly disrupt the employer's operation," in PAF's words.

Like your rights under the ADA, your rights under the FMLA may vary a good deal, depending on your employer and your situation. "Standards aren't out there on what qualifies under the FMLA and what doesn't," says Janine McMillion, a job discrimination lawyer for PAF and herself a young survivor who was diagnosed with breast cancer at age 29. "It's still a fairly new law, so there are not a lot of case studies on it. But if you have a strong chronological diary, you have a leg to stand on. It also seems to be guided a lot by the states. There are some states in which the employers tend to be harsher than in others." McMillion stresses, however, that PAF is always available to help women sort through both their employment and their insurance issues.

COBRA

The Consolidated Omnibus Budget Reconciliation Act (COBRA), passed in 1986, is a federal law that, among other things, requires your employer to continue your group health coverage even after you leave your job, although you have to pay your own premiums. If you choose continued coverage, you will have to pay both the employee and the employer portions of the premium, plus a 2 percent service charge. The law prevents your COBRA cost from exceeding 102 percent of the premium cost for the full employee rate.

COBRA covers anyone working for a company with 20 or more employees. When you leave your job, your employer must notify you about COBRA and then give you 60 days to either choose COBRA or lose your rights to COBRA benefits. COBRA coverage usually lasts for 18 months. However, if you are the spouse of an employee and you lose coverage because of the death of the employee or because of divorce, you can continue coverage for 36 months. And if you are the dependent child of an employee and you lose coverage because you have passed the age limit for dependent children, you can continue the coverage for 36 months. COBRA coverage can be denied only to employees who are fired for "gross misconduct."

HIPAA

The Health Insurance Portability and Accountability Act of 1996 restricts insurance companies from refusing you coverage because of a preexisting condition, such as breast cancer. It also bans discrimination against you on the basis of your health status and guarantees that you will not be charged a higher premium for any reason related to your health status. HIPAA also guarantees other rights that are specific to women, including protections for mothers and newborns and certain benefits for mastectomy patients, including coverage of breast reconstruction and related services.

For more details on how HIPAA applies to your particular situation, contact PAF.

Looking for a New Job

Just as the ADA protects you from being fired or harassed at your current job, it also protects your right to be hired at a new job. And again, a new employer may find apparently legitimate reasons not to hire you that are really cover-ups for unwillingness to take on a cancer survivor.

You're the only one who knows what the right answer is in this situation. If an employer is reluctant to hire you because of your breast cancer, it will probably be difficult for you to prove that you've been discriminated against—and in any case, you may not have the time or energy to bring a lawsuit, which is your only legal recourse. Once your new employer has hired you, of course, he or she is then obliged to make reasonable accommodations under the ADA or state law (if he or she has enough employees to be covered under the law).

Coping with Perceptions

Even if you're fairly confident that you can keep or get a job, you may be concerned about being taken seriously at work. As a young woman, and perhaps as a new employee, you may have been eager to prove yourself to your coworkers and your employer even before you got your diagnosis. Now you have breast cancer, a disease that most people associate with weakness and fragility. How do you cope with people's fears and assumptions about your illness?

Cynthia Rubin, Partner in a Law Firm

I think these are big issues for newly diagnosed young women: who to tell, how to tell them, when to tell them. There's no road map for that. And I found that to be very difficult. I'm a lawyer, and 21 days before I was diagnosed, I'd become a partner at my law firm. So it was good timing, I think, but I was also at a jumping-off point to really go with my career, and I had concerns about it. "Do I tell my clients? Will they think I can't do my job? Will I be able to do my job? What am I going to do if I have to be in court the day I have a chemo treatment? Do I say to the judge, 'I'm on chemo, and I have a treatment that day?'"

Once I found out how I reacted to the chemotherapy, it was much easier for me to figure things out. But there were uncomfortable moments also.

I know women who really didn't tell a lot of people in the workplace. I did. It spread in the community of lawyers I work with. And then you get this feeling that every time you walk into the room, everybody's looking at you and thinking, "Oh, poor Cynthia." And that wasn't my persona at all.

I didn't want people feeling sorry for me or whispering behind my back, "How's she doing?" And sort of wondering, "Is that her real hair?" People knew, and I wasn't shy about talking about it, but I never complained about it. I tried not to use it as an excuse.

But then, on the other hand, you're thinking, "Nobody's asking me how I'm feeling today!"

My friend Meg gave me very good advice. She said, "Tell as few people as possible until you know exactly what you're doing." It's hard to tell people, "I have breast cancer, and I don't know what I'm doing about it yet." And then you realize you have to call 18 people back every day, because they all want to find out if you've made any decisions. It's much better to go at it, "I was diagnosed with breast cancer, and I found a terrific doctor, and I've decided on X treatment, I'm going to have surgery on this date," so people know you're in control of the situation.

Kelly, for example, works in the toy industry. She associates wearing a wig with being a stodgy older woman, not at all with her own "quirky, artsy" image as a designer. Left to her own devices, she'd prefer to "go bald." But she worries that her coworkers will see her baldness not as a fashion statement but as a symbol of disease.

Tips for Coping with Perceptions at Work

- *Remember that the ways in which you view yourself, your responsibilities, and your rights are the most important of all.* If you feel you're not living up to your own standards, draw on your support system and your inner resources to question yourself. Do you need to try harder? Are your standards too high? Do you need to adjust your idea of what's realistic in response to your new situation? In the end, what matters most is whether you believe you've done what you thought was right.

- *Do a reality check.* Try not to let your imagination get the better of you. If you think people are viewing you in a particular way, and if you believe that's affecting your treatment at work, see if you can find out more. Speak to a trusted coworker, have a conversation with your supervisor, or just pay attention for a while. You might discover that there really isn't a "perception problem" after all.

- *Consider small solutions first.* If you're already feeling stressed and fragile, you may think that the perception problem is worse than it is. Perhaps it can be solved by simple means, such as slipping quietly out of the office on the days you have chemo, rather than saying good-bye to your coworkers. Perhaps all you have to do is wait it out until your colleagues see how good your work still is. Think of the smallest possible step you might take to solve your problem, and try it out before going on to bigger actions.

- *Draw on your support network.* Use your family and friends outside of work as a sounding board and for moral support. Figure out whose work-related advice you trust, and who consistently sees you as the strong but sometimes vulnerable person that you really are. Enlist these loved ones in helping you to stay focused on a clear, realistic, and loving portrait of yourself—and then brainstorm about some on-the-job strategies with them.

"I don't want to be perceived as weak because I have cancer," Kelly insists. "That's the only thing I don't like about this whole bald head thing. You see a bald woman, you think, 'Oh, cancer, chemotherapy. She's sick.' That's not who I am, and that's not how I want to be perceived."

Being perceived as competent is one issue. But really *being* competent, even while coping with a disease that can drain your energy and impair

Lisa Muccilo, Full-Time Advocate for Young Women with Cancer

I never wanted the disease to take control of my life. I always wanted to continue living my life. And I was always working.

So I'd be sitting at work hearing that the lump on my neck was cancer. I finally said, "What the hell am I doing at work?"

At that point, I think, my whole life changed. I said, "I don't want to do this any more. I'm not going to live forever, and I know that. I don't want my days to be spent like this—breaking my back to do this job. I should be with my family. I should be with people who love me."

So I left that day, and I never went back to that job again. I was home every day spending 3 or 4 hours on the computer, doing whatever I could for the YSC. Then I went to work full time for the Susan G. Komen Foundation.

I think now I'm more thoughtful, more mindful of what I do. I feel like I just soak things up more now. I've done a lot of great things since I was diagnosed.

your concentration, is another matter. Like most young people starting their careers, you may have expected that you would come to work early and stay late, putting in the long hours and extra effort that will demonstrate your value to the company. But the reality of your illness may interfere.

"I'm used to working longer hours at work," Kelly says. "I'll stay late and come home and still be thinking about my job. But when you have cancer, you're not quite all there. You're at work, and you're thinking about cancer. You come home, and you're thinking about cancer. Or you're thinking about what's going to happen with treatment options. And because that shift has happened in my life, I'm more sensitive about telling people I have cancer. I already feel the change or weakness in me, so I don't want someone to have that reinforced."

As a young woman, you may also have a particular stake in focusing on your professional life at work while keeping your personal life out of bounds. Like Cynthia Rubin, you may have worked hard to establish your professional credibility, turning your colleagues' attention away from your youth and femininity and toward your work-related credentials. Now, suddenly, you have breast cancer, a disease that seems to bring your private life into the workplace.

Changing Your Relationship to Work

As we've seen, breast cancer brings lots of changes—including changes in the way young women relate to their work.

"If anything, cancer has kind of kicked me in the butt," says Kelly Douglas. "I'm really easygoing and maybe too complacent. So this has made me focus. I have so many art and music things I'd love to do, and I have only so much time in the world to do them. So maybe cancer has kicked me into getting some things done."

Tracy Pleva Hill, diagnosed with breast cancer at age 32, has actually felt energized at her workplace as a result of her illness, partly because she's been inspired to integrate her professional life with her activism. When she heard at a YSC meeting that the group was looking for office space for Michele Przypyszny, the organization's executive director, "I brought it back to my company . . . and they said, 'Bring her in.' Every time I've asked my company to help with the cause, they've responded positively." Lisa Muccilo's activism, on the other hand, prompted her to leave her long-time job as a telephone engineer to find more meaningful work at the YSC and the Susan G. Komen Foundation. Lisa knew that her decision had been right for her the first time her oncologist called her at her new job to tell her that her cancer had spread.

"But I was at my new job, which meant so much to me," Lisa says, "and all I could think was, 'All right. There's no other place for me to be at this moment. I have everything I need here. I can handle this.'"

CHAPTER 12

"I Just Try to Focus on the Now . . ."

When Cancer Recurs or Metastasizes

Juanita Lyle was diagnosed with breast cancer at age 32. She was given a very poor prognosis when she was first diagnosed, and, indeed, her cancer recurred three times. But today, at age 58, she has raised her two children to adulthood and is still pursuing the activities she enjoys.

"The thing about living with breast cancer is that you have such uncertainty in your life," she says. "I would simply pray and say, 'God, let me see these kids get out of elementary school.' As time went on, I'd say, 'Let me see them get out of junior high.' But I always focused on having fun and making light of things."

Juanita remembers having an enormous amount of fear as she continually wondered what her illness might mean. "Living with the idea of dying is scary," she says. "I'm not going to tell you there weren't times I would cry. Because in the midst of having three recurrences, I also had four biopsies that were scares. There are things that go wrong with you, and the longer you live, the more time you have to have something go wrong."

Still, Juanita says, focusing on the fear doesn't help. "If you constantly think something's wrong every time you get a little ache or pain, that would be too much to take. The way I keep myself afloat is to focus on the now. I put more quality time into relationships, I connect with people, and, most of all, I don't put things off. I never say, 'Oh, I can do that tomorrow.' No, I just do that today."

Nalini Yadla was a 22-year-old medical student living in Baltimore when she was first diagnosed with ductal carcinoma in situ (DCIS), a noninvasive form of breast cancer. She had a mastectomy 3 days after she was diagnosed. Since her lymph nodes tested negative, her margins were clear, and DCIS is considered noninvasive, she thought her ordeal was over. "It happened so fast that I barely had time to think about it," she says. "All I thought about was catching up on all the schoolwork I had missed. I never had a fear of death, or even of actually being sick, and my doctor told me not to worry. So, I didn't."

The following October, Nalini developed a dry cough that somehow never went away. When she had a chest x-ray done that winter, the technician said casually, "You're a med student, right? You want to take a look at this?" As Nalini recalls, "He was probably thinking it would be fun to look together and find a little glob from pneumonia or something." Instead, she says, "When the x-ray came out of the machine, I thought there must have been a mistake. Why were there all these white spots all over my lungs?"

Nalini's cancer had been misdiagnosed. Instead of DCIS, she had a particularly invasive form of breast cancer that had metastasized to her lungs and her brain. After a long, difficult course of treatment, 27-year-old Nalini is back in medical school and looking forward to her future. "Medically, I'm doing very well. My tumor markers are undetectable, and the scans show no cancer activity. Based on what I know about my prognosis, I'm confident I'll live a long life."

⤜⤗

When Beth Brokaw was first diagnosed with breast cancer, she was 37 years old, a teacher and therapist living in the southern California town of Azusa. She had just given birth to her first child a few days before. She responded to her cancer with a lumpectomy—a complicated procedure for a newly lactating mother—and then chemotherapy, and finally a double mastectomy, which, she says, was "essentially prophylactic," to ensure against the possibility of recurrence. On the advice of her physician, noted breast surgeon and author Dr. Susan Love, she chose not to get pregnant again for fear that the hormones released during pregnancy would cause her cancer to recur. Instead, she and her husband adopted a son. Her lump "wasn't huge," and only one lymph node was involved. After all of Beth's precautions, she says, "They gave me a 75 percent chance of its not metastasizing."

But, after 7 cancer-free years, it did metastasize. Learning that her cancer was metastatic, Beth says, transformed her response to her illness—and to her life. "When I was first diagnosed, I kept going with life," she says. "I lived like a survivor." Now, she says, "It's a whole different picture. This is not curable. I'm not living like a survivor—I'm living like someone who wants to get the most life squeezed out in the time I have left. That's a very different way to approach life."

Coping with Cancer That Recurs or Metastasizes

If you have breast cancer and you're reading this book, you are probably focusing on what you can do to survive. And, indeed, you have an excellent chance of living a long and cancer-free life.

Sometimes, though, cancer does recur, and sometimes it metastasizes, or spreads, to other parts of your body. (This chapter is written primarily for women who are facing a recurrence of their cancer or who were initially diagnosed at stage 4.) If you'd rather not consider those possibilities right now, you may want to skip this chapter.

The prevailing view of breast cancer—which is usually correct—is that you'll face a terrible year, and then you'll be able to put it all behind you. If, however, you are facing a diagnosis of breast cancer that has spread to other parts of the body or is locally advanced, you may be afraid of the new treatments and concerned by the prospect that a cure is unlikely. Many survivors of advanced cancer are women who live with breast cancer in their lives and find that arming themselves with knowledge replaces fear with facts.

But for some women, the fight continues. Tracy Pleva Hill, was diagnosed with breast cancer at age 32—and faced the recurrence of her cancer in the lymph nodes of her neck and underarm at age 33. "I still can't believe it," she says. "When you first get the diagnosis, they march out every survivor, and they all say, 'I did it. I survived. This is the worst year of your life. But you get your life back.' Then if it happens to you again, it's like, you can't find anybody. I was so angry. I felt so cheated."

And it's hard, says Tracy, not to blame yourself. "I was trying to rack my brain," she says. "What did I do wrong? Am I such a horrible person? Who did I hurt? And how can I make it better? Because this wasn't in my plan."

If facing breast cancer when you're young is hard, facing recurrence and metastasis is that much harder. "Young women with breast cancer are already an invisible population, and young women with metastatic disease are even more hidden," says Roz Kleban, an administrative supervisor of the Department of Social Work at Memorial Sloan-Kettering in New York City and the leader of a support group for young women with metastatic cancer.

"It turns your world upside down," says Carolyn Messner, director of education and training at the national office of Cancer Care, a group that provides counseling and other services for people with cancer. "It destabilizes your expectations, your feelings of being in control."

Elizabeth Barrett, Ph.D., a psychotherapist in private practice who has treated many young women with breast cancer, including Tracy Hill, agrees that facing death is particularly hard for young women, who thought they had so much of their lives ahead of them. "Particularly for women who have young children," she says, "the thought of not being able to raise them is especially hard. Or for people who want to actualize their career potential, or their academic potential—there are just so many realms in a young person's life that are just emerging."

For Nalini, one of the hardest parts of having metastatic cancer is her sense of being out of step with what society expects for her. "It's important not to get caught up in societal expectations," she says. "To think that we have to get married by a certain age, and have kids by a certain age, and meet all our career goals at the same time. Because that whole fairy tale gets blown away when you have a health problem like breast cancer. You have to take things as they come and not let yourself get beaten down by what you think society expects of you. It's something I still have trouble with."

Roz Kleban agrees. "That's part of what makes this disease so much harder for young women," she says. "They cannot follow the social prescriptions that are out there. And you are reminded of your disappointment a hundred times a day. One of my clients told me, 'Society thinks you're legitimate only if you're married with children.' Older women have had time to work through those expectations. Many younger women have not."

Some observers believe that the difficulties of dealing with recurrence and metastasis are further heightened by the current wave of breast cancer activism, which appears to hold out hope to so many women. What happens, they wonder, when you are not one of the women who has been able to "beat the cancer"?

"My patients have told me that they have felt discriminated against within breast cancer organizations," says Kleban. "I believe that's because it's hard to look at a young woman with cancer. Young people aren't supposed to get breast cancer—and they're doubly not supposed to get metastatic disease. All that you read about are the breast cancer 'winners,' which leaves out an important segment of the population."

Ellen Leopold agrees. Leopold is the author of *A Darker Ribbon: Breast Cancer, Women, and Their Doctors in the Twentieth Century*, the first cultural history of breast cancer. In her view, women whose breast cancer recurs or metastasizes are being given the message that their illness is somehow their own fault. "I do not want a single woman out there to feel responsible for her failure to survive," says Leopold. "That's like trying to kill someone twice. I think that is unspeakable. Everybody's biology is different. Everyone's response to treatment is different. It is a vicious thing to make women feel that they are responsible for overcoming breast cancer when 150 years of medical science has failed to do so."

> **Juanita Lyle, Diagnosed at Age 32, Now Age 58**
>
> *When I first met the young women of the YSC, it just touched me. I get teary-eyed every time I think about it. So much emotion came into my heart. I looked at them and said, "That was me." Because when I first got diagnosed, I wasn't sure if I would make it or not. I didn't even get through 5 years without recurrence—my recurrences came much closer together than that. So I looked at those young women and said to myself, "They need to know about me. They need to know someone is here who has gotten through the worst of it." I talked to every one of them and said, "I know how you're feeling. And I want you to know that even as poor as my diagnosis was—I'm alive and well. And I want you to understand that you can be alive and well too. There is hope. We all have to fight for that hope."*

The issue is further complicated by the fact that there are some women whose breast cancer recurs, even several times, yet who go on to live happy, active lives. Juanita Lyle is an example of such a woman—diagnosed at 32 and still going strong at 58, after three recurrences. Shirley Williams, now 68, was first diagnosed with breast cancer at age 30. Although her cancer metastasized, she, too, has led an active life, working as a teacher and volunteering at the American Cancer Society. Nalini, at age 27, is back in medical school. Similar stories abound.

Understanding Recurrence and Metastasis

As we saw in Chapters 2 and 3, breast cancer initially appears as disease in the breast tissue. What doctors hope is that by removing the lump, with or without the surrounding breast tissue, they can remove all of the cancer from a woman's body. What they fear is that by the time they discover the cancer, it has already spread to other parts of the body, through the lymphatic system and/or the bloodstream. In your initial treatment, your doctors may have performed surgery to remove the cancer from your breast, followed by radiation and/or chemotherapy to eradicate any cancer that remains in your system. Their goal is to destroy the cancer before it takes hold in another part of your body.

When cancer recurs in the breast in which it was originally discovered, this may simply mean that the doctors were unable to remove all of the cancer cells the first time. The cells they left in your body then multiplied, creating a second tumor in the same breast. (Preventing this possibility is one of the reasons why doctors recommend mastectomies.) Sometimes, even if a breast has been removed, the cancer can return to affect the area's skin, in a series of nodules. Cancer in the breast is usually discovered through mammography or when someone detects a lump. Nodules on the skin can simply be felt.

Cancer that recurs in the same breast is known as a local recurrence; this is the easiest type of recurrence to treat, with the most optimistic prognosis. Usually, according to Dr. Bert Petersen, a breast surgeon at Beth Israel Hospital in New York City, locally recurring cancer is treated with additional surgery, and perhaps with additional radiation. The radiation supplements the surgery by attempting to burn out any remaining cancer.

When breast cancer spreads to the area immediately around the breast—the neck, lymph nodes, and the area under the arm—that's considered a regional recurrence. Regional recurrence is somewhat more serious than local recurrence, but doctors still hope to interrupt the cancer before it spreads to other parts of the body. According to Dr. Petersen, regional recurrence in the lymph nodes would also be treated with surgery, along with radiation (to eradicate the cancer at the site) and chemotherapy (to counteract cancer in the bloodstream or lymphatic system). If a woman finds a lump in her neck, however, surgery is no longer an option. "The cancer has spread through the bloodstream," says Dr. Petersen, "so surgery won't be effective at that point." A woman with a lump in her neck—like Tracy Pleva Hill—would be treated with chemotherapy in an effort to interrupt the cancer before it spreads any further.

If the cancer spreads beyond the neck and breast, it's known as metastatic, the most serious stage of cancer. Breast cancer can metastasize anywhere, but it most commonly spreads to the bones (as in Beth Brokaw's case), lungs (as for Nalini Yadla), liver, and brain. Note that breast cancer that has metastasized somewhere else is still breast cancer—it's not lung cancer or liver cancer, even though it may appear in those organs.

Treating Metastatic Cancer: Reason for Hope

For women who have gotten used to the idea that surgery can remove their cancer, it can be upsetting to accept the fact that surgery is no longer an option, says oncologist Dr. Robert Taub of New York Presbyterian Hospital: "Metastatic breast cancer has spread beyond the limits of what the surgeon can do." For a young woman, says Dr. Taub, "This is the ultimate sense of losing control. And it's this loss of control—the fact that they can't somehow make the disease go away—that causes fear."

Lisa Muccilo, Diagnosed at Age 28 and with Metastatic Cancer at Age 29

Initially they were telling me that the cancer I had was stage 1. Then the lymph nodes were involved, and it was stage 2. Now I don't even ask. Five times now I've gotten the news, "You have cancer."

How do I feel when I hear the word metastatic? *"It's not me," that's what it feels like. It doesn't feel like me. I think it's hard to define yourself as metastatic—you just don't think about yourself that way. It's not like denial. It's just like, "It couldn't be. No way. I feel great."*

Metastatic represents everything you don't ever want to consider. It's almost like the step before the end. That's really terrible to say, and I don't want to think of it like that. More and more people are living longer and longer with metastatic cancer. I don't think it has the same meaning that it once had.

But Dr. Taub encourages his patients to be optimistic. "There are reasons to be positive even about this kind of situation," he says. "First, we have been able to change the overall survival of people with metastatic disease to some degree now, with chemotherapy. A lot of the chemotherapy that we give is much more tolerable than it was years ago. Even after we give strong drugs, people are still able to work, they're able to cope with their lives."

Moreover, says Dr. Taub, ongoing scientific advances offer much reason to hope. "What I need to do," he says, "is help my patients hang on for a year or two until we can give them the kinds of things that we are really hoping for—therapy that will either eradicate the disease or convert it into something chronic that will go on for an indefinite period." Fortunately, many of the new drug treatments that are now available enable young women both to survive and to preserve their quality of life. For example, when a cancer spot appeared on the spine of Lisa Muccilo, whose metastatic breast cancer was diagnosed when she was 28, Dr. Taub prescribed Xeloda (capecitabine) for her. Xeloda is an oral chemotherapy agent that has more tolerable side effects than other medications, so that Lisa was able to continue with all the activities that mattered to her. The Xeloda did not cure Lisa, but it did allow her to maintain an active and satisfying life and did not cause her to lose her hair.

Moreover, Dr. Petersen points out, women with metastatic cancer are surviving longer than ever before. "My experience shows that there

James and Theresa Muccilo, Parents of Lisa Muccilo

James: *Lisa started with chemo and a stem cell transplant, and then the radiation—and that all took about 8 months. And then you say, "We did everything, we did the best we could, we took the most aggressive treatment." And we walked out of there and said, "It's over. We're done. It's over, Lisa."*

Theresa: *We all believed that. The whole family thought that was it. We thought it was over.*

James: *Then maybe 9 months to a year later, she found a lump in the same breast.*

Theresa: *She found it, even though she had just been to the oncologist. When she called me, I tried to reassure her. I said, "It's probably nothing; don't get upset." And we went back to the doctor, and it was cancer, and this time they had to take the breast off. She was only 28. That was our next step. She had to have the breast removed.*

James: *We were hoping, of course, that Lisa's cancer was confined to the breast, but no, she had five positive lymph nodes. And then she went through various treatments, some of which at this point I would categorize by saying that they didn't work. And so when you get that news as you go down the line, you get smacked down.*

Theresa: *You do a lot of crying with the family.*

James: *And then you pick yourself up and you get refocused, and you say, "What's the next step; what are we going to do now?" And you do it.*

James: *I think about it [death]. How can you not? But what's the sense of thinking about it? We try to keep a good attitude. We try not to think about it—but that bogeyman is always there.*

Theresa: *And it doesn't want to go away.*

seems to be a trend toward women living longer with metastatic disease because of the newer drugs that have come on the market," he says. "There's a whole class of new drugs on the market that allow women to live longer."

Unfortunately, just as breast cancer tends to be more aggressive among younger women, so does metastatic cancer. "It's not uncommon for women in their late seventies or early eighties to have metastatic breast cancer that has spread and is no longer removable, but that just simply stays there and doesn't interfere with their lifestyle and is more easily controlled," says Dr. Taub. "But in a young woman, most of the time, the cancer just continues to grow—and grow rapidly. Not in every case, but we do see that."

Dr. Petersen agrees that learning the statistics about metastatic cancer can be overwhelming. But he also argues that these statistics exist only to help doctors evaluate various treatments. They have "absolutely no bearing" on an individual woman's chance of survival.

"I think it's a mistake to put any emphasis on the numbers," he says. "Physicians don't have a crystal ball. We know the average survival rates, but you have to put that into context. Those numbers mean nothing to you as an individual—really, they don't. And they shouldn't be used to judge what you do."

Making Treatment Decisions

When you were first diagnosed with breast cancer, you figured out one set of treatment options. But getting the news that you have a recurrence or metastasis means that you've got to start the process all over again. The strategies you used the first time may serve you perfectly well this time through, or you may want to develop a new approach. Here are some options you might consider:

- *Look for a second opinion.* Check out "Tips on Getting a Second Opinion" in Chapter 2, and remember Dr. George Sledge's reassuring words: "Doctors should not only not be offended, they should routinely offer to let patients have a second opinion. . . . If your doctor makes you feel bad about asking for a second opinion, that's great evidence that you really do need a second opinion."

- *Consider the possibility of participating in a clinical trial.* Remember, clinical trials are the arena in which new drugs and treatment protocols are tested before they are made available to the general public. If your condition has not been responsive to standard chemotherapy, perhaps you are a good candidate for a new treatment. Ask your doctor about what clinical trials might apply to your condition, or call the National Cancer Institute. (For more information on clinical trials, see Chapter 3.)

- *Call the YSC, American Cancer Society, Y-ME, or another such organization to find a woman who has had a similar diagnosis.* A survivor who's been through your stage of cancer will be able to offer you practical suggestions and emotional support, as well as her own perspective on the medical treatments that may be in store for you.

Whatever decisions you make about treatment, remember that there's probably no need to rush. Although in some cases a diagnosis calls for immediate action, usually a recurrence or metastasis has been growing for some time. Taking another week or two in order to get a second opinion and to discuss options with your loved ones is probably a good idea.

Defining "Quality of Life"

One of the major factors that will help you make decisions about your treatment is your definition of "quality of life." Since there is no known cure for metastatic breast cancer, most medical treatments for the condition are aimed at prolonging your life as long as possible—partly in the hope that, as Dr. Taub explained, you can take advantage of the cure when it becomes available.

Some women, particularly those with children, have as their primary goal prolonging their lives on virtually any terms. Other women are more concerned with pain management, with continuing as many of their former activities as possible, or with remaining alert and aware until the end. No treatment is equally effective in achieving all of these goals, so knowing your priorities and being able to communicate them to your doctor is of utmost importance.

Doctors have different skills and personalities, just like any other group of people. Some doctors excel at laying out choices and talking through them with their patients. Others may be perfectly willing to share information, but the patient may need to be the one who asks the questions or expresses the concerns. It may not be enough to tell your

Questions for Your Doctor about Treatment

- What goals do you have for this treatment?
- What other treatments might be available? Why is your choice preferable?
- What are the possible risks and side effects?
- What can I do to minimize or respond to risks and side effects?
- What happens if I choose not to receive treatment?
- What kinds of symptoms should I expect from the cancer I have?
- How will my life be affected by my illness and treatment? Can I continue with work, child-rearing, and other important activities?
- How will you evaluate my treatment? When will you do it? What will you consider a successful treatment?

doctor what your priorities are; you may also have to find out more about what options are available and discover his or her reasons for recommending a particular choice. The very factors that lead your doctor away from a particular choice may lead you toward it, so be sure that you've talked with your physician about what you really want and what your options are.

Finding the Strength to Deal with Recurrence

For many women, hearing that their breast cancer has recurred brings on enormous fear. "It's the most overwhelming thing that can happen," says Roz Kleban. "You've been living with a prayer, a wish, a desperate hope that it will not come back. For women for whom it does come back, it's the worst of all possible things—and it's happened."

What these women need, Kleban says, is "to be shown that recurrence is not a death sentence. A chronic illness, perhaps. A death sentence, no." Women whose cancer has recurred or metastasized, in Kleban's view, must make sure to continue living their lives.

Indeed, Juanita Lyle found that it was crucial not only to continue with her old life but also to commit herself to new activities. "It was important for me when I was going through chemo—the first time and the second time—to do things that proved to myself that I was embracing life," she says. "During my first round of chemo, I started running. My mother said, 'What in the world are you doing?' There were just things I felt I needed to try to do each time something was going on. Then when I was on chemo the second time, I decided it was time for me to look at getting back in the workforce. So I decided, 'Hey, I'm going to get a job.' And I did. I didn't have any hair. So, I went out and found a wig and got a job."

Nalini Yadla credits her passion for medicine with getting her through a long, discouraging course of treatment. "I want to be a pediatrician more than anything in the world," she says. "I can't wait. I think children are just so precious and so important. I want to help children become healthy adults—that's what keeps me going." Although medical school is often tiring for Nalini, it continues to provide her with immense satisfaction. "When I was going through treatments, I had a lot of time to think about what I wanted to do with my life, and in the end, all I wanted to do was come back to school," she says.

Shirley Williams is an advocate of such commitment. "The one thing I would say to young women who are living with metastatic breast cancer—and this might sound clichéd, but it became meaningful to me—is to try to live each day to its fullest," says Shirley. "That was very impor-

Juanita Lyle

Going for that second course of chemo really took a lot. It took so much for me to get my mind set and say, "Oh, boy, here I go again." I thought, "What have I put off doing? What can I achieve?" Each time it was a process of coping with chemo and cancer and even challenging myself with something that maybe I'd put off or wanted to try. Although it seems crazy to create another challenge when I was already going through such a big challenge, it worked for me. I think what it was about for me was holding on to life. I said, "I'm not letting this life go yet."

tant to me." Like Juanita, Shirley was especially eager to boost her morale before and after chemotherapy.

"On the day when I had the chemo, I would be sick as a dog," she recalls. "And the next day, I would wake up and wear my highest heels, put on makeup, and try to look my very best. This is silly and embarrassing, but I always used to say, 'My creditors are not going to let me die if I owe them money,' so I'd go shopping and charge clothes. I also tried never to go to bed being angry or carrying a grudge. I thought, 'Maybe tomorrow I won't be here, and I won't have a chance to say I'm sorry.' And I tried to do other good things for myself. I even used to try to see one play a month."

Looking back from her vantage point as a woman of 68 who was first diagnosed with breast cancer at age 30, Shirley suggests "finding something to hold onto. It doesn't have to be a man or a person or a child. Many people get pets or go to school or travel. It's very, very important to have something to hold onto. If you do nothing, the anger is there, and you start to feel sorry for yourself."

Roz Kleban strongly recommends that women with metastatic or recurrent breast cancer find some kind of counseling and/or support group to help them cope with the experience. Even women with supportive friends and families, she suggests, may need the kind of comradeship that can come from a group of fellow survivors. "It's important to be with other people who are feeling like you are," she says. "Often people want to be helpful, but they don't know what to do."

Facing Treatment a Second Time

For Juanita, as for many other women, one of the hardest parts of having her cancer recur was knowing that she had to face yet another course of chemotherapy. Most women find their first round of chemotherapy to be a harrowing experience, and for many, the prospect of a second treatment can be overwhelming. Yet William Worden, Ph.D., a psychiatrist who taught at Harvard Medical School, has discovered that many people actually find their second encounter with chemotherapy less upsetting than their first. Dr. Worden studied 102 patients whose cancer had recurred—both people with breast cancer and people with other types of cancer—and compared them with 102 newly diagnosed patients who had been studied earlier. He discovered that some 30 percent of the patients whose cancer had recurred "found the experience less traumatic than their original diagnosis. These were patients who were less surprised by the recurrence, who had not let themselves believe that they were cured, and who, in some respect, were living under the proverbial Sword of Damocles."[1]

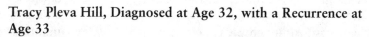

Tracy Pleva Hill, Diagnosed at Age 32, with a Recurrence at Age 33

It's not the thought of going to chemo that unnerves me. It's the thought that the doctor is going to touch my neck and go, "It's over. We have to do something else. It's not working." There's always this fear that I'm going to go in there, and it's going to be worse.

I will not touch my neck. I won't touch it. I get dressed in front of the mirror every day, and it's so easy for me to cock my neck and see if things are changing. But I know if I do it on a daily basis, I won't notice a difference or I'll perceive that it's bigger. So I force myself not to look. Denial can be good. I try to be realistic, but only to the point where I can keep my sanity. To the point where I can get out of bed every day.

It's amazing what you can come to terms with. It's amazing how much power your body has to adjust. When the doctor touched my neck and said, "We gotta take these out," I just curled up in a ball. He let me lie in an exam room for 2 hours and cry. I didn't think I'd ever smile again. I thought I'd spend whatever time I have left sad and scared. But I'm not. I have those periods, and I have them quite a bit. But you can't go backward. You have to go forward. And if you're going to go forward, then you might as well be happy. Take the moments as they are. I feel like I've made a lot of progress in just a couple of months. I can keep going. Oh, God, I gotta keep going!

Coping with Limitations

As the women quoted in this chapter discovered, a profound commitment to getting on with your life is often the best response to living with recurrence or metastases. Sometimes, though, the illness makes it impossible to go on as before. Although Nalini is now back in medical school, she feels that she's not as strong a student as she was before her cancer. Not only did she have to drop out for a while, but her stamina and concentration are not as good as they once were. "It was really hard for me to adjust to having a daily routine and to feel competent enough to do things right," she says. "I was putting a lot of pressure on myself to be the person I was before the cancer diagnosis, and I was comparing myself to other students who didn't have a 3-year break. I got through it day by day, week by week. I'm not the A+ student I used to be. But I think being a B student is pretty good right now."

Beth Brokaw thinks of the cancer-related changes in her life as permanent. She lists the things she'll never again be able to do: pick up her children, teach, work as a therapist (though she does continue to see a few patients). Although she is now in only a moderate amount of pain, she says, "The fatigue and the lack of energy are as problematic as the pain. I sleep a lot. I sleep about 10 to 12 hours a day. I just have to take it real easy."

Beth has found, though, that even as metastatic cancer deprived her of many aspects of her life that she loved, it has also brought a new richness and depth to her relationships. "More than anything, I've continued to be a friend, and my relationships have flourished, and they have kept me alive," she says. Beth's friends have come through for her and her husband, driving her to the hospital, cooking for her family, and taking care of her children. Beth also draws strength from her Christian prayer group. "We are very close anyway, but this is times ten," she says. "The intensity of the situation multiplied the level of intimacy—walking through suffering together is a very powerful experience. I feel like the spirit of God has descended upon my life."

Juanita believes that her own faith helped her live far longer than any of her doctors ever thought she could. "People don't always understand that process," she says. "We need to focus on how do we get through this, how do we keep our quality of life? It's very important that you understand who you are. And even if your doctor tells you that he or she knows what your diagnosis may be, don't stop there, don't say, 'This could be over.' Say, 'I'm going to look beyond the circumstances and focus on this as an opportunity.' That's what I always tried to do. I could

Beth Brokaw, Diagnosed at Age 37 and with Metastatic Cancer at Age 44

I had incredible encounters with people in the radiation waiting room. Someone would be discouraged, and we would compare stories. I might offer a word of hope, and you'd see a light go on in their eyes. One mother I met had cancer all through her brain. She was still going. She said, "I have to live"—and I thought, "I can live, too. I can keep going." These are moments that cut through any surface trivialities and go right to the heart of what we're going through.

Cancer is such a leveler. It's like when I was pregnant: People identify, and it pushes through all the cultural and age barriers, and there's instant bonding. Cancer is the same way. It has no regard for who you are. Our color, age, and intellect don't matter—we all have cancer together. And that creates an immediate way for us to connect on a very genuine human level.

see that good was going to come of this, and I felt strongly that this was part of my life's purpose."

Tracy Pleva Hill went through a similar spiritual strengthening. "You live by faith," she says. "Everybody goes through their daily lives thinking they are going to be fine. And September 11 changed that for a lot of people. The blinders are off, and a lot of people walk around now with complete faith. Because you have to have faith to get through your day. And that is the true spiritual path. I don't have any delusions about what can happen on a day-to-day basis. But life is for the living, and I am sitting right here."

Difficult Decisions

It's hard—though crucial—to remember that death comes to us all. So whether you have 1 year left to live or 60, you may want to spend some time thinking about how you'd like to face your final days and communicating your decisions to your loved ones. Roz Kleban says that many women focus on practical aspects of dying during the course of their cancer.

"Women are afraid they're going to die," she comments. "And they start to think about how they are going to be buried, where they are going to be buried, if they want to be viewed, what music they want at the funeral. And all of that is normal. I think what you have to do, though, is to make your plans, and then put them away. Put them away. Spend your time living. Not dying. Attend to it. Then put it away."

Dr. Barrett's Imagery Exercise for Expressing Anger

You might read through this exercise, invite a friend to read it aloud to you, or create a tape and go through the exercise as you listen. You might also use this exercise as a model to create your own visualization.

Imagine that you're building a fire. Pile up the kindling, put in some paper. If you like, take a little charcoal fluid and flame it up. See the fire burning and burning. It's becoming a huge fire. And you know that it's your anger. Experience your anger. Be the fire. Feel the fire inside you raging. What does it feel like to be the fire? What color are you? What other details do you notice?

Now, throw a little water on it. It's sizzling. Throw some more water on it. It's so big you may need to bring several hoses. Finally, the fire is beginning to go out. There's still some smoldering. Put it all out. It's completely out.

Now dig a hole. Scoop up all the ashes, put them in the hole, cover the hole with dirt, and plant your favorite flower.

After you've completed the exercise, take some quiet time to think about how you felt when you were going through it, and how you feel now. You might write about your feelings in your journal, express them to a friend, or use them as the basis for a poem, song, or picture.

Dr. Elizabeth Barrett agrees that every woman faces death in her own way. It's currently fashionable, she says, to insist that we all face the prospect of death boldly and without "denial." But, says Dr. Barrett, "I've had my eyes opened. At first you think that everyone needs to talk about death, and you worry that it's something health-care providers run away from—and I think there's some truth to that. But then you find that there are people who prepare for death in a different way. Some people need to talk about dying. Others don't want to. There's no one right way.

"There was one woman I worked with who was very well prepared for death, but she didn't want or need to talk about it. She always talked about something positive. She didn't complain, even though she suffered greatly. It wasn't her way. But I think she was very ready to go when she did."

Although Dr. Barrett thinks that every woman has her own emotional journey, she also believes that when women feel anger or resentment—a common response to recurring or metastatic cancer—it's best to express

Taking Charge

- *Where do you want your last days to be spent?* Some people like the idea of passing their final days at home, surrounded by their loved ones. Others would prefer to have access to the facilities of a hospital. For still others, the right choice is hospice care. Hospice care can help with pain management and spiritual support. A hospice team—physicians, nurses, aides, social workers, counselors, and therapists—visits the patients at home or cares for them in the hospital.

- *How do you want to spend your last moments?* If pain is involved, some women would choose to be medicated heavily, whereas others would prefer to be alert. Some women would like every possible heroic medical measure to be taken to prolong their lives; others might choose to let nature take its course, or would agree to some medical measures, such as feeding tubes and hydration, but not others, such as resuscitation or a ventilator. Advance directives tell your doctor what kind of care you would like to have if you become unable to make medical decisions. Laws about advance directives vary from state to state.

- *Who should make decisions for you?* Choosing a proxy who can ensure that your wishes will be followed is a crucial part of preparing for your death. You'll want to have spoken at length with this person about your choices and to have told other people close to you that this is the person who will eventually speak for you. You may also want to specify who should not be involved in any decisions.

- *How have you communicated your wishes?* A living will is a type of advance directive in which you can specify your choices, name a proxy, and otherwise communicate your decisions about the kind of death you want to have. Different states have different laws concerning the treatment of dying patients, so consider working with a lawyer.

- *Who can help you think about these issues?* A lawyer, counselor, or advocate may help you think through both the medical situations that might arise and the legal means of safeguarding your wishes. Local cancer groups may be able to give you some referrals.

it. Women may speak their anger in words; express it through creating a poem, picture, sculpture, or song; or release it through physical exercise. "I'm talking about working out with the intention of pumping out this anger," Barrett explains. "Every step on the treadmill you think, 'I am getting rid of my anger.'"

Imagery and visualization are also powerful tools, according to Dr. Barrett, enabling women to create mental pictures that express their anger and then allowing them to release it. "You experience your anger, and then you experience relief from it," she explains. "You always need the relief. But anger definitely needs to be expressed." She urges women to yell and scream, to take a tennis racket and hit the bed, or even to use a punching bag. "Visualize at the same time," she counsels. "Visualize what you are hitting. See it. Maybe it's seeing a red, flaming fire. The more severe your anger is, the more work it'll take to get rid of it."

Taking It Day by Day

Although the women in this chapter have had widely varying experiences, they all agree on one piece of advice: Take it one day at a time. "I couldn't be angry that metastatic cancer stopped my life because I'm never going to let it stop my life," says Juanita. "I'm going to do this life in the grandest style I can—whether it's for 4 more months or 40 more years. I believe that no matter what happens to you—no matter what diagnosis you get—you go out with grace. And that's what I feel—I'm going to go out in grace and with a big party."

"I would like my life to be an inspiration to others," Shirley acknowledges. "It's why I went to great lengths to be just that." But if she is an inspiration, Shirley feels, it's because more often than not she's been able to follow her own advice: "Hold onto something, live each day to the fullest, and keep busy."

CHAPTER 13

"I Was Looking for a Way to Fight"

A Guide to Getting Active

"I like the word fight,*" says Lisa Muccilo. "This feels like a fight. And it feels like you never want to run out of ammunition." Lisa was diagnosed with breast cancer at age 27. Five years later, after numerous treatments, her cancer has recurred several times and is now metastatic. Certainly Lisa continues to do everything she can to combat her own breast cancer. But for her, a key part of her personal battle is the political fight. Indeed, after her first recurrence, Lisa left her job as an engineer with a telephone company to become a full-time activist.*

"I wanted to feel like I was making a difference. For myself and for others," she says. "My whole focus shifted. And I knew I had to help find the answers all of us as young women need."

For Dr. Laurie Goldstein, an obstetrician/gynecologist and a breast cancer survivor who was diagnosed at age 39, it's crucial that young women come together to identify what's important to them. "I think that the people in medicine and research mean well, but they don't always realize that issues they may dismiss as trivial are very important to the patient."

For Karen Sattaur, a 36-year-old mother of two, the most important reason to be a breast cancer activist is that it's fun—and it creates a sense of purpose. Karen recalls taking two Fridays off to sit with a 31-year-old woman during her chemotherapy. Her oncologist thought that she was being altruistic at her own expense. "He said, 'What are you doing? Do you want to relive your chemo? Go home this weekend, relax, and don't talk to one person who has breast cancer,'" Karen recalls. "And I thought, 'Oh, no. Am I doing the wrong thing here? Am I jeopardizing my health? Am I hurting my family?'"

Karen thought long and hard about her activism—the meetings and seminars and fundraisers she had organized, all the women she had reached, the friends she had made, and the triumphs she had enjoyed. Finally, she wrote her oncologist a letter. "I said, 'I have to do this because it's helping me—not hurting me,'" she reports. "'And I'm not stopping.'"

Thinking about Getting Active

For many young women with breast cancer, making personal decisions about treatment is only the first step. The second step is connecting with other young breast cancer survivors. And looking for a way to fight back.

Tracy Pleva Hill got involved with the national Young Survival Coalition after being diagnosed with breast cancer at age 32. She went on to become the group's public relations cochair. "You've had your surgery," she explains. "You've had your mastectomy and treatment. And then they turn you loose: 'We'll see you in 3 months.' No, no, that doesn't work for me. I felt like I'd just been dropped out of a plane. I felt like I was completely on my own and I had no way to actively battle the disease any more." For Tracy, becoming politically active was the way to continue her personal battle with breast cancer.

Cynthia Rubin, a successful lawyer who was diagnosed with breast cancer at age 36, had a similar experience. She heard about the YSC and went to a meeting while she was still getting chemotherapy. "I liked the idea of being proactive and doing something to change what happens when a young woman gets diagnosed with breast cancer," she says. "I had tried a support group, and it just didn't fit my personality. I found it much more helpful to say, 'Okay, this is the situation; let's do something about it.'" Cynthia went on to become the YSC's second president.

If You Want to Get Active: Groups You Might Approach

To find out how to contact any of these organizations, see the Resources section.

- *Young Survival Coalition.* The YSC is the only group exclusively devoted to serving the needs of young women with breast cancer. The group is dedicated to helping young cancer survivors achieve representation in the breast cancer and medical communities, by promoting research, educating doctors, and reaching out to health professionals. The group also reaches out to young women through educational programs and organizational partnerships.

- *The American Cancer Society's Reach to Recovery Program.* Reach to Recovery volunteers provide support for women at all stages of the disease. All volunteers receive extensive training in face-to-face and telephone counseling, which, thanks to a new partnership between Reach to Recovery and the YSC in New York, includes specific training in the needs of young women.

- *Living Beyond Breast Cancer.* LBBC is primarily an educational group focused on posttreatment issues. Through large-scale educational conferences, a newsletter, outreach to women who are medically underserved, a help line, a Web site, and a range of publications, LBCC helps women live as long as possible with the best quality of life. The organization also has a young survivors group that focuses specifically on young women. LBBC and the YSC cosponsor the only annual U.S. conference devoted to the needs of young women with breast cancer.

- *Y-ME National Breast Cancer Organization.* Y-ME offers information and support to survivors and their families, reaches out to the medical community and the public, and lobbies for scientific research and survivors' rights. Y-ME–sponsored activities include a Web-based service to help women sort through treatment options.

- *National Breast Cancer Coalition.* The NBCC is a national advocacy group dedicated to ending breast cancer through increased federal funding for research and via collaboration with the scientific community to implement new research models. Among its many activities, the NBCC sponsors Project LEAD (Leadership, Education, Advocacy, and Development), a program that helps train women to influence research and public policy.

- *Susan G. Komen Foundation.* The Susan G. Komen Breast Cancer Foundation supports breast cancer screening, education, treatment, and research, and it also funds community-based grassroots organizations (such as the Young Survival Coalition) through their Race for the Cure events in more than 100 cities nationwide.

- *National Alliance of Breast Cancer Organizations.* NABCO is the leading nonprofit information and education resource on breast cancer in the United States and a national force in patient advocacy. NABCO provides information to medical professionals and their organizations, patients, their families and the media. In addition, NABCO advocates for regulatory change and legislation that benefits patients, survivors and women at risk.

Randi Rosenberg, diagnosed at age 32 and an activist since she began her chemotherapy, says that many young women misunderstand what it means to become active. "*Advocacy* and *activism* are terms that are really misconstrued—it can all be somewhat intimidating," she says. "But it doesn't need to be. The key to advocacy is this: If you can make a difference in one person's life, you are an advocate."

As a young woman with breast cancer, you've got a lot of options for getting active. You might start a support group; give talks about your experience; find ways to help local doctors, hospitals, and cancer centers become more sensitive to the special needs of young women; lobby government officials; or attend a national breast cancer conference. Or perhaps you have no idea of what "getting active" means for you, but you like the idea of reaching out, of doing something to help yourself and others. In this chapter, you'll find a range of resources that can help you make the choices about getting active that are right for you. You'll also learn what other young women have accomplished as they have fought back against breast cancer.

You may not have decided yet how your breast cancer diagnosis may influence your desire to become active in the breast cancer community. It could happen now, in 5 years, or not at all. And whether you're a single mom raising small children or a high-powered career woman, you may find yourself wanting to give back to others and yourself. Finding the time and energy to do so may seem like a challenge, but, as Shirley Williams discovered, it can be rewarding. "It helped me feel energized, like I was living my life to its fullest."

Shirley was diagnosed with breast cancer 38 years ago, at the age of 30. Through the nearly 4 decades since her diagnosis, she has worked as a volunteer for the American Cancer Society. "It's about reaching down and lending a hand to help other women up. That's what I see myself doing. I love volunteering and talking to women. Sometimes women ask me lots of questions, other times they just want reassurance. Whatever they need, I try to give."

Shirley volunteers for Reach to Recovery, a longstanding ACS program that makes information and prostheses available to women recovering from mastectomies. As part of a pilot project in New York, Reach to Recovery joined forces with the YSC to ensure that young women have access to materials relevant to their needs and that the ACS's volunteer training program includes a focus on young women.

According to Elizabeth Tarr, Reach to Recovery's New York director, this partnership "has definitely reenergized the program. It made the staff and volunteers feel like we really are addressing the tremendously broad scope of breast cancer patients. We really are serving everyone."

Tips for Getting Active

- Organize a support group for young women through your local cancer center or hospital.

- Contact a local high school or college and coordinate a breast health seminar. The YSC has a slide show, "Breast Health 101," that you can use. Or ask a local doctor to speak on medical issues, while you share your personal story.

- Bring YSC brochures to your doctor's office so that other young women with breast cancer can learn about available resources. Bring brochures to your local store, boutique, hair salon, bagel store, or coffee shop—young women are everywhere, not just in their doctors' offices!

- Ask your local newspaper to do a story on young women with breast cancer.

- Give a fundraiser for breast cancer research or a breast cancer group.

- Lobby your local congressional and Senate representatives for research funds for young women and breast cancer.

- Encourage local breast health groups to consider young women when planning their programs or their outreach efforts.

- Talk to your company about becoming a corporate sponsor of a local or national breast cancer organization.

- Find out if your company has a corporate giving or foundation program. A local or national group in which you're active can apply for funding from such a program.

- Talk about your breast cancer activism to everyone, wherever you go—you just never know whom you are going to meet or affect!

- Volunteer for a research study focusing on young women.

- Attend the National Breast Cancer Coalition conference, held in Washington, D.C., each spring. The conference is designed to teach women of all ages how to become effective volunteer lobbyists for cancer research and treatment funds.

- Attend the Living Well Today for the Promise of Tomorrow Conference, the only national conference for young women affected by breast cancer, held in Philadelphia each February.

- Register on the YSC Web site to help publicize the large number of young women with breast cancer and to learn more about young women's needs.

Provided by the Young Survival Coalition.

Karen Sattaur, Diagnosed at Age 34

I had been through treatment for 11 months, and I had not seen one other young woman with breast cancer. When I discovered the YSC through their Web site, I couldn't wait to meet them. I went to New York—and I learned very quickly that the YSC was not a support group. But that was what I needed. I told them, "Look, I can't get young women together to kick breast cancer's ass unless I embrace them first."

So when I got home, I went to my social worker at my hospital and said, "I want to start a young women's support group." And we had 11 young women in the first meeting. This social worker was more than happy to start something for us. She just didn't know how or why to do it. I gave her the reason.

It was during our third meeting that I put the YSC brochures out on the table, and the women just jumped at them. So then, at our first Florida YSC meeting, we stopped our support group and started meeting as the YSC. I made myself known to every breast health awareness group and every cancer center. I went door to door with brochures and said, "What do you do for young women?" And they would say, "Not a whole lot." I said, "My name is Karen Sattaur, and I'm 34. I'm a breast cancer survivor, and I want you to give this brochure to any and all young women who walk in the door, whether they are healthy or newly diagnosed. I want to be the one they call."

They said, "Fantastic." They were thrilled that someone was willing and able to address this population that was so in need. They hadn't realized how much they needed me, but once I was there, it all made sense.

Promoting Medical Research on Young Women

One of the biggest problems facing young women with breast cancer is the lack of information. Most research has been done with older women in mind. As a result, young women face a serious lack of information when it comes to choosing a course of treatment.

Lisa Muccilo is particularly frustrated over her own experience with treatment decisions. "It's as though you base all your treatments on knowledge by default," she says. "They tell you, 'Well, this has been shown to be effective for women who are 50.' But what about me? I'm 27! My hormones are a lot different from a 57-year-old's hormones."

Roberta Levy-Schwartz agrees. "Everyone has to make hard decisions about her treatment," she says. "But you'd like to think you're making decisions based on data. And the problem with being a young survivor is that often you're making those decisions without data. Right now, you might as well take a dart and throw it at a board for some of the decisions young women have to make."

Part of the solution, young activists agree, is to lobby for more research. Although in the past it has been difficult to gather enough young women with cancer to carry out significant studies, young women with breast cancer today are both more visible and more organized. Indeed, the YSC has reached out to Mt. Sinai Medical Center to collaborate on a wide-ranging study of young women with breast cancer. Researchers are studying YSC members to analyze the stage and age of diagnosis, treatment received, results of genetic testing, fertility issues, and psychosocial issues. The results will be published in medical journals and presented at national cancer conferences, helping to establish the fact that young women do indeed get breast cancer and identifying the issues that require further study.

But although young women may see the need for more research, they are not always willing to volunteer for clinical trials. "Although," says Randi Rosenberg, "that's exactly what's needed to find answers." Randi has volunteered for several studies and feels an obligation to put herself on the line. "We as young women can help pave the way for other women who come behind us," she says. "To me, it's not optional." (For more on participating in current clinical trials, see Chapter 3.)

Educating Doctors and the Medical Community

Activists say that it's not enough to push for more research. They also want to make sure that the medical community is fully aware of the information that does exist.

"We really don't know how to prevent breast cancer, so the best we can do is find it early," says Cynthia Rubin. "But a lot of our members have similar experiences: They actually felt a lump in their breast, they went to their doctor, and the doctor said, 'Oh, you're too young—don't worry about it.' And somehow we don't know that we should say, 'But I feel this lump,' and 'Too young' is not a diagnosis. I think it's a really important lesson for younger women that doctors are not infallible, and if you think there's something wrong, you should do something about it."

Randi Rosenberg, diagnosed at age 32, had exactly the experience that Cynthia describes. A year before her diagnosis, Randi and her gynecologist had found a lump in Randi's breast. The doctor assured Randi that she probably had fibrocystic breasts and that further investigation was

Reaching Out to Doctors, Hospitals, and the Medical Community

- Get together some other young survivors and visit doctors and hospitals in your area. Tell your stories and ask what can be done to raise awareness about young women with breast cancer.

- Put together a packet of information—medical studies, press clips, personal stories—and mail it to selected doctors, hospitals, and clinics. Then call a week or so later for a follow-up meeting. Ask what the protocol will be for treating young women who report possible signs of breast cancer. (You might also get information from one of the organizations listed earlier.)

- Encourage hospitals, clinics, or local cancer societies to hold a health fair for the medical community that focuses on young women with breast cancer. Help them find young women who can tell their stories.

- Send a letter to your own team of physicians inviting them to register on the YSC's Web site as "medical members." It's a great way for them to find out about the YSC's mission and to make them aware of the YSC as a resource for their other young patients.

unnecessary. One year later, when Randi heard that she actually did have breast cancer, all she could think of was the way her gynecologist had reassured her. "I remember her saying to me, 'I wouldn't worry too much about it—you're *too young* for breast cancer,'" Randi recalls. "And, 'It's not cost-effective to look for it.' When I heard the diagnosis, I remember thinking, 'Cost-effective? I could be dying at 32, and we're talking about cost-effective!' I think that's the first time I had a strong sense of something needing to be done."

According to Roberta, both doctors and young women need to be educated. "When I see those signs on people's back at the Komen Race for the Cure," Roberta says, "and the signs say, 'I'm running for my mother' or 'I'm running for my grandmother,' I want to write a sign saying, 'I'm running for my future. I'm running for myself.' Young women don't realize that it's about *them*."

Reaching Out to Young Women

Concerned about the young women who were not aware of breast cancer, Lisa Muccilo created a scripted talk and slide show called "Breast

Health 101," designed for high school and college students. The 45-minute presentation gives statistics on young women with breast cancer, explains basic medical facts about the disease, and tells women how to look for the breast lumps that are often the first warning signs. If you plan to reach out to schools and community groups, you can get a free copy of "Breast Health 101" from the YSC. (See the Resources section.)

Like Lisa, many women find that getting involved can be an important part of the healing process. Lori Atkinson, who was diagnosed with breast cancer at age 37 and who founded the YSC's Indiana affiliate, says her determination stems from the range of hardships she has faced. After fighting breast cancer, Lori lost her teenage son. "Many women are more

Tips for Outreach and Education

- *Write to teachers, principals, department heads, sororities, women's health centers, women's groups, or anyone else who might be interested.* Start with a target list, perhaps of people you know personally. Explain who you are and why "Breast Health 101" would be a useful program for their students or members. Once you've given the presentation, you can ask people to recommend you to other venues.

- *Do the presentation with a buddy or in a small group.* That way, you've got a range of stories to share with the group, and you can process the experience afterward. You might move on to solo work as you get more comfortable.

- *Practice your presentation first.* Do the presentation at least once before a sympathetic audience—a family member, girlfriend, boyfriend, or fellow activist. Encourage your "audience" to ask you questions, too.

- *Allow time for questions, discussion, and comments.* Frequently people don't really process information until they've had a chance to participate. Start with some limited audience participation—a trivia quiz or a quick show of hands: "How many people here have been affected by breast cancer?" You can also develop some fail-safe questions—for example, "How many people here know someone 40 or under who's been diagnosed with breast cancer?" People who raise their hands can be invited to share their stories. If no one responds, you can say, "Well, now you do!" and introduce yourself. Both openings will give urgency to the rest of your information.

committed some times than at other times. I think I'm more focused. My son was killed in an all-terrain vehicle accident a year ago, and after losing him, this is what keeps me going. I like meeting the women, and I feel I can help them. That's therapy for me."

Lori has had good experiences with outreach. The key, she says, is making it fun. "We do a little trivia test; for example, we ask, 'Which famous athlete's sister was recently diagnosed with breast cancer?' The answer is André Agassi. I give out prizes like candy and highlighters, and then I give them a quick 30-second quiz and let them ask questions." Lori says that it's also helpful to bring breast forms—silicone models of breasts—that include different types of breast lumps. That way, young women can learn by touch the difference between a normal lump and a lump that requires medical follow-up.

Working Locally

As Karen Sattaur found, getting a local group going may be difficult at first. But for her, the rewards ultimately outweighed the hardships. "There were months when it was just me at the monthly meetings," she says frankly. "After all, young women have lives. But I stuck it out, and I'm glad I did. Even when I was there by myself, I knew I was making a difference."

Lori Atkinson also found it challenging to start a local group. She discovered that it was useful to get involved with existing activities, such as the Komen Race for the Cure—not just as a runner, but as a member of various committees. "Little by little, that got my name out," she recalls, "and people started to know who we were." The YSC recommends that before you start a local affiliate, you get involved nationally, to learn from women who are already active and to find out what you're interested in: medical outreach/research, outreach and education, public relations, fund-raising, or advocacy and membership.

Raising Funds and Developing Resources

Raising funds is an effective and enjoyable way to get active. And a fund-raising event can serve several purposes: raising money, involving more volunteers, publicizing your group, linking you up with other organizations. For example, one YSC affiliate has convinced local doctors to offer scholarships for young women to attend various national breast cancer conferences.

Lori points to fundraisers as a time for fun and celebration as well as for raising money: a time when women can bring along their husbands, boyfriends, children, and girlfriends so that they can bond with one another. "Their wife, girlfriend or friend has had breast cancer—so the same

Tips for Planning a Successful Fundraiser

- *Be creative.* Think about events that sound like fun, that will appeal to the people you can reach, and that you will enjoy organizing.

- *Be realistic.* Remember, the goal is to make money. If it takes you hours of work to raise a tiny amount of money, or if you have to invest hundreds of dollars for a $100 profit, it's probably not worth it.

- *Be clear about your goals.* Some events are worth doing just for the fun of it—to build a base of support, to bond, to reach out to new communities. That's fine—just don't confuse those events with events whose primary goal is to make money. Sometimes you can combine a fundraiser with other objectives, and sometimes you can't. Knowing ahead of time what you do and don't expect to accomplish will increase your chances for satisfaction in the end.

bond we feel as women, they feel," she comments. "Even though they're strangers, they can be together and be comfortable."

Publicity

Whether you're trying to promote your events or just to get the word out about young women with breast cancer, the media can be a big help.

October—National Breast Cancer Awareness Month—is an especially good time for coverage, but it's generally possible to get in the news any time of year if you offer an interesting news hook. For example, a Mother's Day event could get you coverage in May, and a Snowman Charity Ball may put you in the press in December.

Lisa Muccilo has enjoyed the public relations work she's done, but says that young women need to be alert when talking to the media. "You always want to try to work a question back in your favor to get your message across," she suggests. "Sometimes I get these really crazy questions. I was on this program on New Jersey public television, and the interviewer said, 'But you look so good. You don't look like you've got cancer.' What do you say to that?" The solution, Lisa advises, is to turn any question into a chance to promote your message. "It's good if you have three main points that you want people to walk away knowing when you're done," she says.

Advocacy and National Conferences

Yet another focus of breast cancer activism is lobbying. Locally, you can approach state legislators and congressional representatives for more breast cancer funding and more attention to young women's needs. You can also lobby Congress through a national group; the primary such group is the National Breast Cancer Coalition, the largest national advocacy group on breast cancer issues.

National Breast Cancer Coalition Conference

Each spring, the NBCC holds an annual conference in Washington, D.C., with the goal of teaching women of all ages to lobby for breast cancer funding. When the YSC began attending that conference, it raised awareness about young women in both the national cancer community and Congress. The YSC also uses the NBCC conference as a way to mobilize and bring together young women from around the country, many of whom get their first taste of political activism—and meet their first large group of young women survivors—at the conference.

YSC cofounder Joy Simha has seen many legislators and their aides respond to young women with profound emotion. "Representatives are very busy people," she says. "But when you go in as a young woman who's been diagnosed with breast cancer, you watch their jaws drop. You can say to a legislator, 'This issue is important to me because my child is at risk for breast cancer at the age of 16,' and that hits home for them. They see their daughter, daughter-in-law, grandchild, all possibly suffering from breast cancer. You don't need anything else. It's very empowering."

Joy encourages young women to remember that in our political system, their elected representatives are supposed to be responsible to them. "A representative might come back and say, 'No, we can't support that because the insurance companies will have my head.' It's great to answer, 'Excuse me, I'm your constituent. I vote. The insurance companies don't.' It's our job to tell our representatives what we think. And it's their job to listen."

Living Well Today for the Promise of Tomorrow Conference

Living Beyond Breast Cancer and the YSC cohost the only annual national conference specifically geared to the needs of young women. Held in Philadelphia, the conference focuses on a wide range of issues, including research updates, tamoxifen, genetic testing, breast reconstruction, dealing with managed care and the insurance system, and advocacy.

Randi Rosenberg, who helps develop the conference agendas, finds the experience inspiring—but also painful. "There is nowhere on this

Tips for Lobbying Your State or National Representatives

- *Be informed.* Know what specific legislation you'd like to see passed or defeated. You can find out more through national or local cancer organizations.

- *Be prepared.* Plan with your fellow lobbyists who's going to say what, and how you're going to use your time. You may not have more than 15 minutes, so make every minute count.

- *Stay focused.* If you do have 15 minutes, you'll probably have time for only three to five women to actually speak. And each woman will have time for one or two points at most. Figure out how to divide up the information among you, and practice sticking to the point.

- *Stay personal.* Other lobbyists can talk about statistics and abstractions. Your biggest weapon is your personal story—how old you were when you were diagnosed, what happened to you, and how more funding might have prevented the problems you've encountered.

- *Be polite.* The watchword in legislative circles is "civility." You'll get further if you treat the legislators like colleagues rather than like enemies. After all, you all have the people's best interests at heart.

- *Take advantage of your resources.* Talk to others who have lobbied before. Attend the NBCC conference for training.

- *Allow time to develop a relationship.* You may not get what you want the first time around, but perhaps you'll do better the second—or the third.

- *Draw strength from numbers.* Back up your visits with letter-writing campaigns, petitions, demonstrations, large-scale events—anything that will show that there is widespread interest in this issue.

planet that you can go and have this many young women with breast cancer all in the same room," she says. "And the impact of that is just monumental. Because on the one hand, you say, 'Wow. Five hundred young women with breast cancer all under one roof!' But then you think, 'Oh, my God. There are 500 young women with breast cancer in one room.' So it makes you that much more impassioned to find out why."

Finding Your Voice

When Cynthia Rubin looks at the future, she hopes younger women become more aware of breast cancer. "A lot of us feel we were uneducated about breast cancer when we were diagnosed, and that it didn't have to be that way," says Cynthia. "We didn't have to catch the disease at such a late stage. Maybe we didn't have to lose our breasts. But we did, because we didn't have the information that we needed."

Now, she says, there is a place for young women in the breast cancer community, and a momentum building among researchers and doctors to study the unique issues young women face. The future of breast cancer research and activism is still being decided, but one thing is sure. A great deal of that future depends upon young women themselves, including those of you who are reading this book.

"We want to make sure that future young survivors have access to information that we never had," says YSC cofounder Lanita Hausman. "I think young women are literally changing the face of breast cancer. We are the unexpected face of breast cancer. We are a force. And because we're young, we're passionate, and we have the energy to do this. Take us seriously.

"Formidable. That's a good word to describe us."

Notes

Chapter 1

1. Barron H. Lerner, *The Breast Cancer Wars: Hope, Fear, and the Pursuit of a Cure in Twentieth-Century America* (New York: Oxford University Press, 2001).

2. Ellen Leopold, *A Darker Ribbon: Breast Cancer, Women, and Their Doctors in the Twentieth Century* (Boston: Beacon Press, 1999), pp. 235–236.

3. American Cancer Society, *Breast Cancer Facts and Figures, 2001–2002* (Atlanta, Ga. 2001).

4. J. A. Petrek, "Breast Cancer Treatment in Pregnant and/or Postpartum Women and Subsequent Pregnancy in Breast Cancer Survivors," in J. R. Harris, M. E. Lippman, M. Morrow, and C. K. Osborne, eds., *Diseases of the Breast*, 2d ed. (Philadelphia: Lippincott Williams & Wilkins, 2000), pp. 691–701.

Chapter 2

1. J. A. Petrek, "Breast Cancer Treatment in Pregnant and/or Postpartum Women and Subsequent Pregnancy in Breast Cancer Survivors," in. J. R. Harris, M. E. Lippman, M. Morrow, and C. K. Osborne, eds., *Diseases of the Breast*, 2d ed. (Philadelphia: Lippincott Williams & Wilkins, 2000), pp. 691–701.

2. In press.

3. N. Baxter and Canadian Task Force on Preventative Health Care, "Preventative Health Care, 2001 Update: Should Women Be Routinely Taught Breast Self-examination to Screen for BC?" *Canadian Medical Association Journal* 164 (13): 1837–1846 (2001).

4. Katherine Russell Rich, *The Red Devil: A Memoir About Beating the Odds* (New York: Three Rivers Press, 1999), p. 138.

5. Young Survival Coalition Web site: http://www.youngsurvival.org.

Chapter 3

1. Joan Bloom et al. "Young Breast Cancer Survivors: A Population Based Cohort," University of California, Berkeley, 2001. NCI grant no. R01CA78951.

2. Ruby Senie et al., "Menstrual Cycle Phase at Time of Tumor Excision Influences Survival of Women with Breast Carcinoma," *Annals of Internal Medicine,* 115: 337–342 (1991); Ruby Senie and D. W. Kinne, "Menstrual Timing of Treatment for Breast Cancer," *Journal of the National Cancer Institute*, Monograph No. 16, 1994, pp. 85–90.

3. Richard Love et al., "Oophorectomy and Tamoxifen Adjuvant Therapy in Premenopausal Vietnamese and Chinese Women with Operable Breast Cancer," *Journal of Clinical Oncology*, 20 (10): 2559–2566 (2002).

4. R. Segal, W. Evans, D. Johnson, et al., "Structured Exercise Improves Physical Functioning in Women with Stages I and II Breast Cancer: Results of a Randomized Controlled Trial," *Journal of Clinical Oncology*, 19: 657 (2001).

5. Christine B. Brezden et al., "Cognitive Function in Breast Cancer Patients Receiving Adjuvant Chemotherapy, Princess Margaret Hospital and the University of Toronto, Toronto, Ontario," *Journal of Clinical Oncology*, 18 (14): 2695–2701 (2000).

6. F. S. van Dam et al., "Impairment of Cognitive Function in Women Receiving Adjuvant Treatment for High-Risk Breast Cancer: High-Dose versus Standard-Dose Chemotherapy," *Journal of the National Cancer Institute*, 90 (3): 182–183 (1998).

7. T. J. Powles, T. Hickis, J. A. Kanis, et al., "Effect of Tamoxifen on Bone Mineral Density Measured by Dual-Energy X-Ray Absorptiometry in Healthy Premenopausal and Postmenopausal Women," *Journal of Clinical Oncology*, 14 (1): 78–84 (1996).

8. L. Cohen, D. J. Rosen, M. Altaras, et al., "Tamoxifen Treatment in Premenopausal Breast Cancer Patients May Be Associated with Ovarian Overstimulation, Cystic Formations and Fibroid Overgrowth [letter]," *British Journal of Cancer*, 69 (3): 620–621 (1994).

9. Valerie Baker et al., "Reproductive Endocrine and Endometrial Effects of Raloxifene Hydrochloride, a Selective Estrogen Receptor Modulator, in Women with Regular Menstrual Cycles," *Journal of Clinical Endocrinology and Metabolism*, 83 (1): 3–5 (1998).

10. B. Fisher, J. P. Costantino, D. L. Wickerham, et al., "Tamoxifen for Prevention of Breast Cancer: Report of the National Surgical Adjuvant Breast and Bowel Project P-1 Study," *Journal of the National Cancer Institute*, 90 (18): 1371–1388 (1998).

11. Francesco Boccardo et al., " Sequential Tamoxifen and Aminoglutethimide versus Tamoxifen Alone in the Adjuvant Treatment of Postmenopausal Breast Cancer Patients: Results of an Italian Cooperative Study," *Journal of Clinical Oncology*, 19: 4209–4215 (2001).

12. P. E. Goss and K. Strasser, "Aromatase Inhibitors in the Treatment and Prevention of Breast Cancer," *Journal of Clinical Oncology*, 19: 881–894 (2001).

13. Aron Goldhirsch et al., "Adjuvant Therapy for Very Young Women with Breast Cancer: Need for Tailored Treatments," *Journal of the National Cancer Institute*, 30: 44–51 (2001).

14. T. R. Rebbeck et al., "Breast Cancer Risk after Bilateral Prophylactic Oophorectomy in BRCA1 Mutation Carriers," *Journal of the National Cancer Institute*, 91: 1475–1479 (1999).

15. National Cancer Institute, "Preventive Mastectomy," *NCI Cancer Facts Sheet*, June 1, 2001.

16. W. Burke, M. Daly, J. Garber, et al., "Recommendations for Follow-Up Care of Individuals with an Inherited Predisposition to Cancer," *Journal of the American Medical Association*, 277: 997–1003 (1997).

17. L. C. Hartmann et al., "Efficacy of bilateral prophylactic mastectomy in women with a family history of breast cancer," *New England Journal of Medicine*, 340: 77–84 (1999).

18. L. C. Hartmann et al., "Efficacy of Bilateral Prophylactic Mastectomy in BRCA1 and BRCA2 Gene Mutation Carriers," *Journal of the National Cancer Institute*, 93(21): 1633–1637 (2001).

Chapter 4

1. Beverly Rockhill et al., "A Prospective Study of Recreational Physical Activity and Breast Cancer Risk," *Archives of Internal Medicine*, 159: 2290–2296 (1999).

2. Beverly Rockhill et al., "Physical Activity and Breast Cancer Risk in a Cohort of Young Women," *Journal of the National Cancer Institute*, 90: 1155–1160 (1998).

3. Leslie Bernstein et al., "Physical Exercise and Reduced Risk of Breast Cancer in Young Women," *Journal of the National Cancer Institute*, 86 (18): 1403–1408 (1994).

4. Rockhill et al., "A Prospective Study."

5. Rockhill et al., "Physical Activity and Breast Cancer Risk."

6. Leslie Bernstein et al., "The Effects of Moderate Physical Activity on Menstrual Cycle Patterns in Adolescence: Implications for Breast Cancer Prevention," *British Journal of Cancer*, 55: 681–685 (1987).

7. W. C. Chie et al., "Age at Any Full-Term Pregnancy and Breast Cancer Risk," *American Journal of Epidemiology*, 151(7): 715–722 (2000).

8. C. Carpenter et al., "Lifetime Exercise Activity and Breast Cancer Risk among Post-Menopausal Women," *British Journal of Cancer*, 80: 1852–1858 (1999).

9. Anne McTiernan, M.D., Ph.D., Julie Gralow, and Lisa Talbott, *Breast Fitness: An Optimal Exercise Plan for Reducing Your Risk of Breast Cancer* (New York: St. Martin's Griffin, 2000).

10. J. S. Brunet et al., "Effect of Smoking on Breast Cancer in Carriers of Mutant BRCA1 or BRCA2 Genes," *Journal of the National Cancer Institute*, 90: 761–766 (1998).

11. E. G. Snyderwine, "Diet and Mammary Gland Carcinogenesis," *Recent Results in Cancer Research*, 152: 3–10 (1998).

12. American Health Foundation, "Dietary Fat: Fatty Acids and Breast Cancer," *Breast Cancer*, 4 (1): 7–16 (1997).

13. E. Esrich, "Dietary Polyunsaturated N-6 Lipid Effects on Growth and Fatty Acid Composition of Rat Mammary Tumors," *Journal of Nutritional Biochemistry*, 12 (9): 536–549 (2001).

14. K. W. Singletary and S. M. Gapstur, "Alcohol and Breast Cancer: Review of Epidemiologic and Experimental Evidence and Potential Mechanisms," *Journal of the American Medical Association*, 286(17): 2143–2151 (2001).

15. S. Zhang et al., "A Prospective Study of Folate Intake and the Risk of Breast Cancer," *Journal of the American Medical Association*, 281 (17): 1632–1637 (1999).

Chapter 5

1. David M. Eisenberg, "Trends in Alternative Medicine Use in the United States, 1990–1997," *Journal of the American Medical Association,* 280: 1569–1575 (1998).

2. Loc. cit.

3. Viktor Frankl, *Man's Search for Meaning* (Boston: Beacon Press, 1959).

4. Michael McCullough, W. Hoyt, D. Larson, H. G. Koenig, and C. Thoresen, "Religious Involvement and Mortality: A Meta-analytic Review," *Health Psychology,* 19 (3): 211–222 (2000).

5. Marianne J. Brady et al., "A Case for Inducing Spirituality in Quality of Life Measurement in Oncology," *Psycho-Oncology,* 8 (5): 417–428 (1998).

6. Luciano Bernardi et al. "Beyond Science? Effect of Rosary Prayer and Yoga Mantras on Autonomic Cardiovascular Rhythms: Comparative Study," *British Medical Journal,* 323:1446–1449 (2001).

7. Susan Nessim and Judith Ellis, *Cancervive: The Challenge of Life after Cancer* (Boston: Houghton Mifflin, 1991).

8. Isaac Cohen, in Mary Tagliaferri, Isaac Cohen, and Debu Tripathy, eds., *Breast Cancer: Beyond Convention* (New York: Pocket Books, Simon & Schuster, 2002), p. 38, notes 1–3.

9. Ibid., p. 38, notes 4–16.

10. Ibid., p. 41.

11. Ibid., p. 51, notes 107–116.

12. *Alternative Medicine: Expanding Medical Horizons: A Report to the National Institutes of Health on Alternative Medical Systems and Practices in the United States,* NIH publication 94–066 (Washington, D.C.: U.S. Government Printing Office, 1994).

13. American Cancer Society, *The American Cancer Society's Guide to Complementary and Alternative Methods* (2000).

14. Michio Kushi, in Tagliaferri et al., *Breast Cancer,* op. cit., p. 119, notes 74–75, and p. 121.

15. B. Trock, L. W. Butler, R. Clarke, et al., "Meta-analysis of Soy Intake and Breast Cancer Risk. Abstract," Third International Symposium on the role of Soy in Preventing and Treating Chronic Diseases, Washington, D.C., October 31–November 3, 1999.

16. D. Ingram, K. Sanders, M. Kolybaba, and D. Lopez, "Case-Control Study of Phyto-oestrogens and Breast Cancer," *Lancet,* 350 (9083): 990–994 (1997); W. Zheng, Q. Dai, L. J. Custer, et al., "Urinary Excretion of Isoflavonoids and the Risk of Breast Cancer," *Cancer Epidemiology, Biomarkers and Prevention,* 8(1): 35–40 (1999).

17. L. J. Lu, K. E. Anderson, J. J. Grady, et al., "Decreased Ovarian Hormones during a Soya Diet: Implications for Breast Cancer Prevention," *Cancer Research,* 60(15): 4112–4121 (2000).

18. S. P. Verma and B. R. Goldin, "Effect of Soy Derived Isoflavonoids on the Induced Growth of MCF 7 Cells by Estrogenic Environmental Chemicals," *Nutrition and Cancer,* 30(3): 232–239 (1998).

19. Bernadette Murphy, *Zen and the Art of Knitting: Exploring the Links Between Knitting, Spirituality, and Creativity* (Avon, Mass.: Adams Media, 2002).

Chapter 7

1. Patricia A. Ganz, Julia H. Rowland, Katherine A. Desmond, et al., "Life after Breast Cancer: Understanding Women's Health-Related Quality of Life and Sexual Functioning," *Journal of Clinical Oncology*, 16 (2): 501–514 (1998).
2. "Breast Cancer in Younger Women," Monograph, National Cancer Institute 16:1–222 (1996).
3. Ganz et al., op. cit., pp. 501–514.
4. Patricia A. Ganz, Katherine A. Desmond, Thomas R. Belin, et al., "Predictors of Sexual Health in Women after a Breast Cancer Diagnosis," *Journal of Clinical Oncology*, 17(8): 2371–2380 (1999).
5. Frances Cerra Whittelsey, "The Secrets about Sex: The Silence about Cancer Treatment's Effects on Sexuality Obscures a Common Source of Pain," *MAMM*, May 1999, pp. 49–53.

Chapter 8

1. Julia Rowland et al., "Role of Breast Reconstructive Surgery in Physical and Emotional Outcomes among Breast Cancer Survivors," *Journal of the National Cancer Institute*, 92(17): 1422–1429 (2000).
2. National Cancer Institute, "Understanding Breast Cancer Treatment: A Guide for Patients," National Institute of Health Publication No. 98–4251 (July 1998).
3. Quoted in Barron H. Lerner, *The Breast Cancer Wars: Hope, Fears, and the Pursuit of a Cure in Twentieth-Century America* (New York: Oxford University Press, 2001), p. 191.
4. *Our Bodies, Ourselves, Her Soul Beneath the Bone*, and Lerner, op. cit., p. 270.
5. Lerner, op. cit., p. 271; Susan Ferraro, "'You Can't Look Away Anymore: The Anguished Politics of Breast Cancer," *New York Times Magazine*, August 15, 1993, pp. 24–27, 58, 61–62.

Chapter 9

1. Alison Venn et al., "Risk of Cancer after Use of Fertility Drugs with In Vitro Fertilisation," *Lancet*, 354 (9190): 1586–1590 (1999).
2. Pat Doyle et al., "Cancer Incidence Following Treatment for Infertility at a Clinic in the UK," *Human Reproduction*, 18 (8) 8: 2209–2213 (2002).
3. A. Surbone and J. A. Petrek, "Childbearing Issues in Breast Carcinoma Survivors," *Cancer*, 79 (7): 1271–1278 (1997).
4. Janet Daling et al., "The Relation of Reproductive Factors to Mortality from Breast Cancer," *Cancer Epidemiology, Biomarkers and Prevention*, 11: 235–241 (2002).
5. National Cancer Institute, "Breast Cancer and Pregnancy," (PDQ) June 2002.

6. H. Jernstrom et al., "Pregnancy and Risk of Early Breast Cancer in Carriers of BRCA1 and BRCA2," *Lancet,* 354: 1846–1850 (1999).

7. A. J. Keleher et al., "Multidisciplinary Management of Breast Cancer Concurrent with Pregnancy," *Journal of the American College of Surgeons,* 194(1): 54–64 (2002).

8. J. A. Petrek, "Breast Cancer Treatment in Pregnant and/or Postpartum Women and Subsequent Pregnancy in Breast Cancer Survivors," in J. R. Harris, M. E. Lippman, M. Morrow, and C. K. Osborne, eds., *Diseases of the Breast,* 2d ed. (Philadelphia: Lippincott Williams & Wilkins, 2000), pp. 691–701.

9. Keleher et al., "Multidisciplinary Management."

10. A. Aviles and N. Neri, "Hematological Malignancies and Pregnancy: A Final Report of 84 Children Who Received Chemotherapy In Utero," *Clinical Lymphoma,* 2(3): 173–177 (2001).

11. J. Russo and I. H. Russo, "Toward a Physiological Approach to Breast Cancer Prevention," *Cancer Epidemiology, Biomarkers and Prevention,* 3: 353–364 (1994).

12. J. R. Daling, K. E. Malone, L. F. Voigt, et al., "Risk of Breast Cancer among Young Women: Relationship to Induced Abortion," *Journal of the National Cancer Institute,* 86: 1584–1592 (1994).

13. Mads Melbye et al., "Induced Abortion and the Risk of Breast Cancer," *New England Journal of Medicine,* 336(2): 81–85 (1997).

14. B. M. Harris, G. Eklund, O. Meirik, et al., "Risk of Cancer of the Breast after Legal Abortion during First Trimester: A Swedish Register Study," *British Medical Journal* 229 (6713): 1430–1432 (1989).

15. B. M. Lindefors-Harris, G. Eklund, H. O. Adami, and O. Meirik, "Response Bias in a Case-Control Study: Analysis Utilizing Comparative Data Concerning Legal Abortions from Two Independent Swedish Studies," *American Journal of Epidemiology,* 134 (9): 1003–1008 (1991).

16. L. Rosenberg, J. R. Palmer, D. W. Daufman, et al., "Breast Cancer in Relation to the Occurrence and Time of Induced and Spontaneous Abortion," *American Journal of Epidemiology,* 127 (5): 981–989 (1988). Published erratum appears in *American Journal of Epidemiology,* 140 (9): 856 (1994).

17. American Cancer Society, *What Are the Risk Factors for Breast Cancer?* (Atlanta, Ga.: American Cancer Society, 2001).

18. National Cancer Institute, *Cancer Facts,* Fact Sheet 3.53, March 6, 2002.

19. P. A. Newcomb, B. E. Storer, and M. P. Longnecker, "Lactation and a Reduced Risk of Premenopausal Breast Cancer," *New England Journal of Medicine,* 330 (2): 81 (1994).

Chapter 11

1. *First My Illness, Now Job Discrimination: Steps to Resolution* (Newport News, Va.: Patient Advocate Foundation, 2000).

Resources

HOW TO CONNECT WITH OTHER YOUNG WOMEN DEALING WITH BREAST CANCER

Organizations

American Cancer Society, 800-ACS-2345 or www.cancer.org. This nationwide not-for-profit organization offers many different types of information and support for people living with cancer. Among the many programs available through ACS is the Reach to Recovery program, which "matches" young women with other young women with a similar diagnosis, type of surgery, and/or treatment. The newly diagnosed woman then receives a phone call from a Reach to Recovery volunteer who is close to her in age and has a similar medical situation.

Young Survival Coalition, 877-YSC-1011, 212-916-7667, or www.young survival.org. This is the only international not-for-profit network of breast cancer survivors and supporters that is dedicated to the concerns and issues that are unique to young women with breast cancer. The Young Survival Coalition offers women the opportunity to connect with peers in a number of ways. Through the YSC Web site, young women can access information on fertility, pregnancy, treatment and reconstruction, quality of life, clinical trials, and existing research. YSC members and affiliates can be found across the United States.

PEER SUPPORT AND GENERAL INFORMATION FOR YOUNG WOMEN AND THEIR LOVED ONES

Organizations

Cancer Care, 212-712-8080 or www.cancercare.org. This national organization provides a wide range of free professional social services, including counseling for patients and their partners, parents, and young children.

Gilda's Club, 212-647-9700 or www.gildasclub.org. This organization has a number of not-for-profit centers that offer a variety of services to individuals who are dealing with any type of cancer and to their family members.

Living Beyond Breast Cancer (LBBC), 888-753-5222 or www.lbbc.org. This not-for-profit educational organization focuses on posttreatment and quality-of-life issues.

The Mary-Helen Mautner Project for Lesbians with Cancer, 202-332-5536 or www.mautnerproject.org. This volunteer organization is dedicated to helping lesbians with cancer and their partners and caregivers. Extensive resources, links, and professional trainings are available.

Men Against Breast Cancer, 866-547-6222 or www.menagainstbreastcancer.org. This national not-for-profit organization mobilizes men who wish to join in the fight against breast cancer. It also provides support to men who are dealing with the breast cancer diagnosis of a significant woman in their lives.

Mothers Supporting Daughters with Breast Cancer, 410-778-1982 or www.mothersdaughters.org. This national not-for-profit organization provides support services designed to help mothers whose daughters are battling breast cancer.

National Alliance of Breast Cancer Organizations, 888-80-NABCO or www.nabco.org. NABCO is the largest educational resource on breast cancer in the United States. NABCO publications cover the range of experiences faced by women with breast cancer, and the organization's Web site is comprehensive.

National Breast Cancer Coalition, 202-296-7477 or www.stopbreastcancer.org. This grassroots organization focuses on ending breast cancer through action and advocacy. NBCC's main goals are to increase federal funding for breast cancer research and to collaborate with the scientific community to implement new models of research. Members include breast cancer organizations and individuals around the country.

Sharsheret, 866-832-9909, 201-837-8793, or www.sharsheret.org. This organization is dedicated to addressing the unique challenges facing young Jewish women living with breast cancer.

Susan G. Komen Breast Cancer Foundation, 800-I'M AWARE, 972-855-1600, or www.komen.org. Komen is the largest private funder of breast cancer research in the United States as well as the organizer of Races for the Cure.

Y-ME National Breast Cancer Organization, 800-221-2141 or www.y-me.org. This nonprofit organization provides information and support to individuals with breast cancer as well as to their family members and the significant people in their lives.

Publications and Online Sources

Confronting the Cow: A Young Family's Struggle with Breast Cancer, Loss and Rebuilding, by C. B. Donner (Durham, N. C.: Moonlight Publishing LLC, 2000). Written from the perspective of a husband who lost his wife to breast cancer at age 36.

Cancer in Two Voices, by Sandra Butler and Barbara Rosenblum (Denver, Colo.: Spinsters Book Company, 1996). A moving and honest account from diary excerpts of the authors' identities as lesbian Jewish women living with advanced breast cancer.

A Cancer Battle Plan: Six Strategies for Beating Cancer, from a Recovered "Hopeless Case," by Anne E. Frahm with David J. Frahm (Los Angeles, Calif.: J. P. Tarcher, 1998). Written by a survivor of advanced, metastatic breast cancer. Understand what cancer does to your body; give your immune system the tools it needs to fight disease; choose the treatments that are best for you; learn how to help those who are fighting cancer. Includes resource lists and a complete nutritional battle plan.

www.breastcancer.org This online nonprofit organization provides reliable, complete, and up-to-date medical and personal information about breast cancer. Live chats, transcripts, and booklets are all available by visiting this comprehensive site.

www.imaginif.com This Web site, sponsored by Siemens, is a comprehensive resource for news and information on breast cancer prevention screening, diagnosis, and treatment.

www.mamm.com This Web site is sponsored by *Mamm* magazine, a commercial publication devoted to covering issues of concern to women living with breast and reproductive cancers.

www.susanlovemd.com This Web site provides breast cancer content, personal guidance, chats, and community for women living with breast cancer.

What's Happening to the Woman I Love? Couples Coping with Breast Cancer (Susan G. Komen Breast Cancer Foundation, 2001). This is a general reference covering ways to be helpful and supportive when your partner is coping with breast cancer. Contact The Komen Foundation, 800-I'M AWARE or www.breastcancerinfo.com.

WHEN CHILDREN ARE PRESENT—PARENTING WHILE DEALING WITH BREAST CANCER
Organizations

Kids Konnected, 800-899-2866 or www.kidskonnected.org. This national not-for-profit organization provides age-appropriate books for children dealing with a parent's cancer diagnosis and can connect children with peers. Literature for parents is also available.

KidsCope, www.kidscope.org. This nonprofit organization is dedicated to helping children and their families better understand the effects of cancer and chemotherapy in a parent.

Publications

Kemo Shark, by H. Elizabeth King. Written by a child psychologist who is a breast cancer survivor and her 8-year-old son, this "comic book" is designed to help children with the psychological and physiological changes a family may face when a parent undergoes chemotherapy. Available free through KidsCope, www.kidscope.org.

Michael's Mommy Has Breast Cancer, by Lisa Torrey, illustrated by Barbara Watler (Coral Springs, Fla.: Hibiscus Press, 1999; 34 pages). This book, for children ages 5 to 10, chronicles the feelings that a young boy experiences after his mother is diagnosed with breast cancer.

Moms Don't Get Sick, by Pat Brack and Ben Brack (Aberdeen, S. Dak.,: Medius Publishing, 1990). A powerful firsthand look at breast cancer as told by a mother and her 10-year-old son.

My Mommy Has Cancer by Carolyn Stearns Parkinson (Folsom, Calif.: Solace Publishing, 1991; 916-851-1771). This book is appropriate for young children, ages 3 to 8, who have relatives with cancer.

Our Family Has Cancer, Too! by Christine Clifford (Minneapolis: University of Minnesota Press, 1997). This book, for children ages 5 to 14, talks about one child's struggle to understand and cope with his mother's cancer. Available at bookstores or from The Cancer Club, 800-586-9062 or www.cancerclub.com.

Our Mom Has Cancer, by Abigail and Adrienne Ackerman (American Cancer Society, 2001). Written and illustrated by two sisters, aged 11 and 9, this book relays their experience of living with a mother with breast cancer. Available from ACS, 800-ACS-2345 or www.cancer.org.

The Paper Chain, by Claire Blake, Eliza Blanchard, and Kathy Parkinson (Santa Fe, N.Mex.: Health Press, 1998). This book, for children ages 3 to 8, relays the emotions of two young boys whose mother has breast cancer. Available at bookstores or from Health Press, 800-643-BOOK.

When Someone in Your Family Has Cancer (National Cancer Institute, P619, 1995). This NCI booklet is written for the young person whose parent has cancer. Available from NCI's CIS, 800-4-CANCER.

YOUR BODY AND BREAST CANCER—ISSUES OF RECONSTRUCTION, HAIR LOSS, SKIN CHANGES, AND OTHER PHYSICAL SIDE EFFECTS OF CHEMOTHERAPY AND RADIATION

Organizations

American Society of Plastic and Reconstructive Surgeons (ASPRS), 847-228-9900, 888-4-PLASTIC, or www.plasticsurgery.org. The ASPRS will provide information and referrals to board-certified surgeons in your area. You can find a certified surgeon by calling the ASPS directly or by looking at the society's Web site.

Look Good Feel Better. This program, created by the American Cancer Society, helps women deal with the physical effects of chemotherapy and/or radiation. Groups are led by trained cosmetologists who volunteer their time to teach creative ways to use makeup, accessories, and head coverings to address some of the side effects of treatment, such as hair loss and skin changes. The program is free of charge. To locate a Look Good Feel Better session close to you, contact the American Cancer Society at 800-ACS-2345.

Publications

Cancer-Related Fatigue: Treatment Guidelines for Patients, American Cancer Society and National Comprehensive Cancer Network Version I, 9448.00, December 2001). Available from ACS, 800-ACS-2345.

Coping with the Side Effects of Radiation and Chemotherapy (Cancer Care, Inc., 2001). Available from Cancer Care, 800-813-HOPE or www.cancercare.org.

Managing the Side Effects of Chemotherapy and Radiation Therapy: A Guide for Patients and Their Families by Marylin J. Dodd (San Francisco: UCSF Nursing Press, 2001). Available from UCSF Nursing Press, 415-476-4992 or nurseweb.ucsf.edu/www/books.html.

STARTING A FAMILY AFTER BREAST CANCER— A RANGE OF OPTIONS AND EXPERIENCES

Organizations

Fertile Hope, 888-994-HOPE or www.fertilehope.org. This not-for-profit organization is dedicated to providing support and information to cancer patients dealing with fertility issues before, during, and after treatment.

La Leche League International, 847-519-7730 or www.lalecheleague.org. This organization is a leading source of information on breast-feeding, including information on breast-feeding before and after breast cancer and breast-feeding with implants.

Pregnant with Cancer, 800-743-6724 x308 or www.pregnantwithcancer.org. Pregnant with Cancer is a network of women from across the United States who have been diagnosed with breast cancer during pregnancy. Members lend support, share their experiences, and offer hope.

Publication

Sexuality and Fertility after Cancer, by Leslie R. Schover (New York: John Wiley & Sons, 1997). This book helps survivors and their partners learn to enjoy sex again and make informed choices about having children.

CONCERNS ABOUT WORK AND CAREER

Organizations

Cancer and Careers, www.cancerandcareers.org. This organization's Web site explores issues related to working while dealing with a diagnosis of cancer. Information is also available for those who wish to support individuals dealing with cancer in the workplace.

U.S. Equal Employment Opportunity Commission (EEOC), 800-669-4000 or www.eeoc.gov. This government agency provides detailed information on Americans with Disabilities Act provisions and instructions on how to file a charge of discrimination. To reach your local EEOC office, look in the phone book under "U.S. Government" or call the number given here. In addition to having federal protection under the ADA, you may be protected by state laws. The EEOC can also help you find the right state agency for more information on state protection.

Job Accommodation Network (JAN), 800-526-7234 or www.jan.wvu.edu. This service of the U.S. Department of Labor provides free advice on making accommodations at work.

Patient Advocate Foundation (PAF), 800-532-5274, 757-873-6668, or www.patientadvocate.org. This national nonprofit organization deploys case managers, doctors, and attorneys to function as active liaisons among patients and insurers, employers, and/or creditors in order to resolve insurance, job discrimination, and/or debt crisis matters relating to the patient's condition.

EXPLORING YOUR TREATMENT OPTIONS, RESEARCH, AND CLINICAL TRIALS

Organizations

National Cancer Institute (NCI), 800-4-CANCER or www.nci.nih.gov. This U.S. government office and its Web site provide information on various types of cancer, different treatment options, and current clinical trials. Cancer information specialists can help callers locate information on clinical trials that are appropriate for specific diagnoses, by phone.

Publications

Breast Cancer: The Complete Guide, by Yashar Hirshaut and Peter I. Pressman (New York: Bantam Books, 2000). This is a comprehensive resource of medical information and practical advice on breast cancer.

Dr. Susan Love's Breast Book, by Susan M. Love and Karen Lindsey (Cambridge, Mass.: Perseus Books, 2000). This book is an excellent general reference for all aspects of breast cancer.

HER-2: The Making of Herceptin, a Revolutionary Treatment for Breast Cancer, by Robert Bazell (New York: Random House, 2001). This is the story of the creation of Genentech's Herceptin, the monoclonal antibody that is the first gene-based therapy for breast cancer.

Patient's Guide to Breast Cancer (New York: Beth Israel Medical Center, 2000). This booklet clarifies the complex terms and procedures involved in diagnosis and treatment. Available from Beth Israel Medical Center, 212-844-8468 or www.wehealnewyork.org.

Tamoxifen: For the Prevention and Treatment of Breast Cancer, by V. Craig Jordan (PRR, Inc., 1999). This concise textbook reviews the issues surrounding tamoxifen therapy for breast cancer treatment and risk reduction. Available from PRR, Inc., 631-777-3800 or www.cancernetwork.com.

Things to Know About: Aromatase Inhibitors (NABCO, June 2001). This one-page fact sheet explains the current role of aromatase inhibitors in treating breast cancer. Available from NABCO, 888-80-NABCO or www.nabco.org.

Things to Know About: Estrogen Receptor Status and Breast Cancer (NABCO, October 2001). This one-page fact sheet explains the role of estrogen receptor status in breast cancer treatment. Available from NABCO, 888-80-NABCO or www.nabco.org.

Understanding Breast Cancer Treatment (National Cancer Institute, P458, July 1998). This NCI booklet contains lists of questions that will help a patient talk to her doctor about all aspects of breast cancer. Available from NCI's CIS, 800-4-CANCER.

Understanding Chemotherapy (American Cancer Society, 9458.00, 1999). This booklet provides an introduction to chemotherapy and explains its benefits and side effects. Available from ACS, 800-ACS-2345 or www.cancer.org.

Understanding Radiation Therapy (American Cancer Society, 9459.00, 2001; 36 pages). This booklet provides an introduction to radiation therapy and explains its benefits and side effects. Available from ACS, 800-ACS-2345 or www.cancer.org.

Understanding Your Pathology Report (Y-ME National Breast Cancer Organization, 2001). This brochure outlines the purpose of a pathology report and defines the many elements that compose it. Contact Y-ME, 800-221-2141 or www.y-me.org.

COMPLEMENTARY AND ALTERNATIVE MEDICINE
Organizations

American Academy of Medical Acupuncture (AAMA), 323-937-5514 or www.medicalacupuncture.org. The American Academy of Medical Acupuncture promotes the integration of concepts from traditional and modern forms of acupuncture with Western medical training. A search engine on the AAMA Web site can direct you to an AAMA physician near you.

The Center for Mind-Body Medicine, 202-966-7338, www.cmbm.org. This organization has become a leader in promoting complementary cancer care, the term used for approaches that combine standard treatments with alternative methods.

International Academy of Compounding Pharmacies (IACP), 800-927-IACP, 281-933-8400, or www.iacprx.org. This international, nonprofit association promotes pharmaceutical compounding. You can look for a compounding pharmacy near you through the IACP Web site's referral service.

National Center for Complementary and Alternative Medicine (NCCAM), 888-644-6226, http://nccam.nih.gov, or info@nccam.nih.gov. NCCAM is one of the 27 institutes and centers that make up the National Institutes of Health (NIH). Its mission is to support rigorous research on complementary and alternative medicine (CAM), to train researchers in CAM, and to disseminate information to the public and professionals on which CAM modalities work, which do not, and why.

Publications

The Alternative Medicine Handbook: The Complete Reference Guide to Alternative and Complementary Therapies, by Barrie Cassileth (New York: W. W. Norton, 1998). This book gives an overview of more than 50 therapies, with a discussion of the origins of each therapy, any scientific evidence for its efficacy, and locations that offer that treatment.

American Cancer Society's Guide to Complementary and Alternative Cancer Methods, by David S. Rosenthal (American Cancer Society, 2000). Written in an encyclopedic format, this guide covers specific complementary and alternative modalities. Available from ACS, 800-ACS-2345 or www.cancer.org.

Choices in Healing: Integrating the Best of Conventional and Complementary Approaches to Cancer by Michael Lerner (Cambridge, Mass.: MIT Press, 1996). This book is useful for those who are interested in considering alternative therapies in conjunction with standard medical treatment.

Comprehensive Cancer Care: Integrating Alternative, Complementary, and Conventional Therapies by James S. Gordon and Sharon Curtin (Cambridge, Mass.: Perseus Books, 2001). This book provides sound medical knowledge on alternative and complementary therapies, with an emphasis on tailoring treatments to individuals.

Zen and the Art of Knitting: Exploring the Links Between Knitting, Spirituality, and Creativity by Bernadette Murphy (Avon, Mass.: Adams Media, 2002; www.zenknitting.com). This book explores the act of knitting as a powerful form of meditation. It is a collection of essays that unite Eastern and Western philosophies through art and medical science.

LYMPHEDEMA RESOURCES
Organizations
The Lymphology Association of North America, www.whidbey.com/lana. This organization certifies medical professionals who offer lymphedema management services and maintains a database of certified lymphedema therapists.

The National Lymphedema Network, 800-541-3259 or www.lymphnet.org. This nonprofit organization provides information about the prevention and treatment of lymphedema to patients and health-care professionals, as well as to support groups.

Publications
Coping with Lymphedema by Joan Swirsky and Diane Sackett Nannery (New York: Avery Books, 1998). This book is a practical guide to understanding, treating, and living with lymphedema. Available from Avery Books, 800-788-6262.

Lymphedema: A Breast Cancer Patient's Guide to Prevention and Healing, by Jeannie Burt and Gwen White (Alameda, Calif.: Hunter House Publishers, 1999). This book describes the options that women have for treating lymphedema. Available from Hunter House Publishers, 800-266-5592.

Lymphedema: Results from a Workshop on Breast Cancer Treatment–Related Lymphedema and Lymphedema Resource Guide, by Jeanne A. Petrek, Peter I. Pressman, and Robert A. Smith (1998). This booklet contains presentations and recommendations from the ACS's 1998 national workshop on lymphedema. Available from ACS, 888-227-5552.

GENETICS AND YOUNG WOMEN
Organizations
Facing Our Risk of Cancer Empowered (FORCE), 954-255-8732 or www.facing ourrisk.com. This not-for-profit organization provides support and information to women who are at high risk for developing breast cancer and to their families.

The Genetic Alliance, 800-336-GENE or www.geneticalliance.org. The Genetic Alliance supports individuals with genetic conditions and their families, educates the public, and promotes consumer-informed public policies.

The National Society of Genetic Counselors, 610-872-7608 or www.nsgc.org. The NSGC helps women decide if they can benefit from genetic counseling, and helps them find genetic counselors in their area.

Publications and Online Sources
http//cancer.gov/search/genetics_services The Family Cancer Risk Counseling and Genetic Testing Directory offers a list of cancer risk counseling resources and genetic testing providers throughout the country.

Genetic Testing for Breast Cancer Risk: It's Your Choice (National Cancer Institute, 1997). This booklet provides a general overview on testing for breast and ovarian cancer risk. Available from NCI's CIS, 800-4-CANCER.

The National Cancer Institute's Breast Cancer Risk Assessment Tool (National Cancer Institute, PC version: TO71, Mac version: TO72, September 1998). The "risk disk" is an interactive patient education tool that can help to assess an individual's risk of developing breast cancer. Available from NCI's CIS, 800-4-CANCER.

CONCERNS OF YOUNG WOMEN WITH ADVANCED BREAST CANCER
Organization
The NABCO Recurrence Project, www.nabco.org. This project was created for women who are learning about or living with recurrent and advanced breast cancer and their family, friends, caregivers, and health-care professionals.

Publications
Advanced Breast Cancer: A Guide to Living with Metastatic Disease by Musa Mayer (Sebastopol, Calif.: O'Reilly and Associates, Inc., 1998). This updated, retitled edition of the author's 1997 work *Holding Tight, Letting Go* helps women lead everyday lives while coping with advanced disease. It contains a good resource section. Available at bookstores. Also visit www.patient centers.com/breastcancer for excerpts from this book and updated articles.

I Still Buy Green Bananas: Living with Hope, Living with Breast Cancer (Y-ME National Breast Cancer Organization, 1997). This booklet offers practical advice and personal stories on coping with a diagnosis of advanced breast cancer and living life fully every day despite having cancer. Single copies of the booklet are available free. Available from Y-ME, 800-221-2141 or www.y-me.org.

The Red Devil: A Memoir about Beating the Odds by Katherine Russell Rich (New York, Three Rivers Press, 2000). A young woman's bold, witty, and extraordinarily personal account of her diagnosis of advanced-stage breast cancer. Available in bookstores.

When Cancer Recurs: Meeting the Challenge Again (National Cancer Institute, P129, 1996). This booklet details the different types of recurrence, types of treatment, and ways to cope with cancer's return. Available from NCI's CIS, 800-4-CANCER.

www.livingwithit.org This is an online support program for women with recurrent breast cancer. The site was created by Aventis Pharmaceuticals.

INSURANCE ISSUES
Organizations
ASCO, www.asco.org The American Federation of Clinical Oncologic Societies provides basic criteria to be used in searching for and choosing a health insurance plan that will provide quality cancer care.

Patient Advocate Foundation (PAF), 800-532-5274 , 757-873-6668, or www.patientadvocate.org. The Patient Advocate Foundation is a national nonprofit organization that deploys case managers, doctors, and attorneys to function as active liaisons between patients and their insurers, employers, and/or creditors in order to resolve insurance, job discrimination, and/or debt crisis matters relating to the patient's condition. Reference handbooks are available.

Health Insurance Association of America, 888-869-4078, 202-824-1600, or www.hiaa.org. HIAA is a prominent trade association representing the private health care system. HIAA publications provide information on various types of insurance: health insurance, managed care, long-term care, and disability, and a special guide for business owners. Numerous publications are available by calling or visiting the Web site.

Publications

The National Financial Resources Guidebook for Patients (Newport News, Va.: Patient Advocate Foundation, 1999). This valuable resource provides listings of federal and state resources for obtaining financial assistance for a broad range of needs. Available from Patient Advocate Foundation, 800-532-5274 or www.patientadvocate.org.

What Cancer Survivors Need to Know about Health Insurance (Silver Springs, Md.: National Coalition for Cancer Survivorship, 1999). This pamphlet provides a clear understanding of health insurance and how to receive maximum reimbursement for claims. Available from NCCS, 877-NCCS-YES or www.cansearch.org.

Index

Ablation, ovarian, 69–73
Abortion, 226–228
Activism, 285–298
  for educating medical community, 291–292
  history of, 6–10
  for lobbying legislation, 296–298
  local, 294–296
  for medical research, 290–291
  and national conferences, 296–298
  tips for involvement in, 289
  for young women's outreach, 292–294
Acupuncture, 126–127
ADA (*see* Americans with Disabilities Act)
Advocacy, 141, 296–298
Affirmations, 138
Age myth, 2–5
Aggressive breast cancer, 12
Alternative medicine:
  Ayurveda as, 127–129
  homeopathy as, 129
  naturopathy as, 129
  traditional Chinese medicine as, 125–127
Alternative Medicine Handbook, The
  (Barrie Cassileth), 109
American Cancer Society, 32, 105, 287
Americans with Disabilities Act (ADA),
  253–258
Anger expression, 282
Aromatase inhibitors/inactivators, 68
Art therapy, 120
Atypical hyperplasia, 31
Axilliary node dissection, 53
Ayurvedic medicine, 127–129

Baldness (*see* Hair loss)
Barrett, Elizabeth, 269–270, 282–284
Benign results, 31–33
Benson, Herbert, 117, 145
Bernardi, Luciano, 117
Bernstein, Leslie, 90–92, 94
Beyond Convention (Mary A. Tagliaferri),
  134
Biopsies, 29–31
  core, 29
  excisional, 29
  fine-needle, 29
  incisional, 29
  mammotome, 29, 30
  positive, 35–38
  sentinel node, 53
  stereotactic, 29
Black, Shirley Temple, 8

Blum, Diane, 10
Bodai, Ernie, 6
Body image, 12, 164–181
  changes in, 166–169
  coping with issues of, 165–166, 172
  and dating, 173–175
  and hair loss, 170–173
  and sex/sexuality, 176–181
BRCA1 gene, 70, 73–78, 222
BRCA2 gene, 73–78, 222
Breast cancer, 1–19
  and age myth, 2–5
  causes of, 23–25
  history of treatment/activism for, 6–10
  need for screening tool for, 11–12
  questions about, 12–16
  symptoms of, 25–26
  types of, 33–34
  in young women, 10–12, 16–19
Breast Cancer: A Personal History and In-
  vestigative Report (Rose Kushner), 8
Breast Cancer: The Complete Guide
  (Yashar Hirshaut and Peter
  Pressman), 4
Breast cancer gene, 70, 73–80
  and genetic research, 78–80
  genetic testing for, 74–78
  passing on the, 222–223
Breast Cancer Wars, The (Barron H.
  Lerner), 207
Breast-feeding, 229
Breast Fitness (Anne McTiernan), 89
Breast forms (*see* Prostheses)
Breast reconstruction (*see* Reconstruction,
  breast)
Breast replacement(s), 182–208
  going without, 183–184
  prosthesis approach to, 184–186
  reconstruction approach to, 186–208
Breast self-examination (BSE), 27
Breasts, 5–6
Brinker, Nancy, 10
BSE (breast self-examination), 27

CAM (*see* Complementary and alternative
  medicine)
Cancer as a Turning Point (Lawrence
  LeShan), 116
Cancer Journals, The (Audre Lorde), 208
Cancervive (Susan Nessim), 119
Cassileth, Barrie, 109, 113–115, 119–120,
  135, 138

CBE (clinical breast examination), 27
"Chemo brain," 64
Chemotherapy, 7, 14, 59–65
    decision making about, 64–65
    and fertility, 212–213
    side effects of, 61–64
Childbearing decisions, 218–219
Children, 13, 230–248
    caring for your, 231
    cognition levels of, 234, 236, 239–244
    and daily demands, 244–246
    journaling for, 246–248
    talking with, 231–234
Chinese medicine, 125–127
Clinical breast examination (CBE), 27
Clinical trials, 81–82, 275
COBRA (see Consolidated Omnibus
    Budget Reconciliation Act)
Cognitive-behavioral therapy, 121
Cohen, Isaac, 115, 125, 127
Coinsurance, 43
College of American Pathologists, 31
Communication:
    with children, 231–234, 245
    with family, 155–159
    with friends, 159–163
    about last wishes, 283
    with spouse, 148–149, 244
    with supervisor, 258
    about test results, 37
Complementary and alternative medicine
    (CAM), 15, 109–138
    alternative medicine approach to,
        124–129
    designing your approach to, 138
    and meaning of life approach to, 115–124
    mind/body approaches to, 135–137
    nutritional/herbal approaches to,
        130–136
    questions about, 114
    and standard medical care, 111–115
Conferences, 296–298
Consolidated Omnibus Budget Reconcilia-
    tion Act (COBRA), 260–262
Copayment, 43
Coping:
    with body image issues, 165–166, 172
    with breast reconstruction, 205–207
    with health insurance, 44–46
    with medical procedures, 141
    with recurrence, 269–271, 277–279
    with workplace issues, 250, 252–253
Core biopsies, 29
Creativity, 119–120
Crile, George "Barney," Jr., 8

Daling, Janet, 27
D'Andrea, Alan, 78, 79
Darker Ribbon, A (Ellen Leopold), 6, 270
Dating, 13, 173–175

Daydream exercise, 98–99
DCIS (see Ductal carcinoma in situ)
De Michele, Angela, 69
Death, facing, 281–284
Deductible, 43
Development, child, 234, 236, 239–244
    age 2 or younger, 236
    ages 3 to 5, 236, 239
    ages 6 to 8, 239–241
    ages 9 to 12, 242–244
Diagnosis, 20–47
    biopsies for, 29–31
    and causes of breast cancer, 23–25
    and decision making, 47
    and doctor selection, 39–41
    and insurance companies, 42–47
    and pathology report, 31–35
    of positive biopsy, 35–38
    screening tools for, 26–29
    and second opinion, 38–39
    and symptoms, 25–26
Dietary recommendations, 105–106
Diseases of the Breast (Jeanne Petrek), 225
Doctors:
    and breast reconstruction, 189–192,
        197, 198
    educating, 291–292
    primary-care, 43
    selection of, 39–41
Dominant lumps, 25
Double-blind studies, 81
Dr. Susan Love's Breast Book (Susan Love),
    4, 62, 195, 207
Drains, 57, 58
Dream work, 120
Ductal carcinoma in situ (DCIS), 17, 33

Educating medical community, 291–292
EEOC (see Equal Employment Opportu-
    nity Commission)
Eisenberg, David, 112–113
Employment (see Workplace issues)
Equal Employment Opportunity Commis-
    sion (EEOC), 256, 259
Estring, 180
Estrogen, 90–92
Estrogen receptor, 34
Excisional biopsies, 29
Exercise(s), 88–101, 104–105
    and body fat, 93, 94
    contraindications for, 97
    decision making about, 94–96
    and estrogen, 90–92
    hand clasp exercise, 99
    hand leaning exercise, 98
    postsurgery, 96–101, 104–105
    snow angel exercise, 99
    tips for starting to, 100–101
Expanders, implants with, 194
Expression, anger, 282

Fair Employment Practices Agencies (FEPAs), 256, 259
Family Medical Leave Act (FMLA), 258–261
Family support, 155–159
Fanconi's anemia, 78
Fat, body, 93, 94
FDA (Food and Drug Administration), 82
Fears, posttreatment, 82–86
Fee-for-service insurance, 43
Feminist movement, 7
FEPAs (see Fair Employment Practices Agencies)
Fertility, 14, 211–219
    and chemotherapy, 62, 212–213
    and childbearing decisions, 218–219
    and tamoxifen, 213–215
    treatment procedures for, 215–218
Fibrocystic breast condition, 31–33
Fine-needle biopsies, 29
First, You Cry (Betty Rollin), 8
Fisher, Bernard, 7
Fitness, 14–15, 87–107
    exercise for, 88–101, 104–15
    and nutrition, 101–107
    and smoking, 103
Flap reconstruction, 198–203
    pedicle vs. free, 201–203
    pros and cons of, 200–202
FMLA (see Family Medical Leave Act)
Food and Drug Administration (FDA), 82
Ford, Betty, 8
Frankl, Viktor, 115
Free flap reconstruction, 199, 201–203
Friends, support from, 159–163
Frozen section analysis, 31
Fund raising, 294–296

Genetic research, 78–80
Genetic testing, 74–79
GnRH (gonadotropin–releasing hormone) analogues, 70
Goldhirsch, Aron, 35, 56, 68
Gonadotropin-releasing hormone (GnRH) analogues, 70

Hair loss, 170–173, 251–252, 263, 264
Halsted, William, 6–7
Health insurance, 42–47
    coping with bureaucracy of, 44–46
    lack of, 47
    types of, 43–44
Health Insurance Portability and Accountability Act (HIPAA), 260, 262
Heart disease, 62–63
Her Soul Beneath the Bone, 208
HER2neu, 34
HIPAA (see Health Insurance Portability and Accountability Act)
Hirshaut, Yashar, 4

Homeopathic medicine, 129
Hormonal treatment(s), 65–73
    aromatase inhibitors/inactivators as, 68
    ovarian ablation as, 69–73
    tamoxifen as, 65–68
Hormones:
estrogen and, 91
    infertility procedures and, 215
    soy and, 133–134
Hypnotherapy, 122

Imagery exercise, 282
Implants, 193–198
    with expanders, 194
    pros and cons of, 197–198
    silicone vs. saline, 195, 196
Incisional biopsies, 29
Inflammatory breast cancer, 33
Information overload, 41–42
Insurance, health (see Health insurance)
Internet resources, 41–42
Invasive ductal breast cancer, 33
Invasive lobular breast cancer, 33

Journal/journaling, 246–248, 258

Kash, Kathryn, 6, 124
King, H. Elizabeth, 231–234
King, Mary-Claire, 75
Kleban, Roz, 82–85, 270, 277, 278, 281
Knitting, 135–136
Kolb, Thomas, 11, 25–26
Kushi, Michio, 131
Kushner, Rose, 8–10

Langer, Amy, 10
Laws, 253–262
    Americans with Disabilities Act, 253–258
    Consolidated Omnibus Budget Reconciliation Act, 260–262
    Family Medical Leave Act, 258–261
    Health Insurance Portability and Accountability Act, 260, 262
LBBC (Living Beyond Breast Cancer), 287
LCIS (lobular carcinoma in situ), 33
Legislation, lobbying for, 296–298
Leopold, Ellen, 6, 9, 270
Lerner, Barron H., 8
Lerner, Michael, 119
LeShan, Lawrence, 116
Lesnikoski, Beth, 27, 28
LHRH (luteinizing hormone—releasing hormone) analogues, 70
Living Beyond Breast Cancer (LBBC), 287
Lobbying (for legislation), 296–298
Lobular carcinoma in situ (LCIS), 33
Local activism, 294–296
Local cancer, 58
Lorde, Audre, 208

Love, Richard, 56
Love, Susan, 4, 10, 12, 25, 27, 35, 36, 38, 62, 64, 66–67, 80, 195, 207, 220, 222
Lubricants, 180
Luce, Edward, 189, 191, 194, 196–199
Lumpectomy, 50
Luteinizing hormone—releasing hormone (LHRH) analogues, 70
Lymph node removal, 53
Lymphedema, 51

McCray, Percy W., Jr., 118–119
McMillion, Janine, 261
Macrobiotics, 131
McTiernan, Anne, 88–91, 94
Malignant (cancerous) results, 33–35
Mammotome biopsies, 29, 30
Managed care, 43
Man's Search for Meaning (Viktor Frankl), 115
Margins, 33
Mastectomy, 50–53
    modified radical, 51
    partial, 52
    prophylactic, 52–53
    radical, 6–7, 51–52
    total or simple, 51
Matuschka, 208
Meaning, 22, 115–124
    and creativity, 119–120
    in spirituality, 116–119
    and therapy, 121–124
Medicaid, 47
Medical community, educating, 291–292
Medical procedures, 141–143
Medical research, 290–291
Menopause, 62, 63, 66–67
Menstrual cycles, 55–57
Metastatic cancer, 33, 272–275
Metzger, Deena, 208
Micrometastasis, 58
Modified radical mastectomy, 51
Motherhood, 209–229
    and breast-feeding, 229
    and fertility, 211–219
    and pregnancy, 219–228
Mothers Supporting Daughters with Breast Cancer (MSDBC), 156
Murphy, Bernadette, 135
Music therapy, 119–120

National Alliance of Breast Cancer Organizations (NABCO), 9–10, 287
National Breast Cancer Coalition (NBCC), 10, 287, 296
National Center for Complementary and Alternative Medicine, 110, 111
Naturopathic medicine, 129
Nausea, 62

NBCC (see National Breast Cancer Coalition)
Nessim, Susan, 119
Newman, Beth, 75–76, 79–80
NHS (see Nurses' Health Study)
Node involvement, 33
Note taking, 141
Nurses' Health Study (NHS), 88
Nurses' Health Study II (NHSII), 88, 91
Nutrients, 134–136
Nutrition, 101–107
    dietary recommendations for, 105–106
    and macrobiotics, 131
    and nutrients/supplements, 134–136
    and phytohormonals, 106
    and soy, 132–134
Nutritionists, 102

Ohsawa, George, 131
Oncogenes, 34
Oophorectomy, 69–70
Oktay, Kutluk, 211–212
Our Bodies, Ourselves, 208
Ovarian ablation, 69–73
Ovarian cancer, 69

Paget's disease of the breast, 16–17, 33
Paresthesia, 51
Partial mastectomy, 52
Pathology reports, 31–36
Patient Advocate Foundation, 46, 47
Pedicle flap reconstruction, 199, 201–203
Permanent section analysis, 31
Petersen, Bert, 51–53, 79, 86, 272, 273, 275
Petrek, Jeanne, 10, 62–63, 211, 220–222, 225
Physical therapy, 100
Phytohormonals, 106
Plastic surgeons, 189–192, 197, 198
Positive biopsies, 35–38
Postsurgery exercises, 96–101, 104–105
Pregnancy, 219–228
    and abortion, 226–228
    breast cancer during, 224–228
    and breast cancer gene, 222–223
    and parenthood, 223–224
    risks of, 219–224
Pressman, Peter, 4
Primary-care physician, 43
Prophylactic mastectomy, 52–53
Prostheses, 14, 184–186
Pruthi, Sandya, 74
Przypyszny, Michele, 266
Psychoanalysis, 121

Radiation, 14
    ovarian ablation through, 72–73
    and reconstruction, 203, 205
Radical mastectomy, 6–7, 51–52
Raloxifene, 66, 68

Reach to Recovery Program, 287
Rebbeck, Timothy R., 70
Reconstruction, breast, 186–208
  coping with, 205–207
  decision making about, 186–187,
    207–208
  flap, 198–203
  with implants, 193–198
  and plastic surgeons, 189–192, 197,
    198
  pros and cons of, 193
  questions about, 204
  and radiation, 203, 205
Recovering from Breast Surgery (Diana
  Stumm), 96
Recurrence, breast cancer, 16, 267–284
  coping with, 269–271, 277–279
  and facing death, 281–284
  fears of, 85
  and limitations, 280
  metastatic cancer, 272–275
  treatment decisions for, 275–277
  types of, 271–272
Red Devil, The (Katherine Russell Rich),
Referrals, 43
Rennert, Sharon, 257, 258
Research, genetic, 78–80
Rich, Katherine Russell, 35
Rockefeller, Happy, 8
Rockhill, Beverly, 26, 88, 91, 92, 94, 101–103
Rollin, Betty, 8
Rosenthal, David, 110–112
Rowland, Julia H., 192
Rubin, Cynthia, 27

Salamone, Jeannine, 196, 205
Saline implants, 195, 196
Schover, Leslie, 165–166
Screening tool(s):
  for breast cancer, 26–29
  genetic testing as, 74–79
  need for, 11–12
Second opinions, 38–39, 275
Self-examination, 27
Senie, Ruby, 56
Sentinel node biopsy, 53
Sex/sexuality, 5–6, 13, 176–181
SHARE, 18
Side effects:
  of chemotherapy, 61–64
  of radiation, 73
  of tamoxifen, 66
Silicone implants, 195, 196
Simple mastectomy, 51
Sledge, George, 12, 31, 38, 54, 56–57, 73,
  224–226
Smoking, 103
Soy, 132–134
Spear, Ruth, 10
Spirituality, 16, 116–119

Spouses and partners, 145–155
  communication with, 244
  support for, 154–155
  support from, 145–154
  working things out with, 148–149
STAR (Study of Tamoxifen and Raloxifene), 68
Stereotactic biopsies, 29
Study of Tamoxifen and Raloxifene (STAR), 68
Stumm, Diana, 96
Supplements, 134–136
Support, 13, 139–163
  being open to, 143–145
  for body issues, 172
  for child care issues, 244
  for diagnosis, 22
  from families, 156–159
  from friends, 159–163
  getting, 140, 141
  for medical procedures, 141–143
  for reconstructive surgery, 207
  for partners, 154–155
  from partners, 145–154
  for workplace issues, 252, 264
Support groups, 123, 148
Surgery, 14, 50–59
  aftermath of, 57–58
  decision making about, 53–55
  exercises for post-, 96–101, 104–105
  lumpectomy, 50
  lymph node removal, 53
  mastectomy, 50–53
  and menstrual cycles, 55–57
  questions about, 55, 57
  treatment after, 58–59
Susan G. Komen Foundation, 287
Symptoms (of breast cancer), 25–26
Systemic therapy, 59

Tagliaferri, Mary A., 115, 132–134
Taking charge (of last days), 283
Tamoxifen, 14, 65–68, 213–215
Tarr, Elizabeth, 46
Taub, Robert, 12, 149, 272–274
Test results (*see* Pathology reports)
Testing, genetic, 74–79
Testosterone cream, 180
Therapy:
  art, 120
  cognitive-behavioral, 121
  hypno-, 122
  music, 119–120
  systemic, 59
Thomson, J. Grant, 191, 197–198, 201,
  203, 205
TNM (Tumor size, Node involvement, and
  Metastases), 33
Total mastectomy, 51
Traditional Chinese medicine, 125–127
Transverse Rectus Abdominis Muscle
  (TRAM) flap, 199

Treatment(s), 48–73, 80–86
  after surgery, 58–59
  chemotherapy as, 59–65
  clinical trials as, 80–83
  ending, 82–86
  with herbal remedies, 123
  history of, 6–10
  hormonal, 65–73
  with psychotropic medications, 122–123
  radiation, 72–73
  surgery as, 50–59
Tripathy, Debu, 46, 112, 115
Trock, Bruce, 132
Tumor size, 33

Vaginal estrogen, 180
Vickery, Carlyn, 189, 191, 200, 202, 203, 206, 207
Visualization, 136–137

Weiss, Marisa, 180
What Women Should Know About the Breast Cancer Controversy (George Crile, Jr.), 8

Whole grains, 103
Wiesel, Elie, 115
Wigs (*see* Hair loss)
Winer, Eric, 24, 25, 42, 69–70, 226
Worden, William, 279
Workplace issues, 13–14, 249–266
  coping with, 250, 252–253
  and labor laws, 253–262
  and new jobs, 262
  and perceptions, 262–265
  and work identity, 266

Y-ME National Breast Cancer Organization, 287
You Can Fight for Your Life (Lawrence LeShan), 116
Young Survival Coalition (YSC), 6, 16–19, 27–29, 38, 55, 58, 65, 67, 69, 72, 81, 124, 196, 207, 265, 266, 275, 286
YSC (*see* Young Survival Coalition)

Zen and the Art of Knitting (Bernadette Murphy), 135

ABOUT THE AUTHOR

Beth Murphy is an author, documentary producer, and university professor. As the founder and president of Principle Pictures, she has spent the past two years writing this book and producing and directing the acclaimed Lifetime TV documentary, *Fighting for Our Future*. Murphy's award-winning documentaries, many of which have aired on PBS, focus on stories of hope and social justice, tackling nationally and internationally important topics. An adjunct professor at Suffolk University and a visiting professor at American University Paris, she earned a B.A. in History from the University of Connecticut and an M.A. in International Relations and International Communications from Boston University. Her articles have appeared in *The Boston Globe* and *San Francisco Chronicle*, among other publications.

ABOUT THE AUTHOR

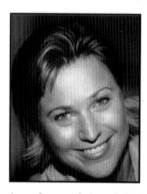

BETH MURPHY is an author, documentary producer and university professor. As the founder and president of Principle Pictures, she has spent the past two years writing this book and producing and directing the acclaimed Lifetime TV documentary, *Fighting for Our Future.* Murphy's award-winning documentaries, many of which have aired on PBS, focus on stories of hope and social justice, tackling nationally and internationally important topics. An adjunct professor at Suffolk University and a visiting professor at American University Paris, she earned a B.A. in History from the University of Connecticut and an M.A. in International Relations and International Communications from Boston University. Her articles have appeared in *The Boston Globe* and *San Francisco Chronicle*, among other publications.